UNDERSTANDING ADOLESCENTS' POLITICAL AGENCY

This ground-breaking volume shows that young people largely shape their own political development, and that to understand young people's political development, we must consider their political agency.

Håkan Stattin explores the findings of an extensive longitudinal study of the political socialization of young people in Sweden from the ages of 13 to 28, which shows that, contrary to popular belief, it is not parents, peers, teachers or other key adults who are the primary agents in shaping young people's political development; it is their own self-directed political interest. Given that political interest is both an input and an output, the book examines how political interest affects young people's political interactions with their parents, and why young people and their parents perceive these interactions differently. It covers key issues such as the impact of political-interest-triggering events and civil unrest, the role of school and peers, parental involvement and the path from political interest to future political and civic engagement.

Launching a new field of research internationally, this volume is essential reading for researchers, students, educators, and policy developers interested in young people's political and civic attitudes, engagement, communication, core values and the emergence of intrinsic political sophistication.

Håkan Stattin is Professor of Psychology at Uppsala University, Sweden. He has conducted studies in many areas of adolescent development and has received awards from the European Association for Research on Adolescence (EARA), the European Association for Developmental Psychology (EADP), the Society for Research on Adolescence (SRA), and the International Society for the Study of Behavioral Development (ISSBD).

Studies in Adolescent Development

Series Editor: Susan Branje

The Studies in Adolescent Development series is published in conjunction with the European Association for Research on Adolescence and is committed to publishing and promoting the highest quality of writing in the field of adolescent development.

The series aims to respond to the recent shifts in the social and ecological environment of adolescents and in the new theoretical perspectives within the social science by providing a range of books, each of which deals in-depth with an aspect of current interest within the field of adolescent development.

Each book focuses on a specific aspect of adolescence and provides either a clear picture of the research endeavours which are currently serving to extend the boundaries of our knowledge and understanding of the field, or an insightful theoretical perspective of adolescent development. The editors encourage publications which represent original contributions to the field.

Also available in this series:

Youth in Superdiverse Societies
Growing Up with Globalization, Diversity, and Acculturation
Edited by Peter F. Titzmann and Philipp Jugert

Online Peer Engagement in Adolescence
Positive and Negative Aspects of Online Social Interaction
Edited by Nejra Van Zalk and Claire Monks

Understanding Adolescents' Political Agency
Examining How Political Interest Shapes Political Development
Håkan Stattin

For more information about this series, please visit: www.routledge.com

UNDERSTANDING ADOLESCENTS' POLITICAL AGENCY

Examining How Political Interest Shapes Political Development

Håkan Stattin
together with Silvia Russo, Yunhwan Kim, and Erik Amnå

Routledge
Taylor & Francis Group
LONDON AND NEW YORK

Designed cover image: © Getty Images. Image by Sadeugra.

First published 2024
by Routledge
4 Park Square, Milton Park, Abingdon, Oxon OX14 4RN

and by Routledge
605 Third Avenue, New York, NY 10158

Routledge is an imprint of the Taylor & Francis Group, an informa business

British Library Cataloguing-in-Publication Data
A catalogue record for this book is available from the British Library

ISBN: 978-1-032-44354-6 (hbk)
ISBN: 978-1-032-44355-3 (pbk)
ISBN: 978-1-003-37173-1 (ebk)

DOI: 10.4324/9781003371731

Typeset in Times New Roman
by Apex CoVantage, LLC

CONTENTS

FIGURES

TABLES

PREFACE

Introduction

This book is based on a Swedish longitudinal project on the political socialization of young people (Political Socialization Study [PSP]). It summarizes the thinking behind our studies of the political attitudes, values, and activities of adolescents and young adults in their different everyday contexts. In the book, we attempt to provide an integration across contexts and offer new ways of thinking about young people's political development. We outline the theoretical perspectives that advance our main premise that politically interested young people drive their own political development. The findings we present in this book are consistent with this argument that youths are active producers of their own political development. Politically interested youth and young adults shape their own political lives within the opportunities and constraints of the contextual conditions around them.

Two political scientists, Niemi and Hepburn (1995), in considering the future of political socialization research, advised that

> as a discipline we might undertake a major new socialization study devoted specifically to the study of intergenerational and youthful change and development . . . [with] specific components designed to study the family, teachers, civics and other social studies classes primarily focusing on the age span 14 to 25 years.

The study described in this book is one such endeavor, integrating multiple contexts of everyday life across a broad age range. To the best of our knowledge, there has been no previous project with such comprehensive information to answer the question: Through what mechanisms and processes do politically interested youth and young adults develop their political interactions with others and their political engagement?

This is not a book about political activism among already politically engaged youth (for excellent insights, see Flanagan, 2013). It is a book about the evolution of engagement with political and social issues among representative samples of adolescents and young adults. The longitudinal scope, spanning multiple years for the same individuals and extending from early adolescence into adulthood, has not been reported in political socialization research. It is time to adopt this perspective. Here we look at young people from ages 13 to 28—from those who dislike discussing political issues to those who find them utterly fascinating.

In 2007, a political scientist (Erik Amnå), a media scientist (Mats Ekström), and two developmental psychologists (Margaret Kerr and Håkan Stattin) decided to plan a longitudinal study of young people's political development. We formulated our research questions from the perspective of our respective disciplines and then worked out the points of contact between them. From a literature review of research in education, psychology, political science, and media and communication—covering the roles of family, peers, school, civil society, education, and the media—we formulated eight challenges for research on political socialization. These research challenges formed the backbone of our application for funding from Riksbankens Jubileumsfond and the Swedish Foundation for Humanities and Social Sciences.

These were the goals we set ourselves:

1. Conceptualize young people as active agents in their own socialization rather than passive objects of socializing institutions.
2. Adopt a longitudinal perspective.
3. Focus on processes and mechanisms rather than correlations.
4. Integrate the different contexts of everyday life rather than studying one context at a time.
5. Take seriously the ongoing changes in different contexts.
6. Conceptualize political participation broadly, rather than focusing on formal institutions and narrow electoral aspects.
7. Disentangle general socialization from specific "civic" experiences in explaining differences in civic engagement.
8. Develop new theoretical explanations of political socialization.

In essence, this approach is characterized by (i) a broadened conceptualization of politics, (ii) a political agency perspective aimed at uncovering the mechanisms of socialization, (iii) sensitivity to changes in contexts and conditions, (iv) a longitudinal approach in which political socialization is embedded in more general development, and (v) preparation for theory development. The unifying research question was Through what mechanisms and processes do adolescents and young adults develop their political interest, and how does this political interest affect their political engagement?

About the Data Collections

Most studies of political socialization in the literature have been cross-sectional. Such designs can show associations between political interest and various features of individuals' contexts and behaviors, but they cannot reveal developmental processes. For example, adolescents may develop right-wing orientations as a result of reading right-wing websites (a socialization effect), or they may choose to read these sites because of their preexisting political beliefs (a selection effect). Only longitudinal studies can attempt to disentangle these effects and reveal the future history of current behavior. Moreover, in the political socialization literature, correlations have typically been interpreted as socialization effects, in which adolescents are shaped by their experiences but do not actively seek out experiences in pursuit of their own agendas. Thus, the recognition of adolescents as active agents in their own development has been largely absent.

In this research program, we developed a longitudinal study of adolescent political development in 2009 that aimed to combine different contexts of development. We followed five cohorts of adolescents and young adults between 2010 and 2015. The dataset contains rich data on family and peer relationships and adolescent behavior in the home, school, and leisure contexts, as well as data on certain adolescent characteristics and internal and external adjustment. Our questionnaires focus on political attitudes and behaviors, media use, family and peer relationships, and educational and leisure experiences. We believe that this dataset is unique because it allows us to understand and explain the political socialization histories of young adults from the perspectives of political science, education, media and communication, and developmental psychology. Unless otherwise noted, the measures used in this book were developed as part of the project.

The participants were adolescents from a Swedish city, Örebro, which had about 135,000 inhabitants at the beginning of the study. (Örebro county is the broader region with a population of approximately 275,000 people.) It is a university town. Pilot studies were conducted to examine the psychometric properties of the instruments and to determine which items were difficult to answer and should be deleted or reformulated.

Out of necessity, we were forced to use an accelerated longitudinal design. Following a group of 13-year-olds would require following them for 15 years before they reached the age of 28. Thus, each of the five cohorts at different ages was followed for four or five years. The basic plan was to take a sample of 1,000 people in each of these cohorts (ages 13, 16, 20, 22, and 26) and then follow them for four to five years.

The Two Youngest Cohorts

What the two youngest cohorts have in common is that all data collection up to the age of 18 took place in the participants' schools. The first cohort was recruited from 10 compulsory schools with 38 participating classes, and the second cohort was recruited from 3 upper secondary schools with a total of 57 participating classes, all strategically selected to represent the social and demographic characteristics of adolescents in Örebro, including ensuring that immigrant adolescents were represented.

Data collection took place in the classrooms during regular school hours—two lessons with a break for a drink and a piece of chocolate. The only adults present in the classrooms were our trained research assistants. Parents were informed about the study before the first assessment and were told that participation was voluntary. We used an opt-out procedure in which parents of adolescents in both cohorts were informed about the study before the first assessment and given the opportunity to decide if they did not want their child to participate in the study (less than 2% refused). A contribution of SEK 1,000 (about US$120) to the class fund was made at the first assessment, and participants were compensated with movie tickets at subsequent assessments. The adolescents were informed in advance about the study and their right to refuse to participate and to withdraw from the study at any time. The Regional Ethics Committee in Uppsala approved the data collection.

In addition to self-reports, parents completed questionnaires mailed to the participants' homes. This was done at ages 13, 15, and 18 for the first cohort and at ages 16, 17, and 20 for the second cohort. In all cases, this was done after the school data collection. Based on previous experience with data collection, we did not send separate questionnaires to mothers and fathers. Instead, the questionnaire sent to the parents' home could be completed by the father and mother either separately or together. We asked which parent completed the questionnaire—for cohort 1 and cohort 2 the first wave: mother (48% and 46%), father (9% and 12%), and both (44% and 42%). For many measures, parents had the option of providing separate responses for mothers and fathers. The parent questionnaire was available in six languages.

The Three Older Cohorts

For each of the three older cohorts, we randomly selected samples of 1,000 persons each in the city. Personal identification information was obtained from a register of eligible participants in the region maintained by the government agency responsible for population information (Spar, a Swedish government agency that maintains data from the Swedish Population Register, www.statenspersonadressregister.se/Om-SPAR/In-English.html). These three samples were then followed every two years for a total of three data occasions. At each occasion, a questionnaire was mailed along with a personalized link to an online version of the questionnaire. All participants received a 250 SEK (approximately US$30) gift card as compensation.

Table 0.1 gives an overview of the data collections.

The numbers behind each data collection group indicate the number of participants in the analytic sample, that is, individuals who completed a questionnaire. The numbers in parentheses indicate the total sample size, the target sample.

TABLE 0.1 Overview of data collections.

	2010 (election year)	*2011*	*2012*	*2013*	*2014 (election year)*	*2015*
Cohort 1	13 yrs/7th grade Sample: 904 (960) Parents:564 (960)	14 yrs/8th grade Sample: 883 (987)	15 yrs/9th grade Sample: 843 (954) Parents:450 (954)	16 yrs/ 1st year Sample: 723 (934)	17 yrs/2nd year Sample: 695 (935) Parents: 312 (889) Post-election follow-up: 1125 (1539)	18 yrs/3rd year Sample: 668 (927)
Cohort 2	16 yrs/1st year Sample: 892 (1052) Parents: 584 (1052)	17 yrs/2nd year Sample: 807 (996) Parents:443 (981)	18 yrs/3rd year Sample: 749 (916)		20 yrs Sample: 467 (939) Post-election follow-up: 1125 (1539)	
Cohort 3		20 yrs Sample: 605 (980)		22 yrs Sample: 600 (983)		24 yrs Sample 571 (972)
Cohort 4	22 yrs Sample: 539 (932)		24 yrs Sample: 564 (976)		26 yrs Sample: 537 (970)	
Cohort 5		26 yrs Sample: 606 (990)		28 yrs Sample: 597 (988)		

The target samples in Table 0.1 are those who were on the list of students in the classes reported by the schools (cohorts 1 and 2), and the target samples among young adults are those reported by the Spar agency (cohorts 3, 4, and 5). The analytic samples are the people who responded to our questionnaires.

The 2014 post-election follow-up group in Table 0.1 consists of those who were eligible to vote (aged 18) in the autumn from cohort 1, and those from cohort 4 who completed the regular questionnaire in spring 2014.

We also collected data for the final cohort at age 30. Because this data collection was not ready for use at the time the early studies were published, we will not use this data set here.

Attrition

For the two youngest cohorts, when data were collected at school in a given year, almost all students who were in school on the days of data collection responded to the questionnaires, and 80% to 90% of participants who responded one year did so the next year. In the two younger cohorts, about 50% to 60% of their parents responded to our mailed questionnaires. When we mailed questionnaires to participants in the three older cohorts, about 50% of them returned them. We attribute the higher attrition rate among participants in the three older cohorts to the type of data collection method used: collecting data for all youths attending the schools at the time of data collection versus distributing questionnaires by mail.

Demographic Comparisons

Örebro versus Sweden. Our main distinction is between the city and the country as a whole, as the sample was recruited to be as similar as possible to the demographics of the city. From official information, we know that the city is similar to the country in terms of immigration rate, average annual income, education level (but see below), unemployment rate, and voter turnout in the last election (Statistics Sweden, 2010).

Sample versus Sweden. We found a difference when comparing the family incomes of the first two cohorts with the national figures. The median monthly income of the families in our sample was between 40,000 and 50,000 kronor (US$4,400 to US$5,500) before taxes, which is 8% lower than that in the country as a whole.

Sample versus other countries. It is difficult to compare family income in our sample with other countries. We used parents' and adolescents' perceptions of the household economy to find out whether the economy was a source of concern in families. When parents reported on their household economy, the most common response was that their monthly income covered their expenses and they were not worried (Figure 0.1). A total of 15% of parents reported that their income did not cover or barely covered their monthly expenses. More than three in four adolescents said that their parents rarely or never complained about not having enough money (Figure 0.2). Five percent said that their parents always complained about

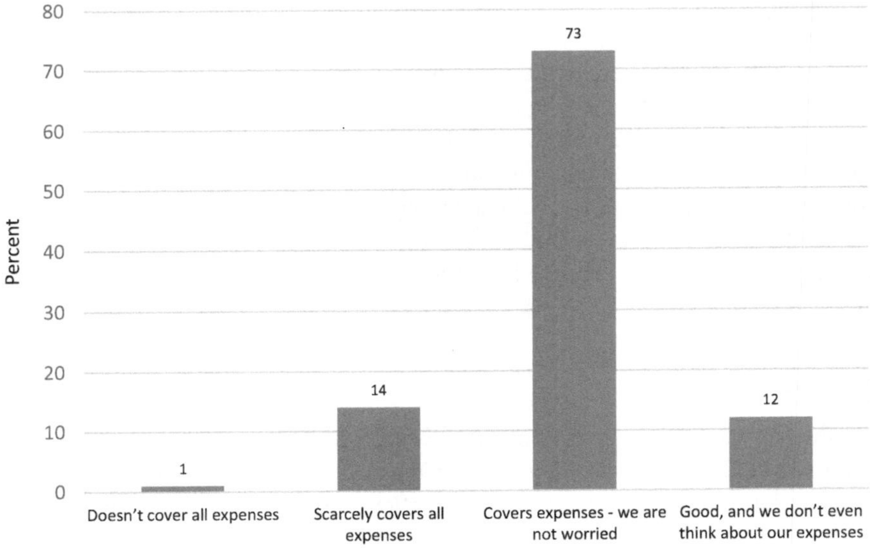

FIGURE 0.1 Household economy (parent reports).

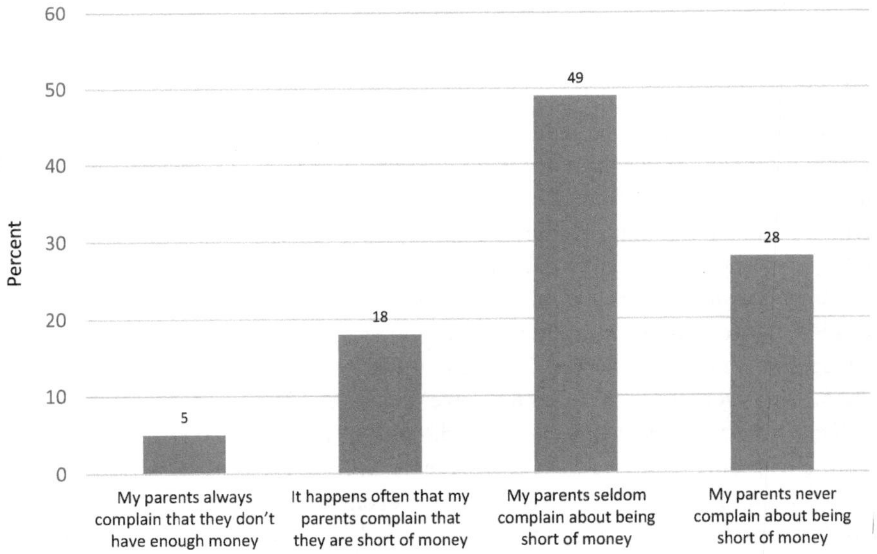

FIGURE 0.2 Adolescents' responses to the question "What are your family finances like?"

not having enough money. In general, the financial situation at home as experienced by most parents and young people seems to be good.

In most OECD countries, women are more likely than men to have completed post-secondary education. As shown in Figure 0.3, mothers in our sample were also more educated than fathers, with an effect size of 0.34. Overall, 54% of mothers and 39% of fathers had a college or university education. These percentages are somewhat higher than the national figures (48% vs. 35%), but comparable to parents living in metropolitan areas or in municipalities with universities and colleges in Sweden. In an international comparison, the percentage of adults with an academic education places Sweden in the middle of countries with higher academic education than the average OECD level (Higher Educations in Sweden, 2018). When comparing the empirical findings in this book with the economic and educational situation of parents in other countries, it is important to note the favorable economic and educational situation of the families in this study.

A Combination of Published Studies and New Information

Some of the chapters include studies that have been published in academic journals, marked with an asterisk (*) in the reference list. We have granted permission to reproduce the tables and figures contained herein. How these studies relate theoretically to each other is outlined here. Other chapters in the book contain new empirical studies and additions to published material. In cases where the studies

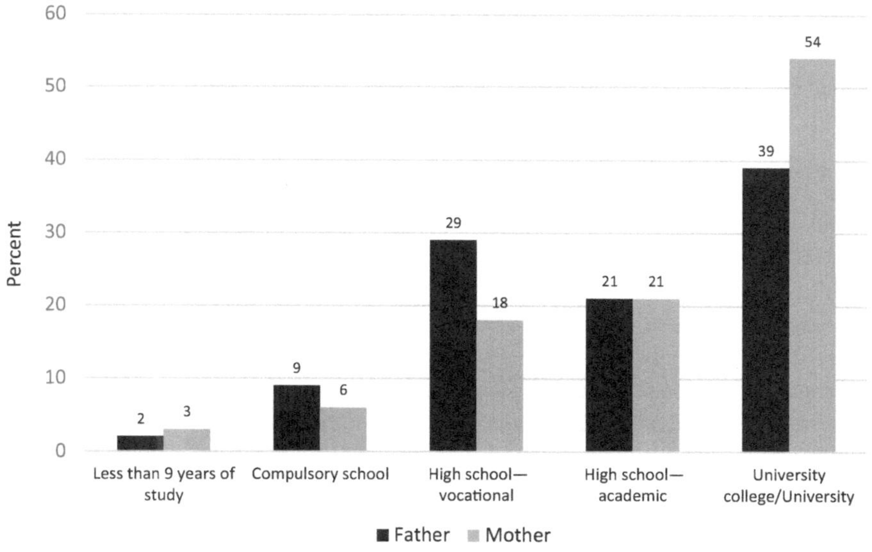

FIGURE 0.3 Parents' education (parent reports).

have been published, we have shortened the Introduction, Methods, and Analyses sections. In these cases, we

- do not report reliability analyses unless the alpha reliability is less than .70,
- do not report attrition analyses unless there is reason to believe that attrition is biased,
- minimize detail in descriptions of advanced types of analyses,
- do not report correlations between measures unless they are necessary for interpretation of the main analyses.

The statistical analyses and choise of covariates are the same as in the published studies. They might differ from reported unpublished material.

Depending on the question, we have used different measures of adolescents' political interest in published studies, ranging from a single item on interest in politics to combinations of this measure with interest in society and the world and feelings about politics. Our reporting of these measures here is as they were in the original publications. We have recalculated the results in most chapters, comparing the different combinations, and found that the results were very similar. The simple question about interest in politics seems to yield the same results as combining this question with other political interest questions.

Chapters containing new empirical studies include all the information typically found in published studies. Given the choice between reporting the original analyses in published studies or reporting potentially more powerful methods in line with more specific hypotheses that have emerged over the course of writing this book, we present the original analyses in most cases. Because the major shifts in political interest occur during adolescence, we focused many of our analyses on the first and second cohorts (ages 13 and 16).

Points of Departure

Political socialization refers to the processes by which young people acquire knowledge about political institutions, their society, and the world, and in the process acquire political beliefs, values, attitudes, and behaviors. The question of why some adolescents become politically interested and curious about society and others do not is likely to involve a combination of genetic, personal, social, and environmental factors. What will stand out in this book is the idea that politically interested young people shape their own political development. They are active agents in their own political development, and their political interactions with others and their search for information shape that political development. This basis for research differs from the theoretical underpinnings of most journal articles, books, and textbooks in the field of political socialization.

Political interest is commonly defined as being personally motivated to pay attention to political issues and experiencing information about politics as exciting, enjoyable, and fun. Genuine political interest is likely to begin with an interest in a particular issue that is perceived as important to the person. What begins as an interest in a specific issue may, over time, become an intrinsic interest in how the world works. There are no well-developed developmental models for understanding what causes a change in political interest, but there are broad outlines of how people's interest typically develops in different domains (e.g., Hidi & Renninger, 2006; Krapp, 2007; Silvia, 2008). According to these models, what was once a situational interest, something that tends to fluctuate in the short term, can evolve over time into a more stable and sustained interest. Thus, an interest that was triggered by an external event can eventually become dispositional, that is, a long-lasting interest in a particular area. Ultimately, interest in politics and what is happening in society is a linchpin in young people's political development and is the classic predictor of political and civic activity (Verba et al., 1995). In the socialization literature, the roots of young people's political and societal interests are supposed to lie in the ideas that their parents conveyed, what their peers tried to influence, what the media and the Internet conveyed, and what their teachers nurtured and motivated in school (Barrett & Brunton-Smith, 2014). We present a different narrative.

Individuals' political interests focus on political processes in which their thinking about what is happening or likely to happen at various levels, their motivations for active participation, and their emotional reactions to what is happening or likely to happen are intertwined. Politics has a powerful influence on the thoughts, feelings, motivations, and behaviors of some people. Perhaps the most distinguishing characteristic of politically interested people is their feelings about political issues. They express this as an intrinsic interest, as something exciting, joyful, and fun—and sometimes frustrating—and that this intrinsic interest is driven by their own curiosity. They are self-motivated to pay more attention to politics than to many other things in their lives; they want to stay informed about what is happening in the world and in their society, and as a result they acquire good political knowledge, from political institutions and parties, to political issues and to policies and ideologies. To stay informed, politically interested young people read and watch news about what is happening in various media. They talk about it with others—parents, friends, classmates, and teachers—and are more likely than other young people to participate in civic and political activities.

Humans are self-interpreting individuals who attempt to create meaningful images of their surroundings. The political views that young people express about politics, political parties, and policies are their social constructions of society and the world. The broad question of how politically interested youth's social constructions align with others in their everyday interactions is central to this book. We will pay attention to how young people view their political interactions with others similarly or differently from how those others view those political interactions.

Young people's political interest, together with their political self-efficacy, is in almost all cases the best predictor of their political interactions with others, their political values and attitudes, and their political behavior. More than other young citizens, politically interested adolescents and young adults

- have an intrinsic motivation to attend to political information (Levy et al., 2016; Moeller et al., 2018; Russo & Stattin, 2017),
- are attentive to news (Erentaitė et al., 2012; Levy, 2013; Shehata & Amnå, 2017; Strömbäck et al., 2013; Strömbäck & Shehata, 2010),
- are politically knowledgeable (Eveland & Scheufele, 2000; Rapeli, 2022),
- perceive that their political-geographical identity goes over and above their national state (Landberg et al., 2018; Šerek & Jugert, 2018),
- believe that their contribution can make a difference in the society (Barrett & Brunton-Smith, 2014; Levy, 2013; Levy & Akiva, 2019; Miller et al., 1980; Russo & Stattin, 2017; Zhu et al., 2018),
- engage in political discussions with their parents and friends (Dostie-Goulet, 2009; Gniewosz et al., 2009; Jennings et al., 2009; Kim & Stattin, 2019; Koskimaa & Rapeli, 2015; Levinsen & Yndigegn, 2015; Mayer & Schmidt, 2004; Oswald & Schmid, 1998; Schmid, 2012; Shehata & Amnå, 2017; Schulz et al., 2010; Stattin et al., 2021; Thorson et al., 2018; Warner & Warner Colander, 2016; Zeglovits & Zandonella, 2013),
- are active on social media (Allen et al., 2013; Moeller et al., 2018; Thorson et al., 2018),
- engage in a variety of offline political activities (Barrett & Brunton-Smith, 2014; Erentaitė et al., 2012; Eveland & Scheufele, 2000; Fieldhouse et al., 2007; Levy & Akiva, 2019; Quintelier & van Deth, 2014; Quintelier & Hooghe, 2012),
- have high levels of environmental engagement (Allen et al., 2013), and
- are likely to vote (Blais & Labbe' St-Vincent, 2011; Eveland & Scheufele, 2000) and increase their political interest during elections (Levy et al., 2016).

There are many specific conclusions to be drawn, but we want to highlight the most general. Politically interested youth seek out political experiences (Prior, 2019). Politically interested adolescents and young adults are better than other adolescents and young adults at finding, understanding, and processing political information, and they are better at translating their political interest into political engagement. Their interest in politics and desire to know more is not limited to a particular developmental context, but generalizes beyond their families, friends, classrooms, the Internet, and social media. This political interest seems to travel easily across these contexts, across native and immigrant samples, and across boys and girls. Any study that examines the links between political discussions, sociopolitical values and attitudes, school experiences, and offline and online political activities is not trustworthy if it does not consider the role that political interest plays in the first place.

How does young people's political interest manifest itself in their political interactions with others and in their political and civic activities? This is the "hot" research question we address.

Answering this question involves the research challenges we have identified. Clearly, a developmental perspective requires longitudinal data. Research needs to move from correlations to developmental processes and mechanisms. We need to explain how political interest emerges and how political interest affects young people's political interactions with parents and other significant others, with civic and political organizations, and with people on social media. On the one hand, few studies have attempted to predict political interest at all (Neundorf et al., 2013; Prior, 2019; Quintelier & Hooghe, 2012). We will address this issue in several chapters. On the other hand, political interest stands out as the most important predictor of political knowledge, engagement, and activity (Prior, 2019; Shani, 2009). Insights into why this is the case are needed. Thus, insights are needed to understand political interest both as an input and as an outcome of predictions.

We will propose that political socialization is different from "normal" socialization. At home, everyday and political conversations between adolescents and parents are influenced by different motivational factors. Normal, everyday conversations about school, friends, relatives, music, etc., depend heavily on the emotional relationship between parents and adolescents. This is not assumed to be the case for political discussions. They depend largely on the political interest of the adolescents and their politically interested parents. In school, it is assumed that adolescents' perceptions of their own political activities in class and their teachers' initiatives to bring up political ideas in class depend on their political interest, not on their affective ties to school, class, or teachers.

Political Agency

Most of the literature on political socialization until the last decade can be described as an input-output model. Parents, friends, teachers, and the media are the inputs. The young person is the output. With respect to the family, much of research has assumed that parents are a certain way and that their stable characteristics shape or mold the political and civic development of their children. With few exceptions (Jennings et al., 2009), these ideas have not been tested. A developmental perspective has been lacking.

One example. Communication is thought to be the most fundamental aspect of political socialization. Parents politically socialize their adolescents through discussions in the home. Many studies have successfully linked the frequency of political discussions at home to various measures of adolescents' political and civic interest, knowledge, and political participation. However, these findings do not preclude the possibility that adolescents play an active role in influencing the frequency and content of these discussions. Indeed, in all of the studies showing stronger associations between political discussions with parents and adolescents' own attitudes and behaviors, it was adolescents, not parents, who reported how often these discussions took place.

In short, the history of political socialization has largely been a story of how external conditions lead young people to become politically engaged. Today, however, the notion of active agency has become more common (Bloemraad & Trost, 2008; Kiousis et al., 2005; McDevitt, 2006, 2015; McDevitt & Chaffee, 2002; Saphir & Chaffee, 2002; Stattin et al., 2017; van den Bulck & van den Bergh, 2005; York, 2019a). According to this view, attending to political issues and engaging in political behavior can be self-directed processes. But - active agency is a presumptive concept. Strictly speaking, in order to confirm active agency, the self-initiated activities of young people must be linked to the intentions they had before engaging in these activities. This direct link is difficult to establish (but see Bloemraad & Trost, 2008). To date, studies have examined how adolescents' interest in an upcoming election, generated at school or in the media, affects family communication patterns (McDevitt, 2006; McDevitt & Chaffee, 2002). Here, newly politically interested children influence their parents' attention to political information and political views through their self-initiated political conversations in the family (McDevitt, 2006, 2015). Young people can also influence their parents in other ways (McDevitt & Chaffee, 2002; Meadowcroft, 1986), for example, to be co-creators of their own development by influencing their parents both actively—through their intentions—and passively—through the way parents respond to their children (van den Bulck & van den Bergh, 2005). Other empirical evidence for self-directed processes stems from the recognition that reciprocal processes operate in different domains. Media use influences people's beliefs, attitudes, and interest and these beliefs, attitudes, and interest in turn influence media use, resulting in media use as both predictor and outcome (Slater, 2007, 2015). Politically interested adolescents pay more attention to political information than other adolescents, and attention to political information positively influences their political interest (Thomas et al., 2021). Politically interested adolescents have more politically triggering experiences than other adolescents, and these experiences further spur their political interest (Stattin et al., 2017). Parents and children mutually influence each other's prejudice and tolerance toward immigrants (Miklikowska, 2015). These are a few examples of the active agency perspective. Overall, the past decades have witnessed a growing number of attempts to understand young people as self-directed agents of their own political development.

This self-directed perspective for understanding young people's political development will run throughout this book. A basic assumption is that *young people's political interests shape their political development*, which we will call a political agency perspective. This is not to underestimate the role of significant others in young people's everyday lives—parents, teachers, friends, classmates, and others.

But political agency is a shift in perspective from mainly assuming that external conditions—such as parents, peers, media, social media, and school—socialize young people's political development. The political agency perspective in this book locates the primary driver of young people's attitudes, values, and behaviors in their intrinsic political interest.

When politically interested youth realize that exciting political conversations and activities are happening around them and that other people and news stories are providing important information about what is going on in the world and in their society, this information tends to go over the heads of young people who are not politically interested. The lack of interest and worldview of politically disengaged youth filters out political processes, but politically engaged youth are more able to see the nuances. They realize that their parents, teachers, and friends communicate with them about political issues. This realization does not reach politically disengaged youth. The ability to recognize nuances in political information in their everyday environment is one of the things that distinguish politically engaged youth from other youth.

What we need to study are theory-driven processes and how young people perceive political interactions with other people. When we interact politically with most other people, we act and react to them (Kiousis et al., 2005; McDevitt, 2006). Why has political socialization research continued to use parents, peers, media, and school as independent variables and youth behavior as the dependent variable? There are many reasons to expect that politically interested adolescents respond to their own social constructions of political interactions with others. We expect that a greater emphasis on adolescent political agency will move the entire field of political socialization research toward more refined theoretical models.

The question is whether an agentic perspective offers a better understanding of the various aspects of young people's political development than a socialization perspective. It is not possible to conduct a specific study that will show once and for all that either an agentic or a socialization perspective is the more correct one. The complexity of the development of young people's political interests, attitudes, values, and behaviors over time requires the simultaneous use of different perspectives. This book presents a juxtaposition of the agentic and socialization perspectives in many areas.

From a political agency perspective, at the level of individual differences, we would expect politically interested young people to see themselves as agents of change in society. They can be expected to do so by:

- *Having a sense of curiosity*: finding exploring politics and society interesting and fun (Moeller et al., 2018; Russo & Stattin, 2017).
- *Paying attention to political information* and being knowledgeable: consider it important to be informed about what is going on in the world and perceive themselves as well informed about politics and society (Shehata & Amnå, 2017; Strömbäck et al., 2013; Strömbäck & Shehata, 2010).

- *Having positive attitudes toward political action*: perceiving that it is a norm to be politically active.
- *Believing in their political self-efficacy*: believing that they can be politically active when needed (Levy, 2013; Levy & Akiva, 2019; Russo & Stattin, 2017; Zhu et al., 2018).
- *Setting civic goals*: having rational goals for future civic engagement (Stattin et al., 2022a). Of course, whether this self-perception as a change agent translates into civic and political action depends on the opportunities available to them.

We operationalized these characteristics (see Table 0.2) and performed factor analyses for members of cohort 1 (age 13) and cohort 2 (age 16). As shown in Table 0.3, one factor was extracted in both age groups. These factors were very stable over time. The correlation between this factor at age 13 and the same factor one year later was .65. The correlation between the factor at age 16 and the same factor one year later was .79. We conclude that political interest is associated with seeing

TABLE 0.2 Operationalization of characteristics associated with self-identification as an agent of political change.

Concept	*Response scale*
Political interest	
How interested are you in politics?	1 (*totally uninterested*) 5 (*very interested*)
Feelings about politics	
People differ in what they feel about politics. What are your feelings?	1 (*loath*) 6 (*great fun*)
Updated and knowledgeable	
Updated:	
Some young people think it is important to keep oneself informed about what is going on in the world. Yet others do not think it is especially important. What do you think?	1 (*No. I am not so interested in keeping myself informed*) 2 (*Yes. I think it is important to keep myself informed. I try to get as much information as I can regarding societal, environmental, and political issues as often as I can*)
Knowledgeable:	
Scale with 3 items: "You could probably describe me as a person who tries to keep oneself informed about what is going on in the world," "I follow the news daily to know what other people are talking about," "I try to keep myself informed about what is going on in the world by following the news." Alpha reliability was .86 in cohort 1 and .87 in cohort 2.	1 (*doesn't apply at all*) 5 (*applies perfectly*)

(*Continued*)

TABLE 0.2 (Continued)

Concept	*Response scale*
Politically active as the norm	
Scale with 4 items: How active should people be on political issues? What do you think? For me it is important to "Join political parties and organizations to bring up the issues that are important to me," "Actively try to influence societal issues," "Make my voice heard on societal issues," "Be involved so that politicians get to know what people think." Alpha reliability was .83 in cohort 1 and .84 in cohort 2.	1 (*not important at all*) 4 (*very important*)
Internal political efficacy	
Scale with 9 items. If I really tried, I could manage to "Write a letter to a newspaper or web editor about problems in my school," "Actively contribute to the work of organizations trying to solve problems in society," "Take leadership of a group to address societal issues," "Help to organize a political protest," "Be an active member of a political organization," "Discuss politics with persons with more experience than I have," "Take part in a demonstration in my home town," "Take on responsibility in a political youth organization," "Convince others to sign petitions about political or societal issues." Alpha reliability was .94 in cohort 1 and .93 in cohort 2.	1 (*I could definitely not manage that*) 4 (*I could definitely manage that*)
Set rational goals	
Some people have set goals for themselves concerning their engagement in societal issues. Have you?	1 (*I'm not interested in issues like this, rather the opposite. I will certainly not commit myself to do anything about them*) 2 (*I'm not interested in issues like this and, as far as I can see, I will not commit myself to getting engaged in them*) 3 (*I will definitely work actively [in organizations or by other means] on issues like this but have not yet committed myself*) 4 (*I will work actively in organizations and I'm already a member of such an organization*)

TABLE 0.3 Principal components analyses of characteristics associated with self-identification as an agent of political change in the two youngest cohorts.

	Age 13	*Age 16*
Political interest	.80	.85
Feelings about politics	.79	.84
Stay updated	.68	.73
Well informed	.66	.68
Politically active as the norm	.69	.72
Political efficacy	.61	.67
Setting rational goals	.63	.74
% variance explained	49	56

oneself as an agent of change, and conversely, not being politically interested is associated with not seeing oneself as an agent of change. The stability over time in perceiving oneself as an agent of change is substantial.

Political Interest Is Both a Push and a Pull in Political Development

Prior (2019) has described the development of political interest as a self-directed process. We seek to explain how young people's political interest can be both a "push" and a "pull" in their political development and in the political interactions they have with their significant others.

For many types of civic and political activities, we should expect politically interested youth to be more politically engaged than youth with less political interest. For some external and internal conditions we can expect reciprocal causation. Politically interested young people seek out political experiences. When they encounter events that they perceive as triggering their political interest, or are perceived by others as politically competent, their intrinsic political interest should be a primary reason. However, the dynamic may also show that encountering these events and being perceived by others as politically competent further increases political interest. Similarly, politically interested adolescents may believe it is important to pay attention to what is happening in the world, and paying attention to this information may increase political interest. In this dynamic process, political interest will be both a push and a pull on political development.

We make specific hypotheses:

Events that trigger political interest. Over the course of, say, a year, some young people experience events that they perceive increase their political interest. We will argue that it was not a matter of chance that they had these experiences with these events. They were prepared to pay attention to political information. More than other adolescents, they had been politically interested for years, followed the news, set personal goals, talked about politics with their parents and others on the Internet, and experienced themselves as politically competent. Moreover, exposure to these interest-promoting events is expected to increase their broader political interest later on.

Importance of staying informed. We will propose that politically interested adolescents and young adults are more likely than other adolescents and young adults to perceive the importance of staying informed about politics, and that this attention to political information increases their political interest over time. Being politically interested and paying attention to current events will both push and pull political development.

A political reputation in the classroom. We hypothesize that some politically interested students will gain a reputation as being politically competent among their classmates. This political reputation in the classroom will increase their political interest and their political involvement several years later.

Finally, in classical political socialization research, parents unidirectionally influence their children's political development by having frequent conversations about political issues at home. This narrative of adolescents' political development as unidirectionally shaped by conversations with parents about politics lacks strong empirical support. We will examine whether there are unidirectional or bidirectional relationships between political interest and political discussion with parents from early adolescence into later early adulthood.

Social Construction of the World, One's Own Society, and Political Interactions With Others

When young people are asked about their political attitudes, values, and political interactions with others, these questions tap into the social construction of young people's encounters with others—the world they perceive as valid for them. In this book, we will devote considerable attention to young people's worldviews and views of political interaction with others. We will show that this worldview does not fit well with their most important people—their parents. Also, perceptions of their political interaction with their parents—for example, how often they have political discussions in the family and how much political support they receive from their parents—differ considerably between the views of young people and their parents. These differences need to be explained.

If parents are the main agents of political socialization, we should expect that the values and sociopolitical attitudes that parents express would be close to the values and attitudes that their adolescent children have. This is not the case. In fact, we have known about this discrepancy for at least 50 years (Connell, 1972; Jennings & Niemi, 1968). Still, political socialization studies have typically proclaimed that young people's sociopolitical values and attitudes are under the unilateral influence of their parents (Beck & Jennings, 1982; Niemi & Hepburn, 1995; Quintelier, 2015).

We expect to show that adolescents' perceptions of their political interactions with their parents do not much resemble parents' perceptions of their political interactions with their adolescents. Adolescents believe that the core values they hold are also the values their parents hold. Parents also believe that the core values they hold are the values their children hold. But we propose that this is not the case. Furthermore, the frequency of political discussions with parents and the extent to which parents support young people's political development are perceptions that we believe differ between young people and their parents. In fact, young people and their parents have quite different perceptions of their joint political interactions. Again, the different perceptions of everyday political interactions between parents and young people do not support the idea that their political views are strongly influenced by their parents.

We make specific hypotheses:

Political interest drives perceptions of political interactions. We propose that how adolescents perceive their political interactions with their parents—how often they have political discussions and how politically supportive their parents are—is strongly related to adolescents' own political interest. Parents' perceptions of their political interactions with their adolescents are also strongly related to their own political interest. However, adolescents' and parents' perceptions of their political interactions are not well aligned.

Explaining the low accuracy between adolescents' and parents' perceptions. Many previous studies show that adolescents' and parents' sociopolitical attitudes and perceptions of their joint political interactions do not match well. We propose that biased perceptions and projections on the part of both parents and adolescents can explain the low accuracy.

Adolescents are open to political communication from significant others. From a classical political science perspective, one would expect that if adolescents experience that the most important people in their lives are politically interested, that these people provide them with political information, that they try to influence them, and that they are susceptible to the views of these people, then these adolescents would be more likely than other adolescents to increase their political interest over time. We suggest that the causal relationships are the opposite. Adolescents' perceptions of important others' (parents, teachers, friends) political views, political interest, political influence and support, and their own susceptibility to others' political communication are all affected by their own political interest.

Along the way, we will use several theoretical models: self-determination theory, theory of planned behavior, value socialization theory, theory of basic human values, and personal reputation theory. They provide the models needed to develop new theoretical perspectives.

Håkan Stattin

ACKNOWLEDGEMENT

In 2009 we started a longitudinal study of young people's political development. Many different publications have emerged, but there comes a time when they need to be summarized, extended and theoretically integrated. This integration is very different from what most of you have seen in the literature. This is the work I have been doing for the past two years. With the help of my colleagues and friends Silvia Russo (chapters 1, 2, 3, 4 and 9), Yunwhan Kim (chapters 5, 6 and 8) and Erik Amnå (chapters 2, 11 and 12), who have spent many hours helping me, this is the result you are holding in your hands. Silvia, Yunhwan and Erik: It was a pleasure to work with you.

Of course I am grateful to all the participants who answered all our questions again and again. Invaluable.

And to Aurora. A center of my spirit.

PART I

The Growth of Political Interest and Action

1

CHANGES IN POLITICAL INTEREST AND CIVIC/POLITICAL ACTIVITY

Highlights

From mid-adolescence onward, young people with high political interest rarely lose this interest, but in early adolescence high political interest may flicker and disappear.

Political interest stabilizes before young adulthood, but there are still fluctuations to consider: Individuals with low political interest may become more interested in politics, but not the most interested, and individuals with average political interest may either lose this interest or become more interested in politics.

Characteristics closely related to political interest—interest in society in general, feelings about politics, internal political efficacy, and attention to news—show roughly the same trends over ages as political interest. The age-related changes in feelings about politics are particularly noteworthy. In young adulthood, between the ages of 20 and 26, one in four finds politics fun, one in four finds politics boring, and one in two finds politics neither fun nor boring. This is different from young adolescents (age 13), where two out of three find political issues boring and only 8% find political issues fun.

Among several measures of political engagement—importance of being politically active, membership in a civic/political association, offline and online political activity—only online political activity increases with age.

Introduction

Historically, researchers have proposed various hypotheses about the growth of political interest among young people. One is the idea that people are open to change throughout their lives and show flexibility in their attitudes in response to changing life experiences. Here, political interest is unstable and fluctuates over time in response to political events. The lifelong persistence hypothesis, on the other hand, holds that political attitudes are resistant to change and that what is learned early in life persists and becomes stable over time (Sears, 1983). Another idea, the impressionable years hypothesis (see Krosnick & Alwin, 1989), is based on attitude research and proposes that individuals form political attitudes, values,

DOI: 10.4324/9781003371731-2

and broader worldviews primarily during late adolescence and early adulthood. This is the period of life when individuals are thought to be most susceptible to socialization influences. Once they have passed through it, they are less likely to change the attitudes and values they have acquired. Thus, political interest is expected to increase during late adolescence and young adulthood and then level off. Different starting and ending ages for the impressionable years hypothesis have been proposed. For example, Jennings and Niemi (1981) suggested that the impressionable years range from ages 17 to 25. Niemi and Hepburn (1995), based on follow-up interviews with high school students, identified the period between age 14 and the mid-20s as the period of maximum change in what people think and how they learn about politics.

Thanks to Markus Prior's pioneering analyses of the stability of people's political interest over time (Prior, 2010, 2019), much has been learned from various panel studies that allow estimating the growth and stability of people's interest in political issues. His research involved large panel and household surveys of the general population in different countries—Switzerland, Germany, the United Kingdom, and the United States. In his 2010 article, Prior convincingly showed that stability rules when it comes to people's political interest. People rarely suddenly change their interest in politics. If they are not interested in political issues, there is little chance that they will suddenly become very interested. Conversely, if people are very interested in political issues, there is little chance that they will suddenly lose that interest. For eample, we will rarely find politically uninterested 25-year-olds who suddenly become highly politically interested. We will rarely find highly politically interested 25-year-olds who suddenly lose that interest. It does not matter much whether it is an election year or not. Stability at the individual level can be reduced to a dichotomy of people: "You either got it or you don't" (Prior, 2010).

Compared to the information that exists on the growth and stability over time of political interest among adults, considerably less information is available for children, adolescents, and young adults. However, in three of the six panel surveys used by Prior (2010), individual-level stability information was available for persons under the age of 22. Expecting lower stability for these younger persons under the impressionable years hypothesis, Prior found little evidence. However, a detailed analysis showed that aging over the life course was associated with a 10- to 15-point increase in political interest on a scale of 0 to 100, and that "this rise occurs almost entirely in adolescence and young adulthood" (Prior, 2019, p. 117).

There are a few empirical studies that have specifically examined the growth of political interest among adolescents and young adults and can provide more nuanced information. In one, Dostie-Goulet (2009) conducted a study in Canada to assess the impact of social networks on the development of political interest, collecting longitudinal data on a group of 14–15-year-old high school students who were surveyed three times at one-year intervals. She found a significant increase in political interest, but the effect size for this increase was small. Dostie-Goulet's study is particularly interesting because it reports on both the students who gained political interest over a year and the students who lost interest over the same period. She reported that about one-third of the students experienced an increase (defined as a change of at least 1 point on a 10-point scale) in political interest one year later, one in eight students showed a decrease in their level of interest, and half of the group remained stable. Surprisingly, this study did not find a profound increase in political interest among high school students.

Neundorf and colleagues (2013) used panel data from a German household database to estimate the developmental trend of political interest for individuals between the ages of 17 and 35. They found that political interest increased from age 17 to 25, an age at which the increase slowed. Despite documenting an increase over time, a closer look shows that the increase in political interest from age 17 to age 35 was not extensive. However, a study that interviewed Belgian youths at ages 16, 18, and 20 found an increase in political interest from ages 16 to 20, with an effect size of about 0.40 (Quintelier & van Deth, 2014). In terms of developmental trends over longer time periods, Wray-Lake et al. (2020) found an increase in political interest from age 18 to 24, which then leveled off until age 30. Growth over time was small.

Our longitudinal study is the only one to date that can shed light on the growth and stability of political interest between the ages of 13 and 28, the period of life commonly considered to be the time of greatest change in an individual's political interest. This chapter addresses the questions of when and how political interest changes over time among adolescents and young adults. The first question, "when," concerns the developmental trend of political interest, and the second question, "how," concerns the direction of change in political interest across age.

The Developmental Trend in Political Interest

Our participants were asked the following question: "How interested are you in politics?" The alternative responses were set as follows: Totally uninterested, Not at all interested, Not particularly interested, Fairly interested, and Very interested. This single question is a standard in research on political interest (ANES, 2014; Verba et al., 1995) and has the advantage of avoiding "complications related to the distinction between interest and behavioral utterances or consequences of interest" (van Deth & Elff, 2000, p. 33).

Figure 1.1 shows the evolution of the mean responses to this question. We used all information for all age cohorts and included data for cross-age cohorts. What stands out in Figure 1.1 is that there was a marked increase in political interest from age 13 to age 18, followed by a slight increase that leveled off by age 24. The increase in political interest was stronger in later adolescence than in early and middle adolescence. Comparing the youngest and oldest ages (13 and 28), there was a nearly large effect size (0.75). The average level of political interest at age 13 was slightly above "not at all interested." The level of political interest for the average young adult was "not particularly interested" in politics. It should be

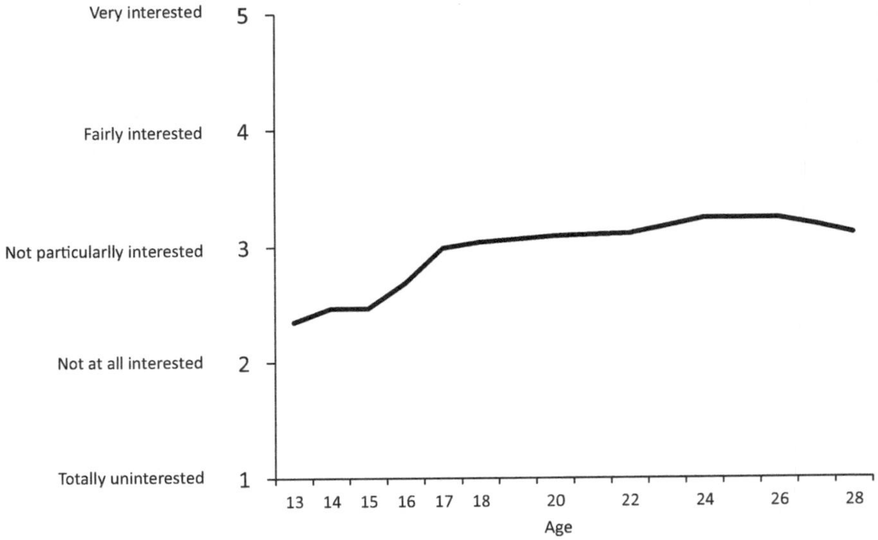

FIGURE 1.1 The developmental trend of political interest.

added that one in eight 13-year-olds were already fairly or very interested, meaning that the onset of high political interest for these individuals occurred at this time or earlier in their lives. Prior (2010) and Berti (2005) place this earliest awakening of interest at around age 10.

We have information on political interest over five years for the youngest cohort. Here we can see in more detail the frequencies for each response option when we look at the same group of adolescents side by side (see Figure 1.2). The most significant changes occurred at the extremes of the scale. As shown in Figure 1.2, at age 13, 28% said they were totally uninterested in politics. Five years later, only 7% said they were totally uninterested. Thus, over the course of five years, individuals move away from the extreme position of being totally uninterested in politics. At the other end of the scale, 3% of participants at age 13 said they were very interested in politics. Nearly five times as many, 14%, were very interested at age 18.

A Latent Change Model

For a direct test, we estimated the direction of change in political interest between T1 and T2 (over two-year intervals) using latent change models (McArdle & Nesselroade, 1994). We examined change over two years for participants in the five age cohorts (ages 13, 16, 20, 22, and 26). By setting all loadings to 1, the latent intercept reflects the mean level of political interest at the first assessment, while the latent slope reflects the amount of linear change that occurred between

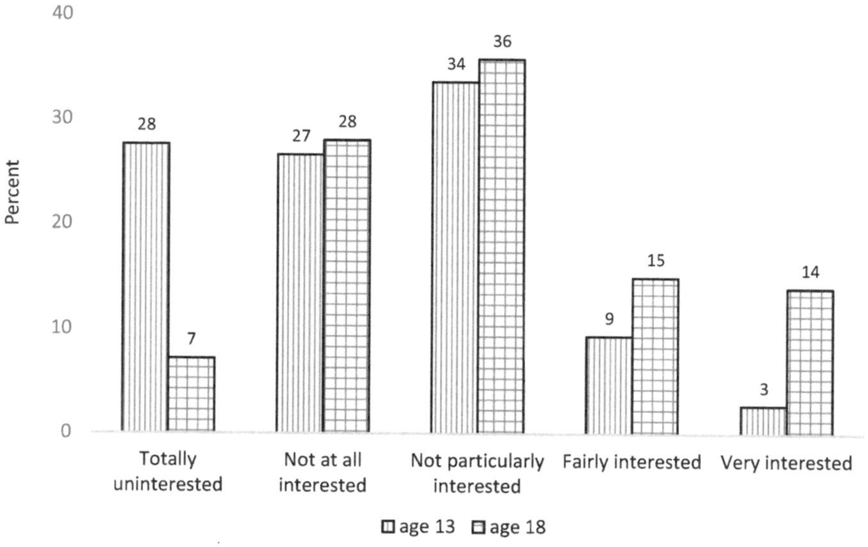

FIGURE 1.2 Political interest of 586 participants at ages 13 and 18 years.

TABLE 1.1 Latent change models of political interest.

Cohort	*Mean intercept*	*Mean slope*	*Variance intercept*	*Variance slope*
13 to 15 years	2.33 (0.042)***	0.12 (0.048)**	1.21 (0.065)***	1.56 (0.084)***
16 to 18 years	2.65 (0.049)***	0.27 (0.043)***	1.43 (0.083)***	1.10 (0.064)***
20 to 22 years	3.10 (0.048)***	−0.06 (0.040) ns	1.05 (0.069)***	0.73 (0.048)***
22 to 24 years	3.24 (0.047)***	−0.04 (0.040) ns	0.88 (0.062)***	0.64 (0.045)***
26 to 28 years	3.21 (0.043)***	−0.06 (0.033) ns	0.88 (0.057)***	0.53 (0.034)***

Note: Entries are unstandardized coefficients (Standard errors in parentheses). ** $p < .01$ *** $p < .001$.

the two time points. Table 1.1 summarizes the parameter estimates of the latent change model for each cohort. The mean slope was positive and significant only for the two younger cohorts, indicating that political interest increased most substantially over two years at these ages. Also important are the significant variance estimates for all parameters, indicating substantial interindividual differences in both initial levels and rates of change in interest. Overall, these results suggest that, at the group level, there is an increase in political interest among adolescents between the ages of 13 and 18. This increase is steeper between the ages of 16 and 18. Political interest is stable among young adults between the ages of 20 and 28.

Stability Coefficients in Each of the Age Cohorts

We analyzed the stability coefficients over two years for the five age groups. Table 1.2 reports different types of correlations: Pearson's product-moment correlation and its value corrected for measurement unreliability according to the procedure suggested by Achen (1975), as well as Kendall's tau-b and Spearman's rho rank correlations. The results clearly show a pattern of increasing stability of political interest across age cohorts, regardless of the type of correlation. The corrected correlation in the oldest cohort had a magnitude (.85) consistent with that reported by Shani (2009) for the Youth-Parent Socialization Study. Between ages 18 and 26, she found a stability coefficient of .87.

The pattern of results is clear. The lowest level of stability in political interest is observed between the ages of 13 and 15. Between the ages of 16 and 18, stability increases, and from the age of 20, the stability of political interest reaches the levels reported in previous studies of representative samples of adults.

We also report the percentages of adolescents who gave the same answer two years later and the percentages who changed by no more than one response category. As shown in the lower part of Table 1.2, the proportion of participants with identical scores over two years increased up to age 20. At this age, approximately 55% had identical scores. This proportion increased to 64% in the oldest age cohort.

Looking at the proportion of adolescents who did not move more than one response level on the 5-point scale, 78% of adolescents in the younger cohort showed stable political interest over time, while the proportion reached 96% in the oldest cohort. It is worth noting that the proportion of stable adolescents in our older cohorts is consistent with the findings of Prior (2010) for the British Election Study panel (18 years and older), in which political interest was assessed using a 5-point response scale. He reported that the proportion of respondents

TABLE 1.2 Correlations between political interest over a two-year period and the percentage of adolescents and young adults giving the same answer or moving no more than one category two years later.

	Ages 13–15	*Ages 16–18*	*Ages 20–22*	*Ages 22–24*	*Ages 26–28*
Pearson's r	.35	.60	.65	.66	.70
Corrected r	.47	.72	.78	.79	.85
Kendall's tau-b r_τ	.31	.52	.60	.58	.67
Spearman's r_s	.36	.60	.66	.64	.73
Identical scores	39.3	44.8	55.3	55.2	63.8
Identical plus ±1 point	78.2	83.4	93.5	94.8	95.5

Note: All correlations are significant at $p < .001$.

who had not moved more than one category two years after the initial survey was over 90%.

Comparing the Youngest and the Oldest Cohort

The trend in political interest aggregates individual differences into an average over time. More information is needed about subgroups on the interest continuum. Before reporting a differentiation of political interest for all age groups, we will compare the youngest and oldest age groups, 13- to 15-year-olds and 26- to 28-year-olds. For ease of visual inspection, we recoded the 5-point measure of political interest into a trichotomy at all ages: One group of people had low political interest (totally uninterested or not at all interested in politics), another group had medium interest (not particularly interested), and a third group had high political interest (fairly or very interested). So first let's consider only the youngest and oldest age cohorts in Table 1.3 (the first three and last three columns).

Table 1.3, which reports the row percentages, show that once young adults are highly interested in politics, they are unlikely to lose that interest. A full 78% of young adults who were highly politically interested at age 26 were still highly politically interested at age 28. Only 2% of highly interested 26-year-olds were not politically interested two years later. There was more instability in the youngest age cohort. Among 13-year-olds, only a minority, 42%, of the highly interested 13-year-olds retained this high interest two years later. High political interest also seems to turn into low interest in these early years. In fact, 26% of politically interested 13-year-olds reported low political interest two years later.

It does not appear to be too late to become politically interested. Although few of the young people moved from low political interest to a high level of political interest (10% of the 13-year-olds and 4% of the 26-year-olds), a significant proportion of them moved from low political interest to at least a medium level of political interest, 29% of the 13-year-olds and 31% of the 26-year-olds. Thus, it does not seem too late to gain political interest (even at age 26)—at least not from low to medium interest. This observation that people can increase their political interest in young adulthood is encouraging news. Politically uninterested young adults may not continue to live with their persistently low political interest. In addition, in both age cohorts, there were individuals who started out with medium levels of political interest. In general, they were just as likely to lose that interest over the course of two years as they were to become more politically interested.

In summary, once young adults have a high level of political interest, they rarely lose it. Also, young adults can still increase their political interest, even if it is from a low level of interest to a medium level, or from a medium level to a high level. Finally, early political interest can disappear. Among 13-year-olds, the majority of those who had high political interest had lowered that high interest in political issues two years later.

TABLE 1.3 Stability of political interest over 2 years in different age cohorts.

	Ages 13–15			*Ages 16–18*			*Ages 20–22*			*Ages 22–24*			*Ages 24–26*			*Ages 26–28*		
T2:	*Low*	*Medium*	*High*	*Low*	*Medium*	*High*	*Low*	*Medium*	*High*	*Low*	*Medium*	*High*	*Low*	*Medium*	*High*	*Low*	*Medium*	*High*
T1:																		
Low	61.3	28.6	10.1	55.1	32.2	12.7	64.5	30	5.5	63.8	27.5	8.7	54.7	36.8	8.4	64.8	30.8	4.4
Medium	36.1	44.7	19.2	23.7	49.1	27.2	23.6	57.9	18.5	16.9	59.3	23.8	11.7	55.6	32.7	18.6	69.6	11.9
High	25.8	32.3	41.9	3.2	19.7	77.1	1.9	25.5	72.7	1.8	27.3	70.9	1.7	15.3	83	1.6	20.2	78.2
Pearson *r*		.32			.58			.65			.61			.65			.71	

Comparing All Cohorts

It is time to add the other three age groups to Table 1.3. Comparing them all at the same time, we come to these conclusions:

1. Across all age groups, both adolescents and young adults with low political interest can change, and when they do, they typically become moderately interested in politics.
2. People with moderate political interest are difficult to predict. When they change, about the same percentage become uninterested as those who become highly interested.
3. With the exception of the youngest age group, adolescents and young adults with a high interest in politics rarely lose that interest.

These findings do not fully support Markus Prior's dichotomy in his seminal 2010 article "“You've either got it or you don't? The stability of political interest over the life cycle." There are not two groups of people: the politically interested and the politically uninterested. It is certainly the case that young adults with a high level of political interest rarely lose that interest. But the opposite tendency, that politically uninterested young adults will continue to have this low interest, needs to be qualified. First, in both adolescence and young adulthood, there is room for increases in political interest from low levels, although these are not always radical changes. For many, it is a move from low to medium political interest. Second, young people with medium political interest—the most common response across all age groups—are just as likely to lose this interest as to gain high interest. We conclude that Prior's "you either have it or you don't" dichotomy is an oversimplification of what happens to young people's political interest over time. The dichotomy gives the impression that there is little change in political interest.

Finally, we should not forget the people who lost political interest over the two years. About one in five people with medium interest lost it over the two years, and between one in five and one in four moved from high to medium or low interest. These are significant percentages. Loss of interest was most common between the ages of 13 and 15.

Other Interest-Related Measures

Now that we know more about when and how political interest changes over time among adolescents and young adults, we will look at trends in other measures related to political interest. These are highly correlated with political interest in the literature:

- *A societal interest:* "How interested are you in what is going on in society?" The response scale ranges from 1 (*totally uninterested*) to 5 (*very interested*).
- *Feelings about politics:* "People differ in what they feel about politics. What are your feelings?" The response scale ranges from 1 (*loath*) to 6 (*great fun*).

- *Internal political self-efficacy:* Nine items, all related to a domain-specific efficacy belief in one's actions to effect change in society (Bandura, 2006). After the stem "If I really tried, I could manage to . . . ," the participants responded to statements such as "take on responsibility in a political youth organization" and "discuss politics with persons with more experience than I have." The response scale ranges from 1 (*I could definitely not manage that*) to 4 (*I could definitely manage that*).
- *Attendance to news:* A single item measure: "I follow the news daily to know what other people are talking about." The response scale ranges from 1 (*doesn't apply at all*) to 5 (*applies perfectly*).

A number of figures will show the developmental trends for these measures. It should be noted that in all age groups these measures formed one factor together with the measure of political interest in the factor analyses. Therefore, it is conceivable that we should expect roughly the same developmental trends for these measures across ages.

A Societal Interest

First, consider the participants' interest in what is going on in society. Are they "outward looking" and paying attention to what is happening outside the immediate environment of family and friends (Amnå, 2012)? This societal interest is a much broader interest than an interest in politics per se. We have considered the developmental trends of political interest and broader interest in societal affairs as two close but not identical aspects of social engagement (Ekman & Amnå, 2022). The comparison is shown in Figure 1.3. The trend in political interest is almost parallel to that in societal interest, with the interest in society being much stronger than the political interest throughout all years. There is a large effect size of 0.99 between the youngest and oldest age group for the societal interest. The increase over ages is one where the average person in the youngest age is "not particularly interested" in societal issues to where the average person in the oldest age is "fairly interested" in what is going on in the society. The mean level differences between the samples may seem small or modest, but they are quite substantial. For example, 40% of the 13-year-olds reported that they had a fairly or very high interest in what is going on in the society. This was the case for 88% of the 28-year-olds. Thus, to be fairly or very interested in societal issues is an overwhelming majority phenomenon in early adulthood.

Feeling About Politics

Political interest has an affective basis (Prior, 2019; Silvia, 2006). We found that feelings about politics gradually increase with age (see Figure 1.4), with the average person in the youngest age group finding politics boring, while the average person in the oldest age group found politics neither boring nor fun. Comparing the youngest and oldest age groups, there was a large effect size (0.94). It should

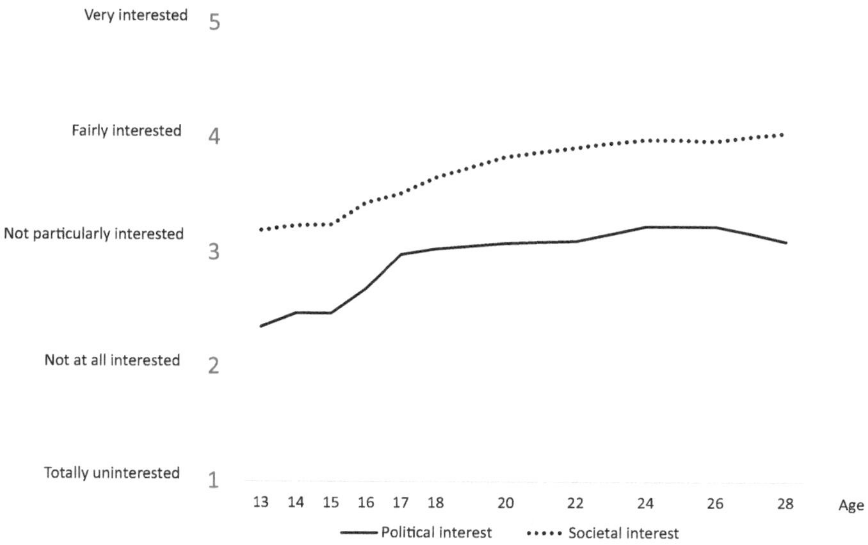

FIGURE 1.3 Trends in political interest and interest in what is going on in society.

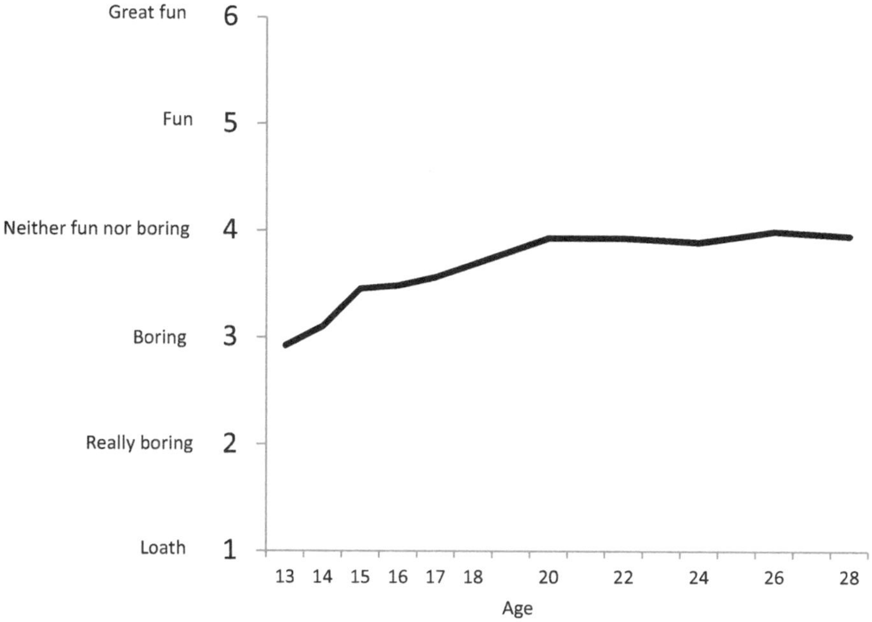

FIGURE 1.4 Trend in feelings about politics.

be noted that in all but one of the five age cohorts (age 13), the correlation between feelings about politics and political interest was .70 or greater.

A simple trend in a sample can hide important information, and this appears to be the case with feelings about politics. We would expect young people to be less likely to be politically engaged if they find politics boring. The likelihood should increase if they find politics fun.

We divided the measure of feelings into three categories:

- *Politics is boring* (the participants reported their feelings about politics was Boring, Really boring, or Loath).
- *Politics is neither fun nor boring* (the participants reported their feelings about politics as Neither fun nor boring).
- *Politics is fun* (the participants reported their feelings about politics as Fun or Great fun).

For simplicity, we used all five cohorts and compared responses to this question for participants at ages 13, 16, 20, 24, and 28. Figure 1.5 shows this comparison. Our conclusions are as follows:

- Profound changes in feelings about politics occurred in adolescence, but less so in adulthood.

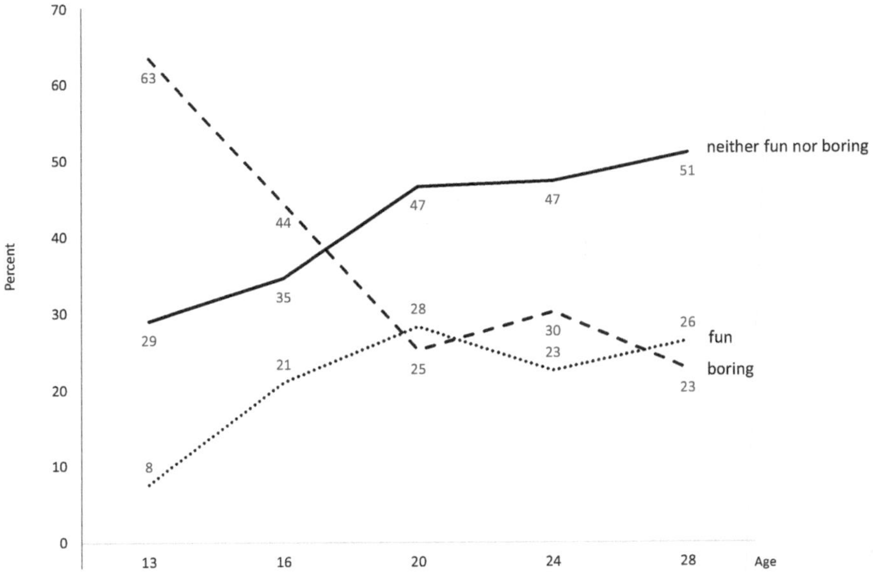

FIGURE 1.5 A trichotomous measure of feelings about politics: changes over time.

- At age 13, almost two out of three adolescents found politics boring. At that age, few had positive feelings (8%).
- This changed over time. In early adulthood—ages 20, 24, and 28—one in four had positive feelings and one in four had negative feelings about political issues. One in two young adults said they had neither positive nor negative feelings about politics.

Political Efficacy

The developmental trend for political efficacy is an increase from age 13 to age 18 and then a leveling off (Figure 1.6). Comparing the youngest and oldest age groups, there was a medium effect size (0.54). The average person moves from believing that they probably could not handle this type of responsibility to somewhere in between believing that they could not handle this responsibility and believing that they probably could. From another perspective, 8% of participants in the youngest age group believed they could (probably or definitely) handle the tasks described in the scale, compared to four times as many, 31%, in the oldest age group.

Attendance to News

Attention to news is the last topic to be examined. As can be seen in Figure 1.7a, attention to the news increased with age, from a level where the average person didn't think attention to the news applied to them so well to a level where it kind

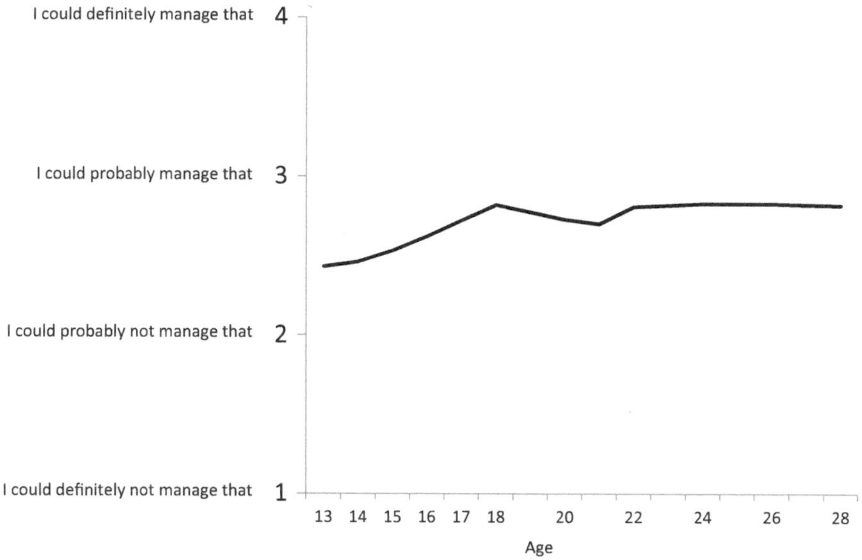

FIGURE 1.6 Trend in internal political efficacy.

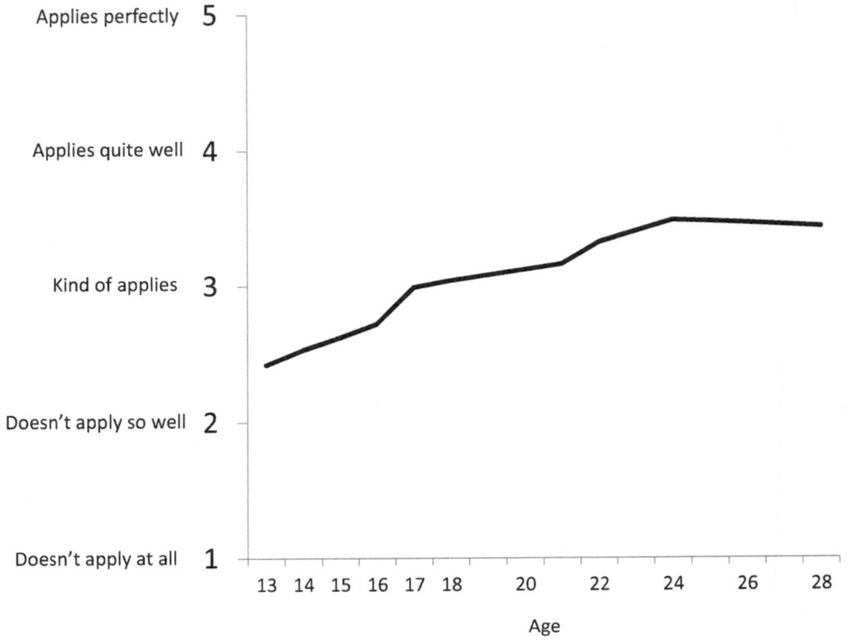

FIGURE 1.7A Trend in news attendance.

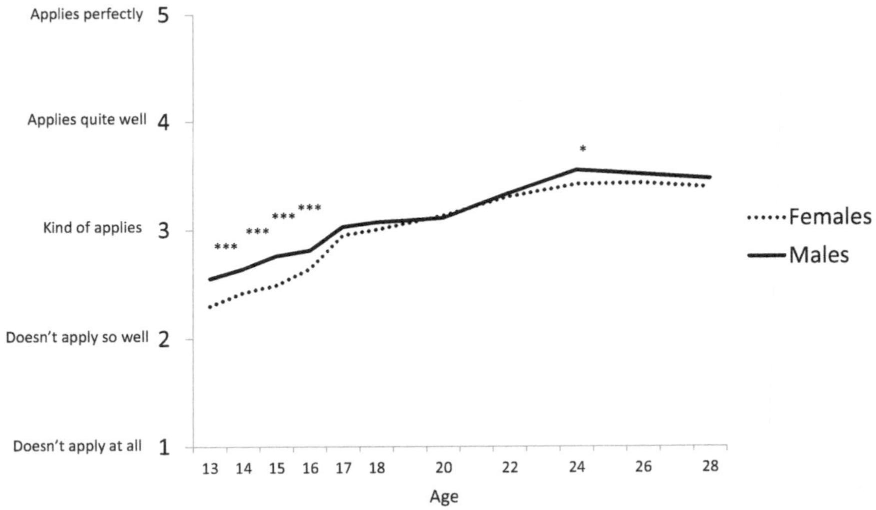

FIGURE 1.7B News attendance: Gender differences.

of did. Only 8% of 13-year-olds said that following the news was a fairly or very accurate description of them, compared to five times as many, 43%, of 28-year-olds. There was a large effect size (1.0) when comparing the youngest and oldest age groups. Attendance at news is the only interest-related measure where we find

TABLE 1.4 Stability over 2 years at different ages for measures political interest measures (Pearson correlations).

	Political-interest-related characteristics		
	Feelings about politics	*Political efficacy*	*Attendance to news*
13–15	.40	.42	.44
16–18	.56	.59	.56
20–22	.64	.64	.59
22–24	.61	.62	.56
24–26	.54	.66	.61
26–28	.66	.63	.64
Average	.57	.59	.57

Note: All correlations are significant at the .001 level.

more substantial gender differences. In the youngest age group (13 to 16 years), more males than females reported following the news. These gender differences disappeared later (see Figure 1.7b).

Table 1.4 shows the stability coefficients over two years for the various interest-related measures at different ages. As expected, the youngest age cohort had the lowest stability, but the stabilities for the other age cohorts were at about the same level—around .60.

Lest it go unnoticed, a final word on gender differences in political interest: For the questions "How interested are you in politics?" "How interested are you in what is going on in society?" and "People are different in their feelings about politics. What are your feelings?" there were no significant gender differences at any age between 13 and 28, except for higher interest in what is going on in society for males at ages 17 ($p = .011$) and 18 ($p = .022$).

From Interest to Participation

The next step was to link interest to participation. More specifically, we wanted to capture changes over time for both civic and political forms of activity. While civic engagement aims to "influence circumstances in society that are relevant to others, outside one's own family and circle of close friends . . . but also outside the formal political sphere" (Ekman & Amnå, 2022, p. 386), political participation refers to "the formal (or institutional) political-parliamentary sphere, with political parties and political decision-making" (Ekman & Amnå, 2022, p. 386). According to much earlier research, "political interest is typically the strongest predictor of the political behaviors that make democracy work" (Prior, 2019, p. 9).

But we are now witnessing what some would call an anomaly, a deviation from the expected, while others would say it is perfectly expected. Young people's political interest is one of the best predictors of their political engagement (Hooghe & Dejaeghere, 2007; Levy et al., 2016; Norris, 2003; Prior, 2019; Strömbäck &

Shehata, 2010). Political interest, like other interest-related characteristics, increases with age. It would be reasonable to expect that young people's political activity would increase with age. This is not the case. (We have added linear trends in the following figures).

We asked, "How active should people be in political issues? What do you think?" Four questions were asked about the importance of civic engagement and political participation: "It is important for me to: Join political parties and organizations to raise the issues that are important to me; Get involved so that politicians know what people think; Actively try to influence societal issues; Make my voice heard on societal issues." The response scale ranges from 1 (*not at all*) to 5 (*very important*).

As can be seen in Figure 1.8, all age cohorts had roughly the same mean scores for the importance of civic and political participation. The mean scores were around 2, meaning that the participants did not consider it particularly important to be involved. Knowing that political interest increases with age, and that political interest is probably the best predictor of political engagement, we might expect to see at least some increase with age in young people's belief that it is important to be engaged. With the exception of an increase from ages 13 to 15, there were no such increases or decreases later. The effect size for the difference between ages 13 and 28 was 0.16.

We asked all participants if they were members of one of three types of civic/political associations: political association; peace or human rights association (peace movement, Amnesty International, or similar); environmental association.

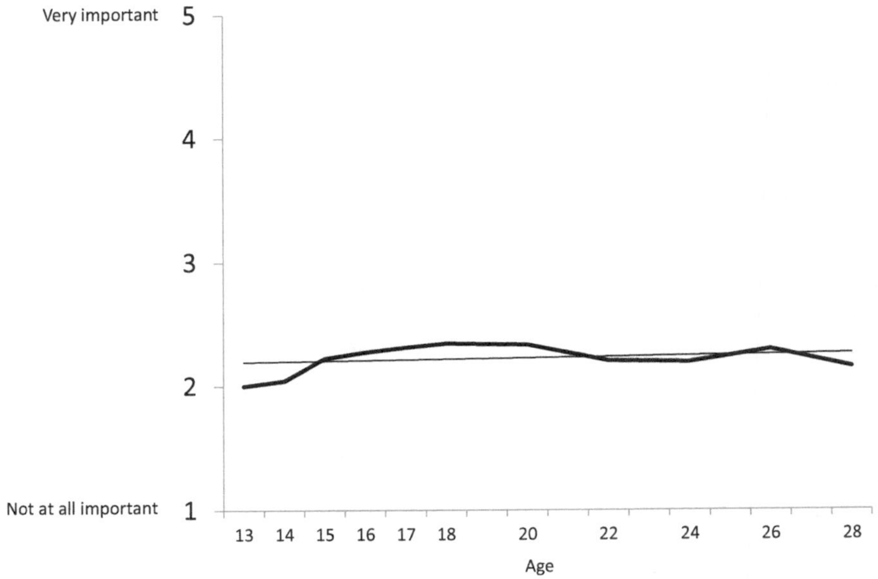

FIGURE 1.8 Trend in the importance of being politically active. A linear trend line is inserted.

The proportion of people who were members of one or more of these types of organizations increased only slightly with age. Three percent of adolescents aged 13 to 20 and 6% of young adults aged 20 to 28 were members of such organizations. Again, there is little evidence of a substantial increase with age. The effect size for the differences between ages 13 and 28 was 0.17.

We also asked participants about their offline civic engagement and political participation over the past year. They responded to seven alternatives: signed a petition; attended a meeting about political or social issues; volunteered for a cause; collected signatures; contacted a politician or public official; donated money to a cause; and attended a concert or fundraiser with a political message. The 3-point response scale was 1 (*no*), 2 (*yes, occasionally*), and 3 (*yes, several times*). Note that the alpha reliability for the three older cohorts was only about .65. As can be seen in Figure 1.9, there was no marked developmental trend over age for this measure of participation in offline civic and political activities. The effect size for the difference between ages 13 and 28 was 0.08.

Finally, we asked the participants about their online civic and political activities with five items: "Discussed societal or political questions with friends on the Internet," "Visited a political website," "Sought information about politics or societal issues on the Internet," "Read about politics in a blog," and "Viewed videos or film clips about societal issues or politics." The 3-point response scale was 1 (*no*), 2

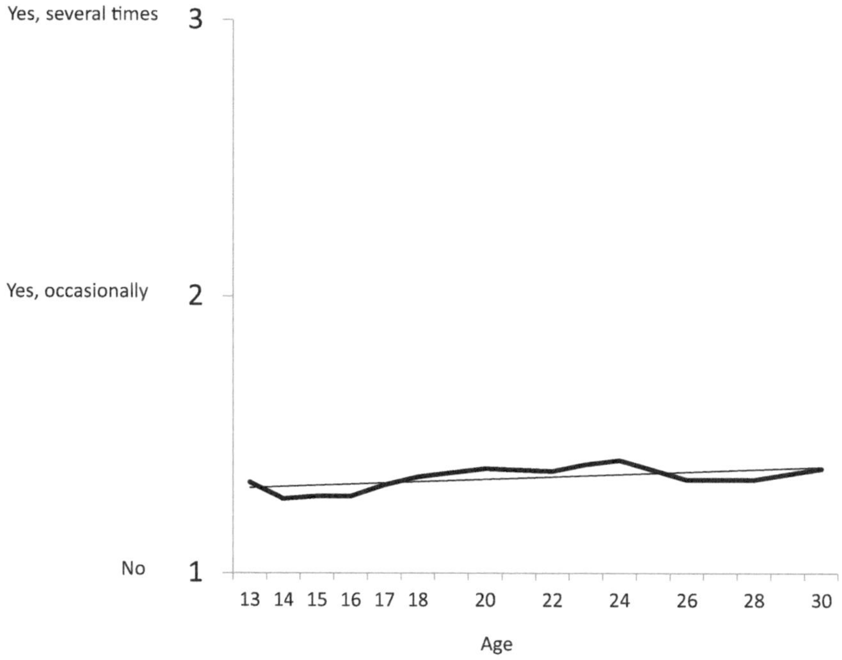

FIGURE 1.9 Trend in offline political participation. A linear trend line is inserted.

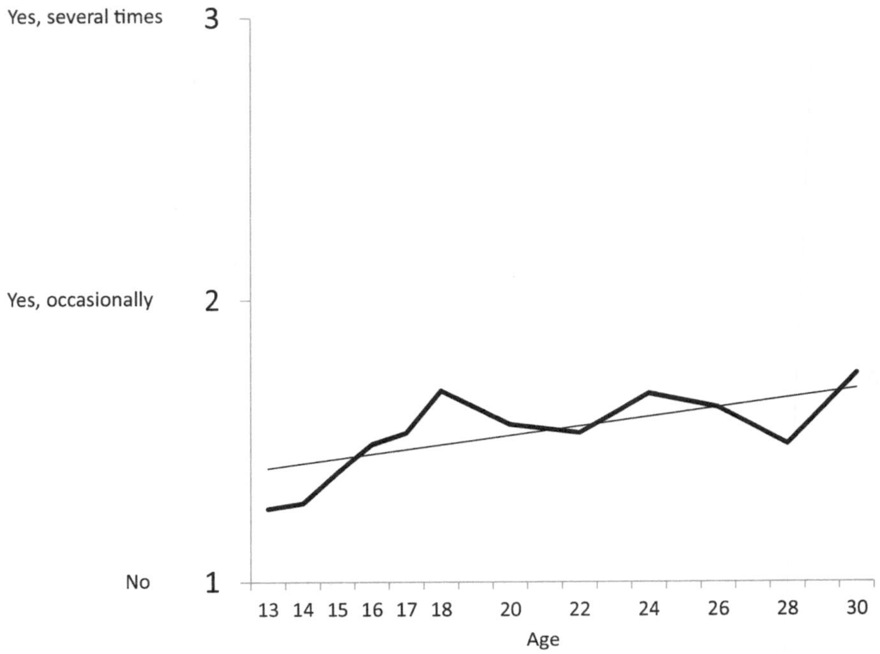

FIGURE 1.10 Trend in political activity on the Internet. A linear trend line is inserted.

(*yes, occasionally*), and 3 (*yes, several times*). As can be seen in Figure 1.10, online political activity increased from ages 13 to 18, but did not change much after that age. Comparing the means for the 13-year-olds and the 18-year-olds, the effect size was almost large, 0.75. The increase in online political activity seems to be the only measure of political activity that shows about the same developmental trend as political interest.

We have taken four examples of young people's attitudes to civic engagement and their actual political participation. With the exception of online activities, young people's civic engagement and political participation do not change much between the ages of 13 and 28. This is notable because the same individuals' political interest increases from early adolescence to late adolescence.

Finally, given that the trends in political interest and other measures related to political interest show much clearer increases over time than the measures of civic engagement and political participation, two-year stabilities were calculated for the activity measures for all age groups. These are summarized in Table 1.5. Two conclusions can be drawn from this table. First, there are mainly low stabilities for the youngest age group. Second, except for the youngest cohort, there are quite high stabilities, consistent with the stability of political interest, for offline and online activities. They are lower for the perception of the importance of being active and for membership in associations.

TABLE 1.5 Stability over two years in different age groups for measures of the participants' views on civic engagment and actual political participation (Pearson correlations).

Age in years	*Important to be active*	*Membership associations*	*Offline activities*	*Online activities*
13–15	.32	.07	.34	.23
16–18	.47	.20	.43	.51
20–22	.53	.40	.50	.66
22–24	.48	.35	.59	.64
24–26	.48	.38	.67	.62
26–28	.55	.43	.57	.71
Average	.47	.40	.52	.56

Note: All correlations are significant at the .001 level except for the stability for membership in political/civic associations ($p = .055$) between ages 13 and 15.

A valid objection to our choice of offline civic engagement and political participation is that some of these activities may be systematically more common among early and mid-adolescents, while other activities may be more valid for capturing the activities of young adults. In light of this criticism, we decided to examine developmental trends for each of the eight measures we originally selected, comparing 13- and 16-year-olds with the early adults at age 28. We found effect sizes as large as .50 for two of these measures. Adolescents were more likely to collect signatures, and young adults were more likely to donate money to a charity. However, excluding or including these two measures did not change the results reported in Table 1.5.

Discussion

The most obvious conclusion from the findings on developmental trends brought up in this chapter is that political interest increases during adolescence, especially in late adolescence, and then stabilizes in early adulthood. Second, the analyses of stability and change at the individual level show that once political interest is acquired, it is maintained. This is true from middle adolescence to the end of early adulthood. Third, political interest does not freeze in early adulthood. Changes do occur, but they are more modest, mainly from a low level to a medium level of interest in politics. It is particularly difficult to predict the future level of political interest for individuals with a medium level of political interest. As their political interest changes, their level of interest may increase or decrease.

We examined measures that have been consistently found in the literature to be strongly associated with political interest—young people's societal interest, feelings about politics, internal political self-efficacy, and news consumption. Overall, there was growth over time for these interest-related measures similar to political interest, and stability estimates over two years were in the range of .60, except for the youngest cohort.

This set the stage for examining whether young people's attitudes toward civic engagement and political participation, as well as various aspects of their activities, followed similar trajectories over time. We asked participants in all cohorts whether they thought it was important for them to be civically and politically engaged. They were also asked about their membership in civic and political associations and about their offline and online activities. With the exception of online activities, there was little evidence that young people's attitudes toward civic engagement and political participation, their membership in political/civic associations, or their offline activities changed from early adolescence to the end of early adulthood.

The massive individual-level change in political interest that we have reported in this chapter suggests that what happens from early to later adolescence is a developmental watershed. For most early adolescents, it is difficult to predict the level of political interest several years later. In the youngest cohort, the 13-year-olds, we had the opportunity to examine their political interest (the trichotomized measure) with their expressed political interest five years later (Table 1.6). Most of the 13-year-olds who had a low interest in politics turned out to have a medium (32%) or high (40%) political interest five years later. The 13-year-olds who had a medium interest in politics were more likely to have a high interest (45%) than a low interest (19%) five years later. When 13-year-olds reported high political interest, most of them (69%) continued to have high political interest at age 18. In short, with the exception that early politically interested adolescents tend to maintain their high political interest, it is almost impossible to predict political interest at age 18 from the political interest participants expressed as 13-year-olds. The correlation between their reports of political interest as 13-year-olds and their reports five years later is only .16 ($p = .014$). Apparently, much happens in the intervening years that changes the level of political interest for the majority.

The changes in political interest before early adulthood, when political interest becomes more stable at the individual level, make it challenging to explain what influences young people's interest in politics in the first place, and how it comes about that young people's political interest has such a strong impact on their

TABLE 1.6 Cross-tabulation of political interest at ages 13 and 18 (row percentages).

Age 18	*Low*	*Medium*	*High*
Low age 13	28.2	32.0	39.8
Medium age 13	18.8	36.5	44.8
High age 13	17.1	14.3	68.6
Pearson *r*	.16[1]		

Note:[1] $p = .041$.

χ^2 (4 df) = 24.50, $p < .001$.

political interactions with others. This is at the heart of the research detailed in this book.

What makes 13-18 the most rapidly changing period of political and social interest? It is probably a combination of factors. One is the cognitive growth of adolescents and the associated communication skills, where they acquire the cognitive abilities to develop general attitudes and values that will have implications for their future lives (Flanagan & Sherrod, 1998; Meadowcroft, 1986; Vollebergh et al., 2001). Another key is education. This is the time when students learn about national and international geography, history, and current information about society, government, comparative politics, democratic and humanistic values, minorities, and gender studies—new information that should fascinate many students. In the words of Niemi and Hepburn (1995), "research seeking to understand how adults form their political ideas and allegiances will be more productive if concentrated on young people in the period of maximum change and maximum concentrated teaching of political material" (Niemi & Hepburn, 1995, p. 11). A third reason is that having a good knowledge of what is happening in society can be a way to achieve a more adult status. Fourth, having knowledge about politics and society is what parents expect their sons and daughters to acquire during these years, and what parents should strive for in their attempts at political socialization. There are other explanations.

In this chapter, we have distinguished between a political interest and a societal interest. Things that are happening in society and the world are what adolescents typically hear about in the news in various media. The words "politics" and "political" are more problematic. When we ask the adolescents questions about "politics" or "political," we have significantly lower frequencies than when we ask about "what is happening in Sweden and the rest of the world" or the like. Perhaps this is to be expected (Fitzgerald, 2013; Görtz et al., 2023). It is quite possible that the word "politics" has a negative connotation among some young people, is misinterpreted into a narrow understanding that politics is strictly about government functions, party preferences, political processes, elections, and voting (and not about human rights and environmental concerns, tolerance, minorities and gender, etc.), or is possibly interpreted differently by adolescents than by young adults. Nevertheless, the temporal trajectories of both political and societal interests have similar shapes, and high coefficients of stability are already present from the ages of 16 to 17.

One final comment. Much of the concern about young people's civic engagement and political participation has been framed in terms of the ideal of active citizenship. However, like Berger (2009), one can ask the question,

> Must citizens be politically engaged all the time or only episodically? Perhaps liberal democracies can flourish with relatively low levels of political engagement if they also feature continuously high levels of engagement which can be channeled into political engagement should the circumstances warrant—and political institutions able to process that episodic engagement and respond satisfactorily.
>
> *(Berger, 2009, p. 345)*

2

PLANS FOR FUTURE CIVIC ENGAGEMENT

Highlights

We hypothesize that adolescents can set rational goals for their future civic engagement. These goals moderate their political interest, and the greatest future political activity will be among adolescents who are both politically interested and have set high goals. The target sample was 16-year-olds. Several types of political activities were predicted four years later: offline political activity, online political activity, membership in a political/civic organization, taking a public stance for a party before and after voting in a national election, and voting. Consistent with the hypothesis, significant interactions were found between political interest and setting societal goals for all future political activities except voting. We conclude that adolescents' early-developed agency in setting goals for their civic engagement has broad predictive utility for their political activities over time.

Introduction

An increase in political interest with age is seemingly not accompanied by a similar increase in political activity or involvement in civic/political associations. What is lacking is knowledge about the early motivational conditions that can potentially transform young people's political interest into future political action. This chapter examines whether politically interested adolescents have goals for their future political engagement and whether such goals influence their future political activities. We hypothesize, first, that adolescents' political interest will be a central predictor of their future political activity and, second, that their goals for future civic engagement can moderate the effect of their political interest. The greatest future political activity should occur among adolescents who are both politically interested and have high goals. Thus, adolescents' early developed agency in setting goals for their civic engagement should have predictive utility for their political activity over long periods of time.

DOI: 10.4324/9781003371731-3

Rational Plans

To our knowledge, only one study in the literature has attempted to answer this question about the role of adolescents' rational plans for future political action (Eckstein et al., 2013). Inspired by Fishbein and Ajzen's theory of planned behavior (1975; Ajzen, 1985, 1991), which later evolved into the theory of reasoned action (Fishbein & Ajzen, 2010), Eckstein and colleagues conducted a three-wave longitudinal study that included the central concepts of the theory of planned behavior: attitudes toward political action, subjective norms, behavioral control, and behavioral intentions. In Fishbein and Ajzen's theory, intentions to act in the future should be the central predictor of their future actions. In their study, Eckstein and colleagues examined whether adolescents' stated intentions to participate in future offline political activities influenced their future political behavior. Adolescents' attitudes toward political behavior, the salience of others' attitudes, and internal political efficacy were also hypothesized to influence adolescents' behavioral intentions. The results supported that behavioral intentions were a significant predictor of later political behavior, but were not significant when individuals' behavioral control (internal political efficacy) was included as a predictor. This is perhaps not surprising. Political efficacy is highly related to political interest and has almost the same predictive power for political behavior as political interest (Levy & Akiva, 2019; Strömbäck & Shehata, 2010).

Eckstein and colleagues' longitudinal study of college students is a good starting point for examining whether goal setting in mid-adolescence affects future political activity. Our consideration differs from Eckstein and colleagues' (2013) study in two main ways. First, in their study, attitudes toward political behavior were measured by items such as "There are not too many, but too few people who are politically active in Germany." In contrast, we argue that adolescents' own political interest should be seen as the most sensitive indicator of their attitudes toward politics. It can be said that adolescents' political interest represents the personal meaning of politics for them and, thus, their political attitudes. Second, in Eckstein and colleagues' study (2013), young adults' attitudes toward politics were treated as a unique predictor of their intentions to become politically involved. In contrast, we do not believe that young people's civic engagement goals are independent of their political interest. Rather, setting civic goals should act as a moderator between their political interest and their future political activities. Political interest will lead adolescents to future political activity, especially if adolescents have set civic goals.

Otherwise, the model we wanted to test followed the Eckstein study. Adolescents' internal political efficacy, that is, their belief in their ability to participate effectively in politics (Craig et al., 1990), was used as a measure of behavioral control, and subjective norm was measured by adolescents' perceptions of their parents' and peers' political interests. Given our goal of making predictions over longer periods of time, goal setting was considered a better label than immediate intentions. We had two hypotheses. First, we hypothesized that adolescents' political interest would be the most important predictor of future political activity. Second, we hypothesized that adolescents' goals for their civic engagement would moderate the effects of political interest on their various future political activities. The model to be tested is shown in Figure 2.1.

The age cohort of 16-year-olds (upper secondary students) survey year 2010 was chosen for a specific reason. At age 20, four years later, they were eligible to vote in a national election for the first time. This made it possible to examine whether the interaction between political interest and goal setting predicted not only general political activity at age 20, but also whether they would take an active public stance for a particular party. At age 20, participants were mailed a questionnaire twice that year (before and after the election in September 2014: April/May and October) along with a personalized link to an online version of the questionnaire.

The target sample at age 16 (T1) consisted of 1,052 individuals. The analytic sample with data on the study measures at T1 was 869 (83% of the target sample). Of the analytic sample, data were available for 463 individuals (53%) at age 20, when the adolescents had left high school (upper secondary school), and for 385 individuals (44%) at follow-up.

Outcome Measures

The following political behaviors were measured at the age of 20:

- *Political activities offline*. The participants were asked if they, during the previous year, had been involved in 10 political activities, such as "Taken part in a

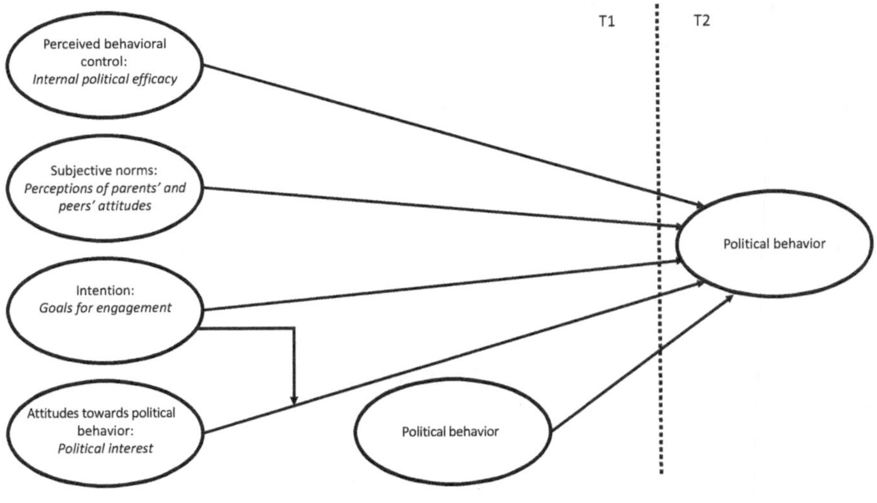

FIGURE 2.1 Outline of the tested model.

legal demonstration or strike" and "Collected signatures." The response scale ranged from 1 (*never*) to 3 (*several times*).

- *Political activities online*. The participants were asked if they had engaged in 15 different political activities online in the last 12 months, such as "Written about politics or societal issues on my own blog or website" and "Taken part in an internet-based protest" (items that represented searching for political information on the Internet were excluded). The response options ranged from 1 (*no*) to 3 (*yes, several times*).
- *Membership in a political/civic organization*. Participants were asked if they belonged to one of three types of organizations: a political organization (4%), an environmental organization (1.4%), or an organization for peace or human rights (the Peace Movement, Amnesty International, etc.) (2.3%). These organizations were among the three most common types of organizations reported by 16-year-olds in pilot tests. Membership in these organizations was summed.

These questions were asked before (in April and May) and after (in October) the national election, which took place in September 2014:

- *Taking a stance in public in the national election*. Before the election, the participants were asked if they would take an active stance in public in various ways: "Use the internet to support the parties I like," "Follow and 'like' parties on social networks, such as Twitter and Facebook," "Work pro-bono for a party in the national election, for example by handing out leaflets for the party," and "Support a party by wearing their badge or t-shirt." The response items were 1 (*I will definitely not do that*), 2 (*I will probably not do that*), 3 (*I will probably do that*), and 4 (*I will certainly do that*). In the post-election questionnaire, the participants were asked again about taking an active stance in public. Here the stem question was "What did you do before the national election?" for the same items, and the response options were 1 (*no*) and 2 (*yes*).
- *Voting*. The participants were asked if they had voted in the election: 1 (*no*) and 2 (*yes*).

Predictors

Setting goals for one's future civic/political engagement was measured with a single item: "Some people have set goals for themselves concerning their engagement in societal issues. Have you?" with the response options:

(1) *I'm not interested in such issues, quite the opposite. I will certainly not commit myself to doing anything about them,*
(2) *I'm not interested in such issues, and as far as I can see, I'm not going to commit myself to doing anything about them,*

(3) *I will definitely work actively (in an organization or otherwise) on such issues, but have not yet committed to doing so*, and
(4) *I will be active in an organization, and I'm already a member of such an organization.*

Because the last response option includes "I am already a member of such an organization," the long-term predictions would, strictly speaking, include individuals who were already members of such organizations at age 16. To account for this, we controlled for the aforementioned membership in a political/civic organization at age 16 when predicting offline and online political activity at age 20 (and, of course, when predicting future membership in civic/political organizations). Other measures of the theory of planned behavior at age 16 were as follows:

- *Attitudes toward political behavior.* Attitudes toward political behavior was a measure of political interest. The level of political interest was measured using two questions. First, "How interested are you in politics?" The response options ranged from 1 (*totally uninterested*), to 5 (*very interested*). Second, the participants' emotional reactions to politics were investigated by the following question: "People differ in how they feel about politics. What are your feelings?" Responses were on a scale from (1) *loath* to (6) *great fun.* The feeling question was rescaled to a 5-point rating scale and the two items were aggregated.
- *Subjective norms.* The adolescents responded to the statements "My parents (friends) are interested in what is going on in the world" and "My parents (friends) keep in touch with the news." The response scale ranged from 1 (*doesn't apply at all*) to 4 (*applies perfectly*).
- *Behavioral control* was measured by the adolescents' internal political efficacy, covering nine items which refer to a domain-specific efficacy belief in the capacity of one's own actions to effect change in society. After the stem, "If I really tried, I could manage to . . ., " the participants responded to nine statements, such as "Take on responsibility in a political youth organization and "Discuss politics with people with more experience than I have." The response scale ranged from 1 (*I could definitely not manage that*) to 4 (*I could definitely manage that*).
- *Covariates.* We controlled for family economic conditions, immigrant status, and sex. Economic conditions in the family were measured by five items to the adolescents, such as "If you want things that cost a lot of money (e.g., a computer, skateboard, cell phone), can your parents afford to buy them?" with responses scale from 1 (*absolutely not)* to 5 (*yes, absolutely*), and "How often do you and your family go on vacation abroad?" with responses from 1 (*seldom*

or never) to 4 (*we travel once or several times a year*). Immigrant status was a dichotomous measure, differentiating between students whose parents were born outside the Nordic countries (coded 1) and other students (coded 0). Sex was coded 0 = female, 1 = male.

Setting the Stage for Long-Term Analyses

Following standard longitudinal practice, the three types of political activity at age 20—offline political activity, online political activity, and political/civic organization membership—were controlled for by the same measures at age 16 to focus attention on what changed between ages 16 and 20. Because the goals measure included the highest option of already being politically engaged, we controlled for membership in a political/civic organization at age 16 in predicting offline and online political activity at age 20.

We ran moderated regressions using Hayes's PROCESS macro (Hays, 2017) predicting youth political activity at age 20 and taking a public stance and voting in the national election from their political interest, goal setting and political efficacy, peer and parental political interest, and the control variables at age 16. The regressions also included the interaction between political interest and goal setting for civic engagement. All measures were standardized before calculations.

One additional piece of information needs to be reported. Attrition analyses showed that the age-20 and post-election data were weakly gender biased. Males did not participate in the age-20 data collection to the same extent as females. The Nagelkerke R^2 was .06. However, there was no bias in political interest, goal setting, behavioral control, or any of the other measures at age 16.

Results

Table 2.1 reports the predictions of offline and online activities and political/civic organization membership four years after the original data collection at age 16. As reported in the table, political interest was a significant predictor of offline and online political activities at the .05 level, but not of membership in a political/civic organization. Goal setting as a main effect was a significant predictor of offline political activity and political/civic organization membership, but not online political activity. Consistent with the hypothesis, the interaction between political interest and goal setting was significant for all three dependent measures. The moderating role of goal setting on political interest is reported in Figure 2.2 (predicting offline activity at age 20), Figure 2.3 (predicting online activity at age 20), and Figure 2.4 (predicting having a membership in a political or civic organization at age 20). In all cases, high levels of political activity were found primarily among participants who had both high political interest and high goal setting at age 16.

TABLE 2.1 Predicted changes in offline and online activity and membership in a political or civic organization, from ages 16 to 20.

	Political offline activities (N = 352)				*Political online activities (N = 351)*			
	β	t	p	*95%CI*	β	t	p	*95%CI*
Variable at age 16	.15	3.01	.003	0.05–0.25	.38	7.02	<.001	0.27–0.48
Member political/civic organization	.06	1.32	.188	-0.03–0 .16	-.03	-0.59	.559	-0.12–0.07
Political interest	.16	2.57	.011	0.04–0.29	.13	2.21	.035	0.01–0.25
Goal setting	.16	2.70	.007	0.04–0.28	-.02	-0.27	.785	-0.13–0.10
Political interest × Goal setting	.13	3.11	.002	0.05–0.22	.14	3.38	.001	0.06–0.21
Political efficacy	.13	2.31	.021	0.02–0.24	.08	1.52	.128	-0.02–0.18
Peers' interest	-.04	-0.79	.429	-0.15–0.06	.04	0.71	.478	-0.06–0.14
Parents' interest	-.00	-0.08	.936	-0.10–0.10	-.01	-0.11	.913	-0.10–0.09
Sex	-.09	-1.88	.061	-0.19–0.00	.07	1.54	.125	-0.02–0.17
Family economy	.05	1.14	.256	-0.04–0.15	-.01	-0.25	.804	-0.11–0.08
Immigration status	-.01	-0.13	.897	-0.11–0.10	-.01	-0.25	.802	-0.11–0.08
R^2	.26				.33			

	Member political/civic organization (N = 347)			
	β	t	p	*95%CI*
Member political/civic organization	.06	1.10	.274	-0.05–0.16
Political interest	.09	1.28	.203	-0.05–0.22
Goal setting	.14	2.24	.026	0.02–0.27
Political interest × Goal setting	.13	2.77	.006	0.04–0.16
Political efficacy	.06	1.03	.302	-0.06–0.18
Peers' political interest	-.02	-0.26	.736	-0.13–0.10
Parents' political interest	.01	0.12	.903	-0.10–0.11
Sex	-.00	-0.03	.977	-0.11–0.10
Family economy	-.02	-0.30	.768	-0.12–0.09
Immigration status	.05	0.85	.405	-0.06–0.16
R^2	.11			

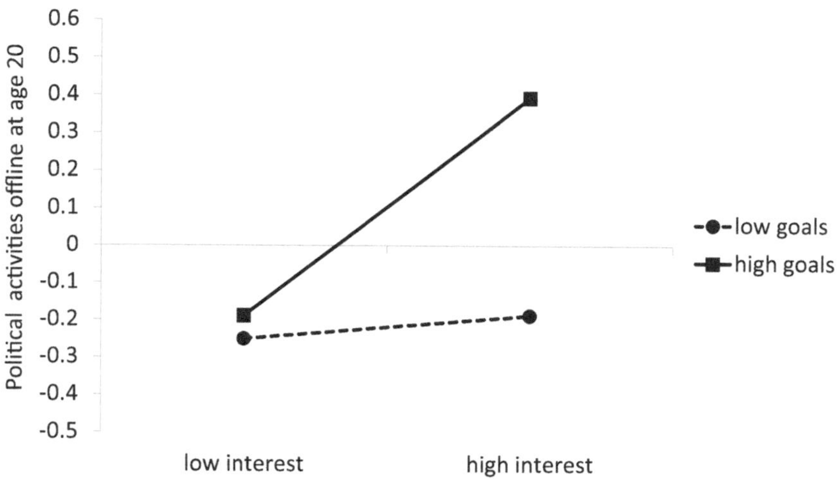

FIGURE 2.2 Interactive effect of political interest and goal setting on offline activity at age 20.

The figure represents the slopes for political interest at high and low values (1 SD above and below the mean) of goal setting. The high goals slope is significantly different from zero ($p = .002$). Predicted values shown here are based on regression parameter estimates reported in Table 2.1 ($n = 352$).

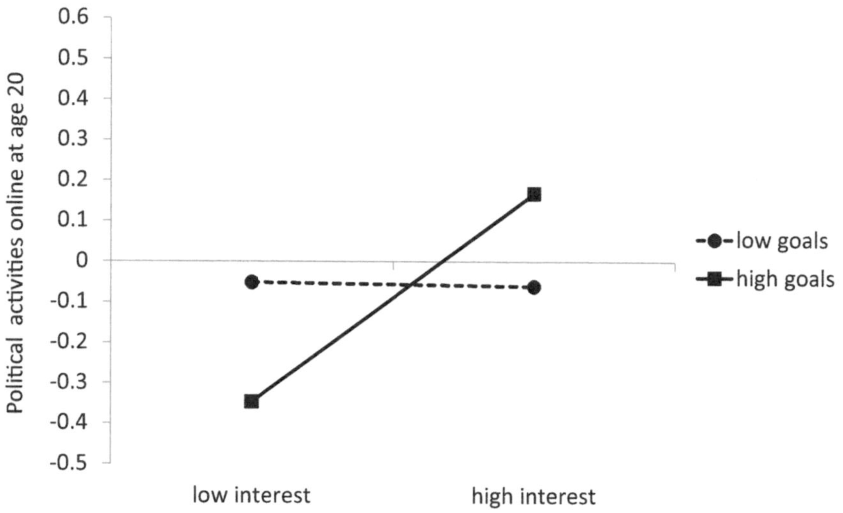

FIGURE 2.3 Interactive effect of political interest and goal setting on online activity at age 20.

The figure represents the slopes for political interest at high and low values (1 SD above and below the mean) of goal setting. The high goals slope is significantly different from zero ($p = .001$). Predicted values shown here are based on regression parameter estimates reported in Table 2.1 ($n = 351$).

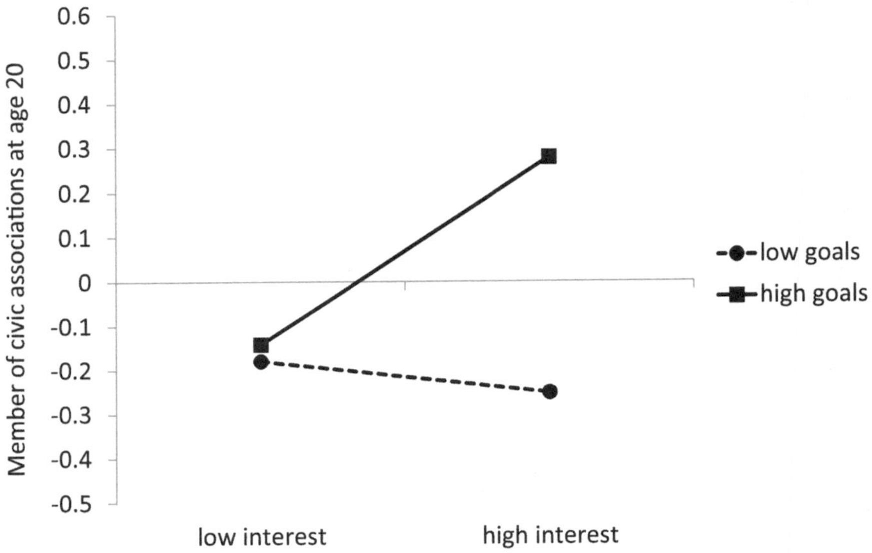

FIGURE 2.4 Interactive effect of political interest and goal setting on having a membership in a political or civic organization at age 20.

The figure represents the slopes for political interest at high and low values (1 SD above and below the mean) of goal setting. The high goals slope is significantly different from zero ($p = .006$). Predicted values shown here are based on regression parameter estimates reported in Table 2.1 ($n = 347$).

Follow-up simple slope tests indicated that political interest was a significant predictor of political activities at high levels (+1 SD) of goal setting (the coefficients ranged from .22 to .30), but not at low levels (- 1 SD) (the coefficients ranged from -.04 to .03). Political efficacy was only a significant predictor of offline political activity at the .05 level.

The same type of regression was applied to the predictors of public support for a political party before and after the election. The results are shown in Table 2.2. Political interest was a significant predictor of public support for a party both before and after the election, and setting goals for one's civic engagement was a significant predictor of taking a public stance for a party before the election. Again, consistent with our hypothesis, the interaction between political interest and goal setting was a significant predictor of both outcomes. As reported in Figures 2.5 and 2.6, high public support both at pre-election and at post-election was particularly true for participants who had both high political interest and high goal setting. Follow-up simple slope tests indicated that political interest was a good predictor of support in public of parties at high levels of goal setting, with coefficients of .37 and .38; significant at the .001 level, but not at low levels of goal setting, with

TABLE 2.2 Predictions of public support for parties before and after the election at age 20.

	β	*t*	*p*	*95%CI*	*β*	*t*	*p*	*95%CI*
	Pre-election support (N = 351)				*Post-election support (N = 292)*			
Member political/civic organization	.04	0.87	.871	-0.05–0.13	.11	2.13	.034	0.01–0.22
Political interest	.17	2.69	.008	0.05–0.29	.19	2.73	.007	0.05–0.33
Goal setting	.23	3.85	<.001	0.11–0.34	.10	1.60	.111	-0.02–0.23
Political interest × Goal setting	.20	4.77	<.001	0.12–0.28	.19	3.88	<.001	0.09–0.28
Political efficacy	.00	0.01	.994	-0.11–0.11	-.00	-0.01	.989	-0.12–0.11
Peers' political interest	.09	1.68	.094	-0.02–0.19	.08	1.41	.161	-0.03–0.20
Parents' political interest	-.05	-1.09	.276	-0.15–0.04	-.12	-2.16	.032	-0.22–0.01
Sex	.06	1.15	.249	-0.04–0.15	-.03	-0.46	.647	-0.14–0.08
Family economy	-.08	-1.70	.091	-0.17–0.01	-.01	-0.21	.834	-0.12–0.10
Immigration status	.05	1.11	.269	-0.04–0.16	-.03	-0.44	.664	-0.14–0.09
R^2	.27				.20			

Note: CI, confidence interval [lower bound, upper bound].

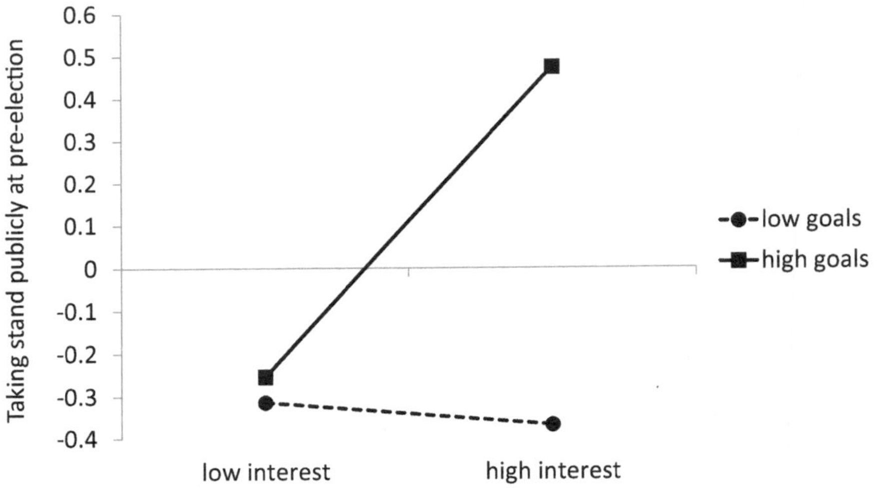

FIGURE 2.5 Interactive effect of political interest and goal setting on public support for a party at pre-election.

The figure represents the slopes for political interest at high and low values (1 SD above and below the mean) of goal setting. The high goals slope is significantly different from zero ($p < .001$). Predicted values shown here are based on regression parameter estimates reported in Table 2.2 ($n = 352$).

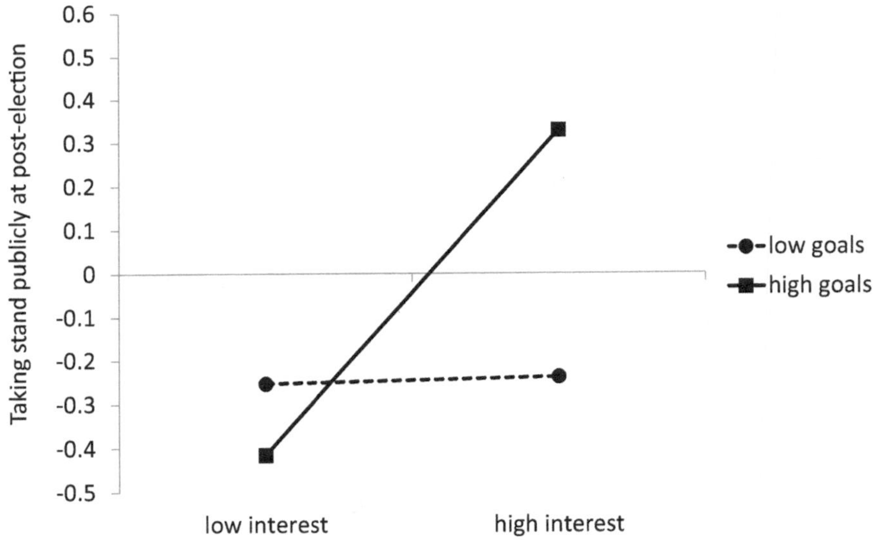

FIGURE 2.6 Interactive effect of political interest and goal setting on public support for a party at post-election.

The figure represents the slopes for political interest at high and low values (1 SD above and below the mean) of goal setting. The high goals slope is significantly different from zero ($p < .001$). Predicted values shown here are based on regression parameter estimates reported in Table 2.2 ($n = 292$).

coefficients as low as -.03 and -01. We were not able to predict voting, primarily due to lack of variability, as 94% of 20-year-olds reported voting.

The highest scale score for goal setting at age 16 was related to both the desire to be involved in the civic activities in the future and being a member of a civic/political organization; "I will be active in an organization, and I'm already a member of such an organization." In control analyses, we excluded all youths who reported the highest scale score on the goal-setting measure and reanalyzed Tables 2.1 and 2.2. For three of the outcome measures, namely offline political activity, membership in a political or civic organization, and taking a public stance for a party reported before the national election, the interaction between political interest and goal setting was still significant. However, it did not reach conventional levels of significance for online activities and taking a public stance reported after the election. This loss of significance was expected due to the limited variability in the independent variable of goal setting. Overall, we conclude that the findings held up well in these control analyses.

Discussion

It is difficult to empirically confirm the existence of a hypothesized interaction term in a regression analysis. Here, we predicted significant interactions between political interest and goal setting in six separate analyses. Five of them (not voting) were significant. This is noteworthy and provides strong support for the hypothesis that rationally setting goals for one's future civic engagement moderates the relationship between 16-year-old adolescents' political interest and their future political activity. Particularly high levels of political activity and taking a position in an election four years later are found among 16-year-olds who have high political interest and high goals for their future civic engagement.

Adolescents appear to be able to set future goals for their political/civic engagement, and these goals are particularly important for those adolescents who are politically interested early on. The results reported here need to be cross-validated, and if confirmed in future studies, these findings have important implications for social policy. They encourage and support various initiatives to channel adolescents' political interest and long-term engagement during their politically formative years. They suggest that the politically oriented organizations of civil society, the political parties and their youth associations, can give voice and direction to young people's future engagement (Pickard, 2019). But they also apply to the provision of forums by public administrations that take advantage of and deliberately develop young people's rationally planned engagement in schools, community planning, participatory budgeting, civic dialogues, and more (Nabatchi, 2014).

This study is based on the theory of planned behavior (Ajzen, 1985, 1991; Fishbein & Ajzen, 1975). This theory, as applied to political behavior, posits that attitudes toward political behavior, subjective norms about that behavior, and people's behavioral control all influence people's intentions to engage in that behavior. These intentions, in turn, should be the best predictor of their actual future political behavior. We have proposed alternative paths. First, attitudes toward political behavior (political interest) were assumed to interact with intentions (goal setting)—not to act as another predictor. Second, in addition to influencing individuals' intentions (goal setting), attitudes toward political behavior, subjective norms about these behaviors, and individuals' behavioral control were assumed to directly influence adolescents' future political involvement four years later. These reformulations of the theory of planned behavior found empirical support.

A note about predicting the actual vote is necessary. Due to the skewed distribution, we were not successful in predicting actual voting. In the study, 94% of participants said they voted in the national election. This is a higher percentage than the 85% of young adults aged 18 to 24 in the region who actually voted, according to Statistics Sweden (2018). It is not uncommon to find a higher proportion of reported voting than actual voting (Ansolabehere & Hersh, 2012; Dahlgaard et al., 2019). One interpretation of the difference found here is that overreporting of first-time voting is particularly high due to a lack of routine among young voters (Gerber et al., 2003). Some of the adolescents may have felt pressured to report in the questionnaire that they had voted in a socially desirable way.

Finally, we relate these findings to what we have learned earlier about the stability and change in political interest over shorter and longer periods of time. These short- and long-term stabilities show that political interest is likely to persist, with the exception of in early adolscence. This does not mean that persistence guarantees engagement in future civic and political behavior. What this study of long-term goal setting adds to the literature is that these goals differentiate the politically interested adolescents who eventually became politically engaged from the politically interested adolescents of the same age who did not translate their political interest into political action.

The main strength of these goal-setting analyses is that they provide empirical support for the idea that young people rationally set goals for their future civic engagement and that these goals help politically interested adolescents in their future political activities. The main limitation of the study is that the sample was found to be slightly gender biased. Approximately equal proportions of males and females participated in the data collection at age 16, but males were underrepresented among the youths who responded to the questionnaire four years later. However, the attrition analysis found no significant effects of any of the other measures used in the study.

Finally, what evidence has been presented in this chapter that young people are active agents in their own political development?

- As early as mid-adolescence, young people set goals for their future civic engagement, and these goals moderate the association between their political interest and political activities of various kinds—offline and online political activities, membership in political/civic organizations, and public support for a party before and after elections—four years later. These goals appear to be early rational plans for future political activism, and early intentions to participate in civic activities appear to be a genuine example of political agency.

PART II

Push and Pull of Political Interest

3

YOUNG PEOPLE'S ATTENTION TO POLITICS

Highlights

Over the course of a year, some adolescents will encounter events that they perceive as increasing their political interest. What characterized these adolescents two years earlier, what are the consequences of these events one year later, and what are the characteristics of these events? We focused on 15- and 18-year-olds. On the basis of self-determination theory, we predicted that adolescents who had experienced such events two years earlier

- *would already be more politically interested than other adolescents, and*
- *would be more likely than other students to engage in behaviors that reflected their needs for autonomy, relatedness, and competence.*

These predictions were largely confirmed. First, a prior interest in politics and engagement in exploratory behaviors that reflect adolescents' psychological needs seem to play a crucial role in understanding why adolescents encounter events in their everyday lives that trigger their political interest. Second, having experienced events that triggered adolescents' political interest was associated with later increases in political interest more broadly.

In terms of the content of events reported by adolescents, many involved national and international issues that were perceived as threatening and that challenged adolescents' beliefs and morals.

There is preliminary evidence that when adolescents encounter events that trigger their political interest, they want to discuss political and civic issues with their parents and friends.

We asked the parents of the younger cohort the same question about whether they had experienced an interest-triggering event. Parents who had experienced such an event in the past year were more politically interested than other parents. Contrary to our hypothesis, they were not more politically interested one year earlier. However, a paired samples test showed that parents who had experienced an interest-triggering event had increased their political interest over the past year, while other parents had decreased their political interest.

Political interest is defined as paying attention to political issues and having an intrinsic motivation for that attention. Political interest as a motivational component has been defined by Lupia and Philpot as "a citizen's willingness to pay attention to political phenomena at the possible expense of other topics" (Lupia & Philpot,

DOI: 10.4324/9781003371731-5

2005, p. 1122), by van Deth (2000, p. 119) as "the degree to which politics arouses a citizen's curiosity," and by Lane (1959, p. 133) as "a sense that it is worth paying attention to a phenomenon" (see also Almond & Verba, 1963; Levy & Akiva, 2019; Prior, 2019, for similar definitions). In these formulations, attention and interest are intertwined. In this chapter, we examine

- whether events that adolescents perceive as triggering their interest are preceded by higher political interest earlier in time and
- whether adolescents' beliefs that it is important to stay informed about social, environmental, and political issues affect their political interest over time.

The analyses also seek to answer the questions of how political interest is related to attention to political issues, and how attention to political issues affects political interest. Are these bidirectional processes that feed off each other? We present two ideas about how attention and political interest are intertwined.

Events That Change the Political Interest of Some Adolescents

In their quest to understand how the world works, adolescents are exposed to an enormous amount of information about society, politics, and the environment on a daily basis. In fact, today's youth are growing up in an "information age" where this information is instantly available and changing. Every day, as they watch television, read newspapers, or surf the Internet, young people are inundated with information about wars, disasters, nuclear threats, terrorist attacks, oil shortages, tsunamis, economic crises and recoveries, political meetings and decisions, and elections. As they talk with their parents, peers, teachers, and others, they learn about issues such as the global financial system, gender inequality, file sharing, refugees and immigration, global warming, and much more. There is a flood of media coverage of events, and information gleaned from conversations with others can be daily eye-openers that spark young people's political interest. How youth are affected by everyday political and civic events has not been much systematically studied.

Of the many new pieces of political information that adolescents encounter in a single day, only small fragments are likely to capture their attention, and only a small fraction of the information they attend to will have longer-term consequences. Nevertheless, some of these events may increase their political interest in the minds of young people. This is the first focus of this chapter. How many adolescents encounter events that they perceive as increasing their political interest, what were the events that changed their interest, and what characterizes these adolescents' years earlier? We will use self-determination theory to develop ideas about what characterizes those adolescents who recognize events that they say have increased their political interest.

We asked the 15- and the 18-year-old adolescents in the first two cohorts the following question: "Has something happened this last year that made you more or less interested in issues concerned with what is going on in Sweden and the world or with political and ecological matters?" (from here labeled events that trigger adolescents' politics interest). The response scale was 1 (*No, I became neither more nor less interested*), 2 (*Yes, I became more interested*), and 3 (*Yes, I became less interested*). They were then asked to describe freely what it was that made them more or less interested.

Relatively few 15- and 18-year-olds reported events in the past year that made them less interested in politics (4.7% of 15-year-olds and 5.2% of 18-year-olds). According to their reports, 18.1% of 15-year-olds had experiences in the past year that made them more interested in politics. Among 18-year-olds, the figure was 23.8%. Is there anything specific, one or two years earlier, that would give us an indication of why some in the two samples of 15- and 18-year-olds encountered events that triggered their political interest while others did not?

Self-Determination Theory

There is no systematic research on whether and how everyday local, national, and global events act as political eye-openers for adolescents. This is unfortunate, because it is precisely these types of events, at various levels of abstraction, that should potentially shed light on how adolescents' political interest grows over time. Historically, researchers have asked what political characteristics people born in one time period have in common and different from people born in another (Jennings & Niemi, 1981; Putnam, 2000). The assumption is that if adolescents are exposed to similar national and international events during their formative years, this will shape their beliefs and attitudes in similar ways in the future. We expect our samples of adolescents to report very different events that increased their political interest, even if they were born in the same year. In short, we are interested in events that are likely to differentiate young people of the same age, rather than events that are likely to affect an entire generation of young people in a similar way.

The reasons why some adolescents experience events that increase their political interest may be highly idiosyncratic, but it can be argued that there are some common features that link them. Here we ask what feelings, perceptions, and behaviors characterize adolescents who encounter events in their everyday lives that increase their political interest. We expect that it will be primarily adolescents who have previously had a heightened interest in politics and positive feelings about political issues who will experience events that trigger their interest in politics. These adolescents who are already politically and socially interested and have positive feelings about politics should be more receptive to these events. Adolescents who have little political interest and some who dislike politics should pay limited attention to political cues in their environment. To identify other antecedents of these adolescents in addition to prior higher political interest and positive feelings about politics, we will use self-determination theory as a guiding theoretical framework.

The socialization perspective has dominated research on youth interest in political and civic issues, but it is based on surprisingly few attempts to formally test the proposed ways in which parents, teachers, other role models, and media influence young people's political development. Another perspective is that some of the thoughts, feelings, and behaviors associated with political interest have their origins in young people themselves (e.g., Strömbäck & Shehata, 2010), rather than in inputs from their interpersonal environments. Thus, an alternative to the classical socialization idea is that young people's political interest can drive their own civic and political development. Self-determination theory (Deci & Ryan, 1991, 2000; Ryan & Deci, 2000, 2006) suggests that young people freely explore things they are interested in and they have intrinsic motivation to engage in things that satisfy their needs. If they are curious and interested in society and politics, they will be motivated to pursue and develop this interest further if the conditions and other people's reactions to them facilitate their exploratory attempts. A basic tenet of self-determination theory is that people are active and engage in activities they are interested in and believe they are good at. In the present study, we use self-determination theory to understand how feelings about politics and society, communication with others about these things, and political self-efficacy can be linked to political interest-triggering events.

In the political socialization literature, youth who are interested in politics are said to have an intrinsic interest in political issues (Shani, 2009; Campbell et al., 1954; Luskin, 1990; van Deth, 1990; Delli Carpini & Keeter, 1996; Althaus, 2003; Prior, 2019). An intrinsic interest, according to major dictionaries, is a genuine, essential, or fundamental interest in a matter that motivates behavior—as opposed to an extrinsic interest, which comes from outside and motivates behavior. In self-determination theory, which is an agentic theory of human motivation, this intrinsic interest is a nexus for people's feelings, desires, and activities. According to this theory, if adolescents have an intrinsic interest in a topic and experience a sense of freedom in exploring it, they will find ways to advance that area of interest if their needs for *autonomy*, *relatedness*, and *competence* are met (Deci & Ryan, 2000, 2008; Ryan & Deci, 2000, 2006). The need for autonomy refers to feeling free to explore and develop personal interests. The need for relatedness refers to feeling connected to and accepted by others. Finally, the need for competence is a sense of confidence that one's actions contribute to the achievement of a worthwhile goal, consistent with Bandura's (2006) concept of feelings of efficacy. Adolescents will seek to satisfy their basic psychological needs in areas where they are intrinsically motivated.

Based on self-determination theory, we identified a set of indicators (behaviors, opinions) that we hypothesized would be important for politically interested adolescents to satisfy their basic psychological needs. These are not the standard needs measures used in the self-determination theory literature because only few studies have applied the self-determination theory framework to the development of political and social interest among adolescents. We hypothesize that these indicators will differentiate those adolescents who later had experiences that triggered their political interest from those adolescents who did not have such experiences.

The need for autonomy is closely related to the concept of intrinsic motivation in self-determination theory, because to be autonomous is to feel a full sense of choice in supporting certain actions and acting out of personal interest (Deci & Ryan, 2002). The need for autonomy, according to self-determination theory, is about feeling free to explore and deepen one's personal interests.

- Following the news to learn about current politics and society should be a core activity for young people who are intrinsically interested in politics. If they feel free to explore what is happening in politics and society, they should find it personally relevant to follow the news.
- Setting personal goals related to the object of interest is a hallmark of autonomy (Deci & Ryan, 2008). We expect that setting long-term goals related to their political engagement earlier in life would be more characteristic of those adolescents who later experience events that trigger their political interest than of other adolescents (see Chapter 2).

The need for relatedness refers to the feeling of belonging to a group of people with similar interests. As indicators of the need for relatedness, we chose to examine political interactions with parents and Internet activities:

- Political discussions with parents. These concerned how often adolescents talked to their parents about politics and what was happening in the world and in their society,
- Adolescent-initiated discussions. If adolescents feel free to express their political views, they should want to initiate political discussions at home.
- Discussions with others on the Internet. Political discussions with friends and others on the Internet were the third indicator of the need for relatedness. Communicating and discussing political and social issues is a shared activity (Shah et al., 2009).

Finally, *need for competence* concerns feeling competent or capable and refers to a sense of confidence in one's own actions rather than an achieved skill (Deci & Ryan, 2002). Here, we examine a specific domain-specific efficacy belief: the internal sense of political competence.

We propose that adolescents who have experienced events that they believe have increased their political interest will differ from adolescents who have not experienced these events in a number of ways. First, they will be more politically interested and have more positive feelings about politics years earlier, and they will years earlier express behaviors and opinions that reflect their needs for autonomy, relatedness, and competence to a greater extent earlier than adolescents who do not experience these events. Second, we expect that an initial and growing interest in politics will be associated with an initial and growing increase in behaviors that reflect adolescents' psychological needs. The study hypotheses are shown in Figure 3.1.

Items and scales are reported in Table 3.1. Covariates were sex and parents' levels of education.

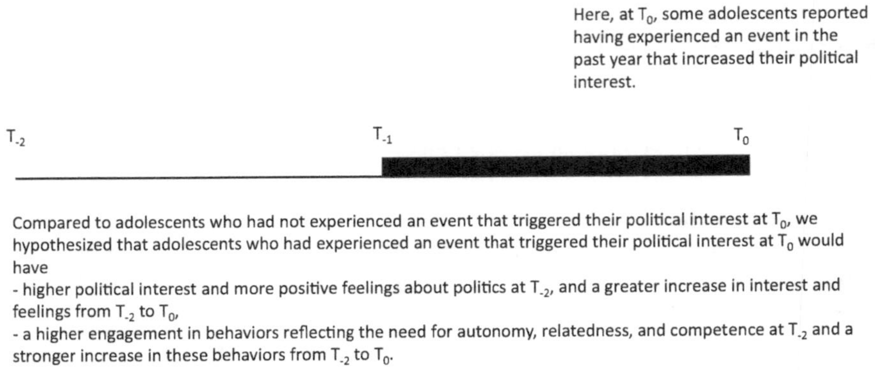

FIGURE 3.1 Study hypotheses.

TABLE 3.1 Scales and items used in the study.

Concept	*Items*	*Response scale*
Political interest		
"How interested are you in politics?" and "How interested are you in what is going on in society?"	2	1 (*totally uninterested)*, 5 (*very interested*)
Feelings about politics		
"People differ in what they feel about politics. What are your feelings?"	1	1 (*loath*) 6 (great fun)
Cognitive and emotional engagement in news consumption [Satisfaction of autonomy needs]		
What is your experience of the following media?. . . Watching or reading the news (on TV, in daily newspapers, or on the Internet)	3	1 (*doesn't engage me at all*), to 6 (*engages me a lot*); 1 (*gives me no new ideas at all*), to 6 (*gives me many new ideas*); 1 (*is boring*), to 6 (*is fun*)
Setting long-term goals [Satisfaction of autonomy needs]		
"Some people have set goals for themselves concerning their engagement in societal issues. Have you?"	1	1 (*I'm not interested in issues like this, rather the opposite. I will certainly not commit myself to doing anything about them*), 2 (*I'm not interested in issues like this and, as far as I can see, I will not commit myself to getting engaged in them*), 3 (*I will definitely work actively (in organizations or by other means) on issues like this but have not yet committed myself*), 4 (*I will work actively in organizations and I'm already a member of such an organization*)

Concept	*Items*	*Response scale*
Perceived family social climate [Satisfaction of relatedness needs]		
Democratic family climate: A four-item scale with items like "Your parents let you take part when you are going to decide something in the family", and "Your parents ask you when decisions are to be made in the family."	6	1 (*don't agree at all*) 5 (*agree totally*)
Attached relations to parents: A five-item scale (separately for father and mother) with items like "I feel comfortable sharing my private thoughts and feelings with my mother (father)", and "I feel like I can try new things because I know my mother (father) supports me"	5 & 5	1 (*definitely doesn't apply*) 5 (*applies very well*)
Parents' attempted understanding: Stem question: "What happens if you do something your mother (father) really dislikes?". Example of items are "Is clear about what she/he thinks, but is open to discussion", and "Honestly wants to understand why you did what you did". The response scales ranged from. The average correlation between the mother and father scales was .65 across ages, so we aggregated the two measures.	5 & 5	1 (*never*), 3 (*most often*)
Parents' warmth towards the adolescents: A six-item scale, separately for father and mother. Example items are "Focuses on the positive and seldom the negative things you do", and "Shows with words and gestures that she/he likes you". Because the average correlation between the mother and father scales was as high as .66 across ages, we aggregated the two measures. We factor analyzed the four subscales, and they produced one factor at all ages with factor loadings ranging from .75 to .88. We used that factor for measuring the perceived family social climate.	6 & 6	1 (*never*), 3 (*most often*)
Discussing political issues with parents [Satisfaction of relatedness needs]		
The participants were asked how often they discussed "What they had heard on the news about what is going on in Sweden and around the world" and "Politics or societal issues", with their parents.	2	1 (*never*) 4 (*very often*)

(*Continued*)

TABLE 3.1 (Continued)

Concept	*Items*	*Response scale*
Initiating political conversations with parents [Satisfaction of relatedness needs]		
Two items: "Are you trying to get your parents to become more aware of what is going on in the world?" and "... more aware of environmental issues?" The average correlation between the two items was .65.	2	1 (*almost never*) 5 *(almost always*)
Political talk on the Internet [Satisfaction of relatedness needs]		
A five-item scale, asking if the participants, during the last two months, had, for example, "Discussed societal or political questions with friends on the Internet", and "Discussed societal issues with people I don't know". The response scale ranged from (1) no, to (3) yes, several times. Alpha reliability averaged .72.	5	1 (*not at all important*) 5 (*very important*)
Internal political efficacy [Satisfaction of competence needs]		
After the stem question "If I really tried, I could manage to...", the participants responded to nine statements, including: "Take on responsibility in a political youth organization", and "Be an active member of a political organization".	9	1 (*I could definitely not manage that*) 4 (*I could definitely manage that*)
Covariates:		
Sex was coded as 0 (*male*) and 1 (*female*). Fathers' and mothers' level of education were aggregated. They were measured on a scale ranging from 1 (*less than 9 years of study*) to 5 (*university college/ university education*).	2	

Participants and Analyses

We use the two youngest age cohorts. In the first cohort, adolescents answered the question about events that sparked their interest in politics when they were 15 years old (n = 836). We have questionnaire information on most of these individuals when they were one year younger (this year's analytic sample, n = 883) and two years younger (n = 909). Participants in the second cohort completed the questionnaire when they were 18 years old (n = 750). Most of them also participated in data collection one year earlier (this year's analytical sample, n = 814) and two years earlier (n = 869).

TABLE 3.2 Reported events that increased adolescents' political interest among the 15- and the 18-year olds at t_0 (2012).

	Age 15		*Age 18*	
	N	*Percentage*	*N*	*Percentage*
Specific issues				
School issues	3	2	5	2.8
Environment and climate change	1	0.7	4	2.3
File sharing	4	2.7	4	2.3
Others	4	2.7	6	3.4
Swedish politics				
Immigration	12	8	13	7.3
Party politics	11	7.3	10	5.6
Others	5	3.3	10	5.6
International events				
Norway	11	7.3	16	9.0
United States	5	3.3	1	0.6
Arab Spring and Middle East	3	2	10	5.6
Greece	4	2.7	1	0.6
Others	10	6.7	10	5.6
Source				
School	14	9.3	14	7.9
Influential teachers	4	2.7	1	0.6
Peers	2	1.3	6	3.4
Media and social media	9	6	14	7.9
Self				
Own development	10	6.7	17	9.6
Voting age	0	0	9	5.1
Could not be coded	38	25.3	26	14.7
Total	150		177	

Which Events Were Reported?

We classified the events reported by adolescents in the two cohorts into 20 categories. Each was reported by at least three people at each age in the two cohorts (Table 3.2). Two raters independently coded all event descriptions into the 20 categories. Inter-rater reliability, Cohen's Kappa, was .79 for the younger cohort and .85 for the older cohort.

The year was 2012, when the 15- and 18-year-olds reported if they had encountered an event the last years which increased their political interest. Participants reported on specific topics such as school issues, environmental issues and climate change, gender inequality, and file sharing on the Internet. They also reported on events specifically related to the Swedish political situation, especially immigration (because an anti-immigration party had entered the Swedish parliament) and party politics (e.g., speeches by party leaders, the resignation of the Swedish prime minister). Other issues related to Swedish politics that were mentioned less frequently (Swedish politics: other) were Swedish arms exports, Internet integrity, and tax policy. Among the international events reported, participants mentioned in particular the tragic shootings on the island of Utøya outside Oslo in Norway, where a right-wing extremist killed 69 and wounded 110 young people at a summer camp in 2011. Participants also reported on U.S. politics (such as the aftermath of the Lehman bankruptcy and the presidential primaries), a regime's bombing of its own people in Syria, the situation in Iraq, the aftermath of the Arab Spring, and the catastrophic budget deficit in Greece. We compared the young people's reports with media reports from the previous year. It seems that most of the national and international events reported by the adolescents were events that had been covered by the media. The way the adolescents formulated these events was close to the way these events were reported in the media.

In some cases, participants did not refer to an explicit issue or national or international event. Instead, they talked about people they had met in the past year that had triggered their political interest, and also about specific contexts to which they attributed an increase in political interest. In terms of contexts, some reported that their civic interest was triggered by assignments they were given at school or by teachers who inspired them. Some also mentioned being engaged and activated by peers and by information and contacts on social media. In some cases, participants did not mention being activated by external sources, but said that one day they realized that they needed to become active on one or more specific issues. Some participants turned 18 in 2012 and were eligible to vote, and they reported this as a triggering event.

This Happened Earlier

To be able to compare the two groups of adolescents over time, we used multigroup latent growth modeling to estimate levels and changes over time in adolescents' political interest and feelings about politics, as well as indicators reflecting needs for autonomy, relatedness, and competence. We first estimated intercepts and slopes in each group, that is, the group of adolescents who experienced an interest-triggering event and the group of those who did not. The intercepts represent the baseline levels of our factors (interest, feelings, and indicators of need satisfaction), that is, their levels two years prior to the triggering event. The slopes indicate the rate of change for each factor over the period considered. Equality conditions were then used to test whether the baseline levels and rates of change differed between the two groups.

The results of the analysis of growth over time for political interest, feelings about politics, and basic psychological needs are shown in Table 3.3 for the first cohort and Table 3.4 for the second cohort. Gender and parental education were controlled.

The equality of the intercepts in the tables tests whether there are significant differences between the youth who reported interest-arousing events two years

TABLE 3.3 Growth in basic psychological needs for younger adolescents (age 15) who experienced interest-triggering events and those who did not.

	Events	*Means and Standard Deviations*[1]			*Intercept*	*Slope*	*Test of Equalities*[2]	
		Age 13	*Age 14*	*Age 15*			*Equality of intercept*	*Equality of Slope*
Intrinsic motivation								
Political interest	No	2.76 (.89)	2.78 (.96)	2.74 (.93)	2.76***	–.02	13.20***	18.33***
	Yes	3.07 (.92)	3.27 (.87)	3.47 (.93)	3.06***	.20***		
Feelings about politics	No	2.84 (1.13)	3.01 (1.24)	3.31 (1.23)	2.82***	.25***	20.21***	10.83***
	Yes	3.3 (1.12)	3.57 (1.15)	4.18 (1.10)	3.28***	.42***		
Autonomy								
Enjoyment in news consumption	No	3.37 (1.28)	3.35 (1.23)	3.5 (1.26)	3.35***	.06*	7.50**	4.66*
	Yes	3.68 (1.24)	3.84 (1.22)	4.09 (1.17)	3.65***	.20***		
Setting long-term goals	No	2.08 (.68)	2.01 (.68)	2.02 (.64)	2.07***	–.03*	5.74*	3.85*
	Yes	2.24 (.76)	2.22 (.70)	2.37 (.71)	2.23***	.05		

(*Continued*)

TABLE 3.3 (Continued)

	Events	*Means and Standard Deviations*[1]			*Intercept*	*Slope*	*Test of Equalities*[2]	
		Age 13	*Age 14*	*Age 15*			*Equality of intercept*	*Equality of Slope*
Relatedness								
Political discussions with parents	No	2.24	2.23	2.36	2.21***	.04*	6.19**	8.10**
		(.69)	(.65)	(.69)				
	Yes	2.36	2.51	2.68	2.36***	.16***		
		(.69)	(.69)	(.77)				
Adolescent-initiated discussions	No	2.44	2.29	2.32	2.41***	–.06*	4.20*	9.14**
		(1.02)	(.91)	(.94)				
	Yes	2.63	2.63	2.81	2.60***	.08*		
		(1.03)	(0.96)	(1.05)				
Talking to others on the Internet	No	1.38	1.4	1.47	1.37***	.05**	8.67**	6.30**
		(.40)	(.41)	(.43)				
	Yes	1.52	1.55	1.78	1.50***	.11***		
		(.49)	(.50)	(.56)				
Competence								
Political efficacy	No	2.40	2.39	2.47	2.39***	.04**	12.35***	9.51**
		(.63)	(.72)	(.76)				
	Yes	2.59	2.77	2.87	2.59***	.14***		
		(.67)	(.69)	(.69)				

* $p < .05$, ** $p < .01$, *** $p < .001$.

1 The values in parentheses are standard deviations.

2 Equalities of intercepts and slopes were tested using equality constraints and subsequent χ^2 difference test. Significant $\chi 2$ differences suggest that statistically significant differences in the estimates.

TABLE 3.4 Growth in basic psychological needs for older adolescents (age 18) who experienced interest-triggering events and those who did not.

		Means and Standard Deviations[1]					*Test of Equalities*[2]	
	Events	*Age 16*	*Age 17*	*Age 18*	*Intercept*	*Slope*	*Equality of intercept*	*Equality of Slope*
Intrinsic motivation								
Political interest	No	2.98 (.91)	3.11 (.94)	3.04 (.99)	2.98***	.12***	18.12***	9.78***
	Yes	3.31 (.90)	3.59 (.85)	3.79 (.82)	3.31***	.25***		
Feelings about politics	No	3.29 (1.24)	3.42 (1.24)	3.49 (1.25)	3.30***	.10***	29.87***	9.92***
	Yes	3.81 (1.15)	4.16 (1.11)	4.30 (1.00)	3.84***	.25***		
Autonomy								
Enjoyment in news consumption	No	3.61 (1.15)	3.84 (1.11)	3.88 (1.14)	3.65***	.10*	8.42**	1.23
	Yes	3.93 (1.24)	4.17 (1.12)	4.30 (1.05)	3.94***	.18***		
Setting long-term goals	No	2.05 (.65)	2.07 (.68)	2.06 (.62)	2.05***	.01	11.27***	18.79***
	Yes	2.25 (.82)	2.45 (.74)	2.58 (.75)	2.26***	.16***		
Relatedness								
Political discussions with parents	No	2.25 (.62)	2.35 (.62)	2.53 (.67)	2.23***	.14***	8.90**	8.02**
	Yes	2.41 (.6)	2.59 (.62)	2.86 (.73)	2.39***	.22***		

TABLE 3.4 (Continued)

		Means and Standard Deviations[1]					*Test of Equalities*[2]	
	Events	*Age 16*	*Age 17*	*Age 18*	*Intercept*	*Slope*	*Equality of intercept*	*Equality of Slope*
Adolescent-initiated discussions	No	2.38 (.96)	2.41 (.90)	2.36 (.92)	2.38***	–.01	24.15***	.97
	Yes	2.82 (.99)	2.85 (.95)	2.88 (.93)	2.80***	.04		
Talking to others on Internet	No	1.54 (.44)	1.58 (.47)	1.66 (.50)	1.53***	.06***	28.31***	3.01
	Yes	1.76 (.54)	1.76 (.57)	1.95 (.59)	1.76***	.10***		
Competence								
Political efficacy	No	2.53 (.69)	2.62 (.74)	2.66 (.75)	2.54***	.06**	16.75***	13.20***
	Yes	2.76 (.67)	2.95 (.67)	3.08 (.67)	2.77***	.16***		

*$p<.05$, **$p<.01$, ***$p<.001$

[1] The values in parentheses are standard deviations.

[2] Equalities of intercept and slopes were tested using equality constraints and subsequent chi-square difference test. Significant test statistics suggest statistically significant differences in the estimates.

earlier and those who did not. As shown in the tables, adolescents who experienced interest-arousing events in both the younger and older cohorts had substantially higher interest in politics and more positive feelings about politics two years earlier, suggesting a genuine intrinsic interest in political issues. The effect sizes were about .35 for political interest and .45 for feelings about politics. The slopes reflect the growth of the measures over time (−2 years, −1 year, present). Tests of equality of the slopes indicate that the adolescents in both the younger and the older cohort who experienced interest-triggering events increased their political interest and feelings about politics significantly more over the two years than did the adolescents who did not experience such an event.

Indicators of autonomy, relatedness, and competence needs were all significantly different between the two groups of adolescents two years earlier in both cohorts (see equality of intercepts). The adolescents who later experienced interest-arousing events showed significantly higher enjoyment of news consumption, set higher long-term goals, had more frequent political discussions with their parents, had more self-initiated discussions with their parents, had more communication with others on the Internet, and had higher political efficacy two years earlier. In addition (see equality of slopes), in the younger cohort, adolescents who had experienced an interest-triggering event showed a significantly steeper increase over the two years for all indicators than adolescents who had not experienced such an event. In the older cohort, three of the seven indicators—setting long-term goals, having political discussions with parents, and political efficacy—showed significantly steeper increases for adolescents who had experienced such an event. Thus, on the whole, the adolescents who experienced an interest-triggering event increased political interest, feelings about politics, and most indicators of autonomy, relatedness, and competence needs at a faster rate, starting two years earlier, than the adolescents who did not experience an interest-triggering event.

This Happened Next

As we have seen in the previous analyses, adolescents who encountered an interest-triggering event had increased their political interest over time more than those who did not (equality of the slopes). This is an indication that encountering events influences youths' political interest. In the latent change models, we also observed that youths who have encountered an event were already more interested in politics than those who did not (inequality of the intercepts). This suggests that the effects between political interest and the exposure to interest-triggering events might be reciprocal. To test this idea more directly, we used a cross-lagged model.

For participants in the younger cohort, we have information on their interest in politics one year after (at age 16) they reported encountering an interest-triggering event. This provided an opportunity to analyze whether exposure to such events subsequently increased these youths' interest in politics more broadly.

We used a cross-lagged panel model and tested these assumptions using data from ages 15 and 16. Note that at age 16, 29.4% of participants reported having experienced such an event, compared to 18.1% one year earlier. We restricted the sample to those who did not report a political triggering event at age 15. Of these young people, 25% reported a politically triggering event at age 16. Similarly, we restricted the sample to those who reported a political triggering event at age 15. Of these, twice as many, 50%, also reported a politically triggering event at the age of 16. Apparently, encountering experiences that trigger one's political interest makes it easier to encounter new such experiences.

The cross-lagged panel analysis revealed, first, stability of political interest from age 15 to age 16 ($\beta = .59$, $p < .001$) and stability for the dichotomous measure of having or not having encountered interest-triggering events ($\beta = .21$, $p < .001$). Second, encountering an interest-triggering event at age 15 affected adolescents' political interest from age 15 to age 16 ($\beta = .11$, $p = .003$). Thus, exposure to an interest-triggering event leads to a more general interest in politics over time in mid-adolescence. In addition, adolescents' political interest at age 15 affected the likelihood of encountering an interest-triggering event at age 16 ($\beta = .22$, $p < .001$). The magnitude of the overtime effect of early political interest and experiencing an interest-triggering event were not significantly different: χ^2 (1 df) = .05, $p = .817$. Apparently, there is a bidirectional relationship between adolescents' political interest and their exposure to interest-triggering events.

Summary

Based on self-determination theory (Deci & Ryan, 2008), we proposed that adolescents who encounter events that they perceive as increasing their political interest would have been more politically interested and had more positive feelings about politics years before encountering these types of events—indicating an earlier intrinsic interest in politics. Adolescents with low political interest and neutral or even negative feelings about political issues were assumed to pay little attention to these types of events. They would be below their attentional radar. We also found that the adolescents who were exposed to political interest events were already more interested in politics and had more positive feelings about politics than other adolescents two years earlier, and their earlier political interest in and feelings about politics increased more over time than the adolescents who were not exposed to such political interest events. These findings suggest that some adolescents were more prepared to encounter political events than others. They had higher levels of interest in these issues earlier. These findings shed light on how interest and attention are related. In their daily perceptions, adolescents who encounter events that arouse their political interest are already more politically interested than other adolescents who do not encounter political interest-triggering experiences—and their broader political interest is affected by encountering these experiences.

There was a wide range of political events that the youth described. What stands out in our thinking is what the youth did not report. None of the adolescents mentioned specific political conversations with their parents that were triggering events for them. Moreover, on a broader level, being interested in political issues does not necessarily mean that these adolescents mentioned "positive" triggering events. In fact, many of them can be described as threatening, dangerous, and challenging to the adolescents' social and moral values of justice and fairness. Political interest, then, is often not aroused by encountering a positive world—local, national, and international—but can be aroused by trying to understand the suffering of others and the conditions that cause that suffering. Negative events apparently can stimulate adolescent thinking and feeling. What seems to motivate some adolescents' political interest are the problems they perceive around them (see Bloemraad & Trost, 2008). From another angle, when Patterson and colleagues (2019) interviewed five- to eight-year-old children before the 2016 presidential election, they found that the majority of children were very interested in this election. At the same time, they were just as likely to express negative opinions about the candidates as positive ones.

Adolescents reported very different events that sparked their interest. There is little evidence in this dataset to suggest that people born at a particular time are influenced by a common set of events that shape their political interest and attitudes (Jennings & Niemi, 1981). Recent work testing the generational hypothesis has found only weak evidence that historical events are responsible for generating generational differences in political interest and civic engagement (Shani, 2009; Prior, 2010; Rotolo & Wilson, 2004). Generational effects may be overstated, which means that critical aspects of how and which specific events influence political interest among different people are neglected. Of course, with the design we have, we cannot say whether the events experienced by our participants were significantly different from those experienced by younger and older generations. We can assume that they are to some extent, but how they affect attitudes and behaviors differently across generations is unknown.

Theoretical frameworks for understanding why some adolescents, but not others, pay attention to and are affected by political and civic events in their development are scarce. Both political science and developmental psychology offer few models. Self-determination theory was used here to provide more detailed insights into how young people's interest in political issues affects their political development. Self-determination theory is not a developmental theory. But the theory is not a static model of human motivation and can predict core processes that are likely to operate over time. Its agentic perspective, with its focus on how people's intrinsic interest is a motivating force for their attitudes and behaviors, complements and goes beyond the classic idea in the political socialization literature that young people's political views, opinions, and attitudes are transmitted in a unidirectional and learning fashion from parents and other socialization agents. In support of the agentic perspective, we found that adolescents' political interest years earlier facilitated encounters with events that triggered their political interest.

Our findings could be understood in terms of several theoretical models other than self-determination theory. For example, the literature on selective attention suggests that, guided by initial cues, some people's attention is drawn to certain information more than others. They are 'primed' to attend to this information because of their previous experiences (Kahneman, 1973; Neisser, 1967). The basic assumption in self-determination theory that people's exploratory behaviors are intrinsically motivated and lead to integration and growth also has its counterparts in the schemas of assimilation and accommodation in Piaget's theory (Deci & Ryan, 2013). The strength of self-determination theory is that this model offers very specific predictions, not only about political interest and feelings about politics, but also concretely about watching the news, setting long-term goals, having political discussions with parents, initiating these political discussions at home, having discussions with others on the Internet, and internal political efficacy: all subsumed under basic psychological needs. Based on self-determination theory, our results show that the encounter with a political interest-triggering event was most common among adolescents who years earlier had had a strong political interest and who years earlier had explored and deepened their political interest by engaging in behaviors related to their needs for autonomy, relatedness and competence in the political sphere. A systematic agentic perspective has not received much attention in the political socialization literature. The agentic feature of self-determination theory seems to provide such a framework.

Finally, we used two cohorts of adolescents: 15- and 18-year-olds. In many ways, the findings reported here were similar for the two age cohorts. Similar types of progression over time seemed to operate in both cohorts, suggesting that our findings reflect robust developmental processes.

Does Encountering a Politically Interesting Event Increase Political Discussions With Parents and Friends?

Because the participants in the youngest cohort report on political discussions with others at ages 15 and 16, it is possible to use these reports at age 16 as the dependent variable and examine whether encountering politically interesting events in the past year at age 16 increased adolescents' political discussions with parents and friends from ages 15 to 16. Thus, the research question becomes one of political agency: When adolescents during one year encounter events that trigger their political interest, does it make them want to talk more with other people about political and civic issues?

We used a simple design and selected all adolescents who had not encountered a political interest-triggering event at age 15. They were 501 adolescents. One year later, about one in four (N = 124) of them reported that they had had such political interest-raising experiences during the year. The other 75% (N = 377) had not. Did the first group of young people increase their political discussions with parents and friends between the ages of 15 and 16 more than the second group?

Here, two issues that we have previously reported on (Table 3.1) were aggregated in the political discussions with parents. The stem question was as follows: How often do you and your parents talk about these things? And the two items were "What you have heard on the news about what is going on in Sweden and around the world" and "Politics or society." The response scale ranged from 1 (*never*) to 4 (*very often*). The alpha reliability for the two items was .76 at age 15 and .73 at age 16. The same items were asked about their friends, with the word "parent" exchanged with "friends." Alpha reliability was .66 at age 15 ($r = .49$) and .72 at age 16.

We used ANCOVAs controlling for gender and level of political discussion with parents and friends at age 15. Partial η^2 effect sizes were calculated, with 0.01 considered a small effect, 0.06 a medium effect, and 0.14 a large effect (Cohen, 1988). Regarding political discussion with parents, gender was not significant, but the ANCOVA showed that encountering an event that aroused one's political interest in the past year at age 16 was associated with having discussed political and civic issues with parents significantly more often at age 16 than at age 15, compared to not having encountered such interest-arousing events in the past year: $F(1, 453) = 11.61$, $p < .001$. η^2 was .03, indicating a small effect size. In the analysis for discussing politics with friends, gender was not significant, and again, having experienced a political interest-triggering event in the past year at age 16 was associated with discussing politics with friends significantly more often at age 16 than at age 15 compared to not having experienced an interest-triggering event in the past year: $F(1, 457) = 41.21$, $p < .001$. η^2 was .08, indicating a moderate effect.

Figure 3.2 reports these results. Apparently, by age 16, having experienced a political-interest-triggering event in the past year motivates adolescents to discuss political issues with their parents and friends more often than if they had not experienced such interest-triggering events.

This is not an ideal design, and it is far from a randomized controlled trial. Our aim was to select adolescents at the age of 15, with one group reporting later at

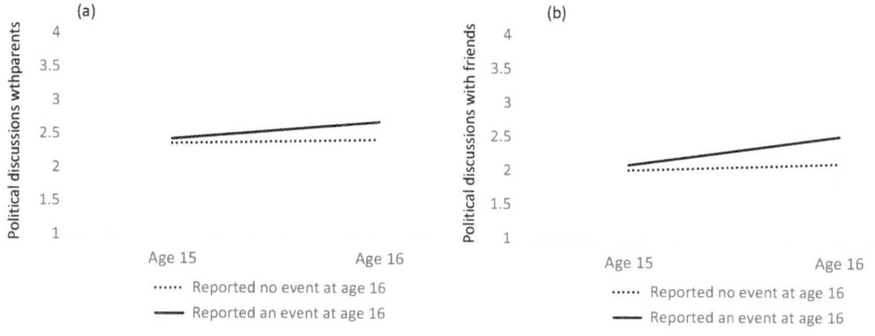

FIGURE 3.2 Comparison of changes in political discussions with (a) parents and (b) friends of 16-year-olds who had experienced an event in the past year that triggered their political interest with 16-year-olds who had not experienced such an event in the past year.

the age of 16 that they had experienced events in the past year that triggered their political interest, and another group having no such experiences in the past year. Did the first group's political discussions with parents and friends increase more over the year than the other group's? They did. Overall, this seems to be important information from a political agency perspective. The results suggest that some young people, as part of their normal development, encounter events that trigger their political interest. As a result of these experiences, they want to talk to other people - parents and friends - about political and civic issues. We see this as preliminary evidence of how political agency may work, evidence that needs to be tested with a more robust research design.We do not have an ideal design. Our aim was to select adolescents at the age of 15, with one group reporting later at the age of 16 that they had experienced events in the past year that triggered their political interest, and another group having no such experiences in the past year. Did the first group's political discussions with parents and friends increase more over the year than the other group's? They did. Overall, this seems to be important information from a political agency perspective. The results suggest that some young people, as part of their normal development, encounter events that trigger their political interest. As a result of these experiences, they want to talk to other people - parents and friends - about political and civic issues. We see this as preliminary evidence of how political agency may work, evidence that needs to be tested with a more robust research design.

. . . *And Parents?*

About one in five adolescents said they had experienced events in the past year that increased their interest in politics. When members of the younger age cohort turned 14, we asked their parents the same question. Overall, 21.4% of parents said they had experienced events in the past year that increased their interest in politics; 2.3% said these events decreased their interest in politics.

A total of 430 parents answered questions about their political interest when the child was 14 years old. The two questions were "How interested is the father in politics or societal issues?" and "How interested is the mother in politics or societal issues?" The response scales ranged from 1 (*totally uninterested*) to 5 (*very interested*). The two questions were aggregated. Three hundred thirty-nine of the parents (79%) also answered the parent questionnaire including the two political interest questions one year earlier. The fact that parents' reports of political interest (when the adolescents were 15 years old, here T_0) were also collected one year before they answered the question about exposure to interest-triggering events gives us the opportunity to examine whether similar changes in political interest can be seen for parents as we have seen for adolescents. We decided to examine the data on political interest and political-interest-triggering events for these two years (T_0 and T_{-1}).

When parents responded to the event question at T_0, those who reported having experienced an interest-triggering event reported higher political interest than parents who had not experienced such an event (political interests: event:

mean = 3.99, SD = 0.63; no event: mean = 3.48, SD = 0.78) (t = 5.74, df = 422, $p < .001$). The effect size was 0.68. We compared parents' political interest one year earlier. At T_{-1}, parents who reported experiencing an interest-triggering event reported higher but not significantly higher political interest than the other parents (event: mean = 3.73, SD = 0.71; no event: mean = 3.59, SD = 0.66) (t = 1.56, df = 337, p = .060). A paired samples t-test separately for parents who experienced an interest-triggering event at T_0 showed a significant increase in political interest from T_{-1} to T_0: t = 3.03, df = 66, p =.002. A similar paired samples test for the parents who did not experience an interest-triggering event showed a significant decrease in political interest from T_{-1} to T_0: t = 2.44, df = 267, p = .008. Figure 3.3 shows these changes in political interest for the two groups of parents. It should be added that the changes reported in the figure are similar for the separate reports of fathers' and mothers' political interest.

We draw both similar and different conclusions about exposure to interest-triggering events for adolescents and parents. Yes, when adolescents and parents report experiencing an interest-triggering event in the past year, both adolescents and parents have significantly higher political interest than adolescents and parents who did not experience such an event in the past year. In the case of adolescents, we proposed and found support for the idea that adolescents who experienced events that triggered their political interest would be more politically interested at a much

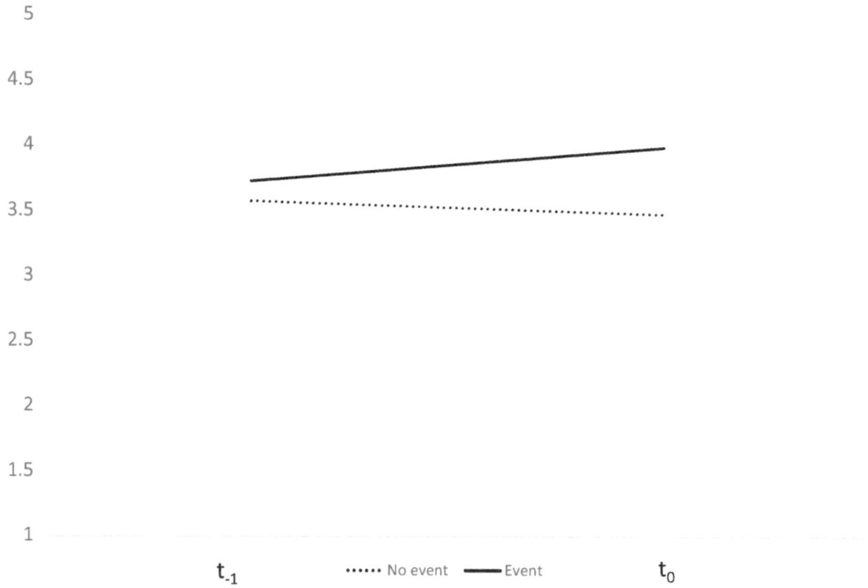

FIGURE 3.3 Political interest 1 year earlier and at the same time, when some parents, but not others, reported encountering an event that increased their political interest.

earlier point in time than adolescents who did not experience interest-triggering events. We found support for adolescents, but not for parents. The political interest of parents who had experienced interest-triggering events was not significantly different from that of parents who had not experienced such events. But the parents who said they had experienced an interest-triggering event showed an increase in political interest from one year earlier to the time they responded to the event question, while the parents who had not experienced these events showed a decrease in political interest from one year earlier to the time they responded to the even question.

From his studies on the stability of political interest, Prior (2019) found little change in political interest among adults around major political events, such as elections, and concluded that political interest appears to be dispositional, "a largely chronic predisposition that does not respond much to short-term bursts of political coverage and campaign hoopla" (Prior, 2019, p. 61). The present findings suggest that some adults (as well as their children) can have event experiences that they perceive as increasing their political interest. And it seems that both the young people and their parents are gaining in political interest.

To Keep Oneself Informed

Perhaps the most direct way to examine the dynamic between political interest and attention to current events is to ask young people themselves: Do you think it is important to stay informed about what is happening in the world? If political interest influences adolescents' beliefs that it is important to stay informed, and if motivation to stay informed influences adolescents' political interest, we should expect bidirectional relationships between interest and attention to emerge over time (cf. Slater, 2015).

All cohort members were asked, "Some young people think it is important to keep up with what is going on in the world. But others do not think it is very important. What do you think?" They could answer 1 (*No. I am not so interested in keeping myself informed*) or 2 (*Yes. I think it is important to keep myself informed. I try to get as much information as I can regarding societal, environmental, and political issues as often as I can*).

As shown in Table 3.5, the proportion of young people who agreed that it was important to keep up with what was going on in the world increased with age. One in three 14-year-olds thought it was important to keep up with current events. By age 28, about two in three young adults thought it was important. This is an effect size (0.49) between the ages of 14 and 28. There was a peak at age 18, perhaps indicating that this was the age at which young people can vote for the first time.

If young people's reports of the importance of keeping up with social, environmental, and political issues are influenced by their political interest, we would expect their own political interest to predict their reported importance of keeping up over time. Conversely, if young people believe it is important to keep up with

TABLE 3.5 Percentage of 14- to 28-year-olds who say it is important to stay informed about what is happening in the world.

Age	*Percentage of respondents*
14	34
16	35
18	54
20	43
22	48
24	49
26	51
28	65

what is happening in the world, this attention to current events may increase their political interest over time. We examined predictions over two years: ages 14 to 16, ages 16 to 18, ages 18 to 20, ages 20 to 22, ages 22 to 24, ages 24 to 26, and ages 26 to 28.

We used latent growth models to examine the relationship between political interest and the importance of being informed about world events over two years. We first estimated baseline levels and latent changes in both political interest and the importance of being informed. We then analyzed the effect of adolescents' initial levels of perceiving the importance of being informed on the growth of political interest over time, as well as the effect of adolescents' initial levels of political interest on the growth of the importance of being informed over time. As shown in Table 3.6, these analyses revealed reciprocal effects for ages 14 to 16 and ages 16 to 18: the perception that it is important to stay informed had a positive and significant effect on the increase in political interest over time (second row) and, in particular, a high level of political interest had a positive and significant effect on the increase in the importance attached to being informed (third row).

The reciprocal effects in the older age intervals could not be estimated because the linear growth function did not fit the data well. This may indicate a lack of change or nonlinear change over time. However, we changed strategy and used cross-lagged models to examine whether reciprocal effects would also be found in all age cohorts. We made predictions over two years at all age intervals. If the same age interval could be examined in two cohorts, both cohorts were included. The results are presented in Table 3.7. As shown in this table, political interest significantly predicted the importance of staying informed at all age intervals. The importance of staying informed significantly predicted political interest over two years in seven out of nine analyses. The first prediction was stronger than the second, but the differences between the coefficients were significant in only two of the analyses.

Taken together, these analyses support the dynamic between political interest and keeping up with world events. Young people's belief in the importance of

TABLE 3.6 Examining the relationship between political interest and the importance of staying updated over two years using latent growth models.

	Ages 14–16		*Ages 16–18*	
	Coeff.	p	*Coeff.*	p
Predicting growth in political interest from				
Initial level of political interest	−.475	<.001	−.218	.162
Initial level in the importance to stay informed	.244	.017	.447	.007
Predicting growth in the importance to stay informed from				
Initial level in political interest	.587	<.001	.706	<.001
Initial level in the importance to stay informed	−.394	<.001	−.264	.103

TABLE 3.7 Cross-lagged analyses testing whether political interest predicts the importance of staying politically updated and whether the importance of staying updated predicts political interest over two years.

Ages	*Staying updated predicts political interest*	*Political interest predicts staying updated*	p *value for the Wald test*
14–16 (cohort 1)	.11	.40***	.02
16–18 (cohort 1)	.39***	.42***	.84
16–18 (cohort 2)	.36***	.36***	.97
18–20 (cohort 2)	.33**	.40***	.64
20–22 (cohort 3)	.16	.50***	<.001
22–24 (cohort 3)	.23*	.44***	.14
22–24 (cohort 4)	.38***	.63***	.07
24–26 (cohort 4)	.34***	.47***	.42
26–28 (cohort 5)	.40***	.53***	.35
Average	.30**	.46***	

Note: * $p < .05$, ** $p < .01$, *** $p < .001$.

keeping up with current events both is influenced by and influences their political interest. This belief in the importance of keeping up with what is happening in the world may ultimately be one key explanation for the growth of political interest over time.

Summary

It is the attention to political information by politically interested adolescents that links the two issues we have raised. Focusing on attention to political information has been a way to find out how political interest develops over time. The results show that political interest predicts encountering events that trigger one's political interest, and these events also lead to a more general interest in politics over time.

Political interest shapes the belief that it is important to keep up with information about what is happening in society and the world, and the motivation to keep up with societal, environmental, and political issues positively affects political interest over time. Bidirectionality seems to prevail. Overall, if we want to understand why some adolescents and not others increase their political interest over time, one answer is that they are more attentive to political cues in their everyday lives. These cues fuel their political interest.

Finally, what evidence is there in this data that young people are active agents in their own political development?

Encountering interest-triggering events:

- It is mostly adolescents who previously had a high interest in politics and positive feelings about political issues who experience events that they perceive as increasing their interest in politics.
- Adolescents who have these interest-raising experiences differ from other adolescents in several ways. Based on self-determination theory, we found 2 years earlier that measures of need satisfaction were higher among the adolescents who had experienced interest-arousing events:
  - Autonomy: They showed greater enjoyment of news consumption and were more likely to set long-term goals.
  - Relatedness: They had more frequent political discussions with parents, more self-initiated political discussions, and more frequent discussions with others about political issues on the Internet.
  - Competence: They had higher internal political efficacy.

For the younger adolescents, this need satisfaction increased over time for all measures compared to two years earlier. For the older adolescents, this increase was found for setting long-term goals, frequency of political discussions with parents, and political efficacy.

Political interest and exposure to events that increase political interest are bidirectionally related. Previous political interest facilitates the perception of events that increase political interest, and exposure to these interest-increasing events affects future political interest.

Overall, we conclude that it is no coincidence that some adolescents, over the course of a year, encounter events that they perceive as increasing their political interest. These adolescents differ in predictable ways from other adolescents one and two years earlier. They are, in a sense, "prepared" to encounter interest-raising events.

About to keep oneself informed

When young people feel it is important to keep up with what is happening in their world, this attention is steered by their political interest and this attention stimulates their political interest.

4

A POLITICAL REPUTATION

Highlights

- *People can acquire political reputations in different contexts. The first part of the chapter examines the individual characteristics and consequences of psychological group processes in the classroom that lead some students to gain reputations for being politically knowledgeable and verbal—a political reputation in the classroom.*
- *Cross-sectional predictions for the 13- and 16-year-olds showed that political interest and internal political efficacy positively predicted classroom political reputation, and social anxiety negatively predicted classroom political reputation for both cohorts.*
- *Having a political reputation predicted increased political interest and political efficacy over the course of a year.*
- *Mediation analyses showed that students' political interest and political efficacy significantly influenced political interest and efficacy one year later via political reputation. This suggests that a political reputation in class may function in part as a booster of these students' initial political interest and efficacy over time.*

The second part of the chapter examines, in the context of a long-term perspective, the role of students' political reputation in the classroom on their future political activity. The measure of political reputation in the classroom at age 16 was used to predict participants' political activity four years later at age 20 and their attempts to take a public stand for a party in that year's national election.

- *Political reputation in the classroom positively predicted future political activity, membership in political organizations, and attempts to take a public stand for a party in the national election at age 20.*
- *The role that political reputation played also depended on other characteristics of these students observed by their classmates (popularity and anger).*
- *Mediation analyses showed that students' political interest and political efficacy at age 16 significantly influenced their political interest and efficacy at age 20 via political reputation. This suggests that political reputation acts in part as a booster of these students' initial political interest and efficacy over time.*

DOI: 10.4324/9781003371731-6

The Emergence of Political Reputation

This chapter is about the political reputations that some students gain in their classes—public recognition as politically competent in everyday settings. By "political reputation" we mean the extent to which students are perceived by their classmates as politically well informed and articulate in class. Behind this political reputation in class should be the political interest and internal political efficacy of some students who are not afraid to bring up their political views in class. Such public recognition of their political sophistication may also shape these students' political interest and political efficacy in the future.

In any group of people, individuals develop reputations based on how they are viewed by others in the group. When group members meet regularly, they have a great deal of information to form opinions about other members' personal characteristics through direct observation, sharing information with each other, and gossip (Baumeister et al., 2004; Foster, 2004). Over time, as they gain more insight, group members are likely to develop a commonality in these opinions.

Reputations are the collective judgments of group members' perceptions of an individual. Emler's (1990, 2013, 2019) theory of reputation enhancement links a person's social identity to social group processes. A person's social identity is the social representation of the self. In various ways, people generate behaviors that are consistent with their social identity and are observable to others. These behaviors are the basis for the acquisition of personal reputations in the group. Over the course of many encounters, people in the group will form collective judgments about each other's social identities, and these judgments will constitute those people's personal reputations. Reputation enhancement theory suggests that people's reputations are both collectively earned and sought. The theory proposes that adolescents can choose a particular social identity, and through the way they behave, talk, dress, prefer certain types of music, and hold certain opinions, they communicate to others a social identity that benefits them. A delinquent identity can also be advantageous for some adolescents (Emler & Reicher, 1995). The way others respond may reinforce or discourage these adolescents' behaviors and opinions.

In the Classroom

A classroom is a social environment with characteristics that are fairly stable over time. It is an ideal setting for the study of reputations. The location is fixed and rarely changes from week to week, the students engage in a narrow range of familiar activities and teacher-student and student-student interactions, and the students in the class rarely change. In class, students often have thousands of hours to observe the ways their classmates think, dress, and act. The regularity of interactions among students in a class maximizes the likelihood that students will reach a high degree of consensus about who has a particular social identity. When they are uncertain, they can validate their own judgments against those of others in the class. In fact, the reputations for certain attitudes and behaviors that are visible to others that students have in one year tend to be much the same reputations that they have the next year. Measures of individuals' social attributes based on the collective judgments of classmates show stability over time that is probably among the highest found in psychological research on the social behavior of children and adolescents, higher than measures of social attributes based on self-reports or individual observer reports.

As early as late childhood and early adolescence, peer nominations of social behaviors reflecting traits such as aggression, popularity, achievement orientation, and immaturity have shown stability coefficients greater than .50 over a one-year interval (Bukowski & Newcomb, 1984), while aggression, shyness, cooperativeness, and leadership have shown stability coefficients in the .60 to .70 range over two years (Aleva et al., 2017), and peer victimization has shown a stability coefficient of .50 over two years (Liu et al., 2014). Peer nominations of other students' social behaviors show considerable stability even in late childhood. This is most likely due to the aggregation of similar opinions from all students in a class, which provides a highly reliable measure of an individual student's characteristics in the classroom.

We measured the political reputation in class by asking all age 13 and age 16 students the following question: "Different types of people are described below. Which of your classmates resemble these people?" The students reported on different descriptions of which two were "Keeps track of what is going on in Sweden and in the world" and "Often starts discussions about societal issues in class". The two-item political reputation measure had alpha reliabilities of .75 for 13-year-olds and .79 the following year. The corresponding reliabilities were .87 for the 16-year-olds and .91 the following year. Stabilities over one year were .72 for the 13-year-olds and .80 for the 16-year-olds. These stabilities are well in line with stabilities previously reported for various social characteristics. It should be noted that we are studying intact classes. The students in a class at one point in time are roughly the same as the students in the same class one year later.

Does Political Interest and Efficacy Precede Political Reputation in the Classroom?

Students' political interest should be an important explanation for their political reputation in the classroom. Also, their internal political efficacy—their belief in their own ability to understand and participate effectively in politics (Craig et al., 1990; Miller et al., 1980)—should influence their political reputation in the classroom. Adolescents' political interest and internal political efficacy are both central markers of their political engagement (Barrett & Brunton-Smith, 2014) and strong predictors of their political participation (Levy & Akiva, 2019; Strömbäck & Shehata, 2010). Having a political reputation among classmates should be a peer group validation that the person has the ability, interest, and efficacy to publicly discuss political issues. Our basic study hypothesis is that political dispositions, such as political interest and internal political efficacy, are predictors of adolescents' classroom political reputation, and that classroom political reputation can act as a booster of these same dispositions over time.

Political reputation in the class is based on social behavior, so other social behaviors may provide additional explanations. One example is *social fear*. Social fear, or the fear of speaking in front of the class, may prevent some adolescents from daring to express their political views and become politically visible among their peers (Musso et al., 2020). Another explanation for political reputations in the classroom is students' *perceptions of their own political activities in the classroom*. Students' political reputations may reflect their own perceptions of how politically active they are in the classroom. According to Emler (1990, p. 190), reputations are "social representations of the self" and should reflect an individual's identity. Thus, how classmates perceive individuals' political behavior in the classroom should, to some extent, be consistent with those individuals' own beliefs about their political activity in the classroom. Perhaps their own perceptions of their political behavior in class should be the most obvious individual characteristic of students with a political reputation in class. This is basically a question of whether the insider's perspective is consistent with the outsider's judgment. We will use both the first cohort (age 13) and the second cohort (age 16) and make cross-sectional and longitudinal predictions over one year, and we control for sex and immigrant background.

It should be noted that the ability to make concurrent predictions may be limited by the psychometric properties of the political reputation measure.

As shown in Figure 4.1, the reputation measure is positively skewed at both ages 13 and 16 (age 13: mean = 4.47, SD = 7.76, skewness = 2.72; age 16: mean = 6.46, SD = 12.47, skewness = 3.00). Thus, the majority of students are not nominated for a political reputation by any of their classmates. This is in contrast to other measures. For example, the skewness of political interest was 0.24 for the 13-year-old students and 0.04 for the 16-year-old students. We used square root and logarithmic transformations to adjust for skewness. We computed all analyses with the original measure of nominations and with square root and log transformations. They yielded very similar results and do not change the overall conclusions. Therefore, we report the original nominations here.

Making longitudinal predictions is even more problematic because of the high stability of the reputation measure over time. As will be seen in Table 4.1, political reputation at age 13 already explained at least 60% of the variance in political reputation at age 14 and at age 17 when other measures entered the prediction equation earlier at ages 13 and 16.

We studied the following:

Political reputation in the classroom (peer nominations). Students were asked to nominate three students who fit each of the two descriptions above. The number of times students were nominated for each of the two descriptions was divided

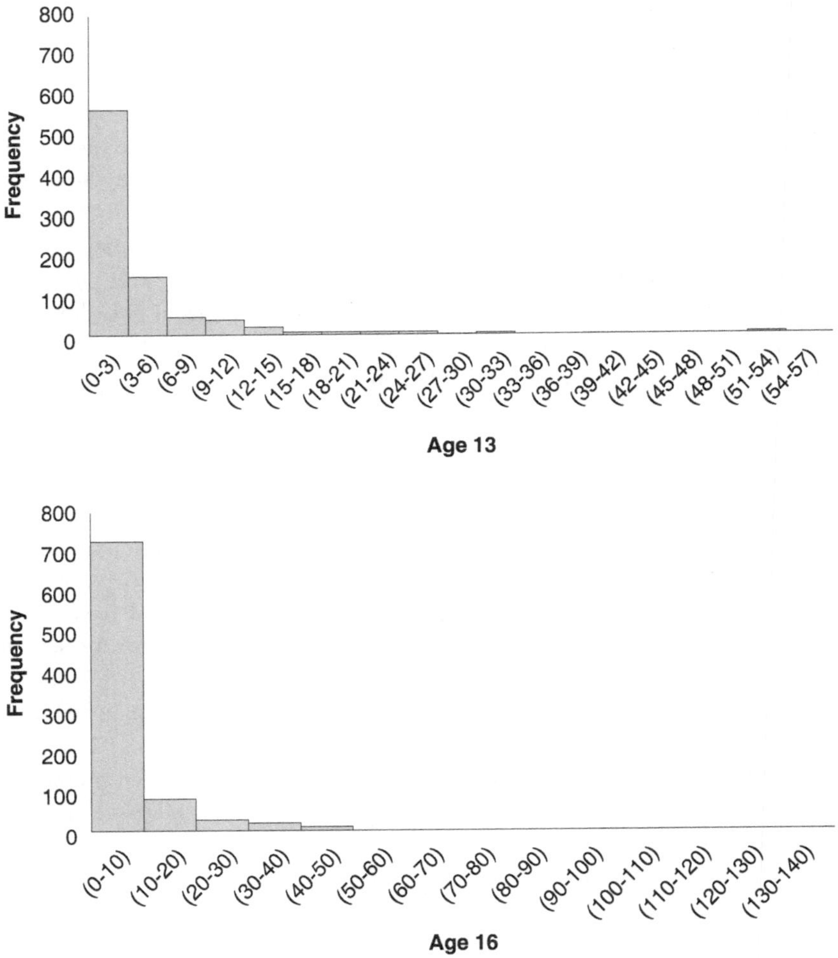

FIGURE 4.1 The distribution of the political reputation measure at ages 13 and 16.

by the total number of students participating on the day of data collection (and multiplied by 100 for clarity), and the two resulting scores were averaged.

Political Interest. Political interest was measured with two questions. "How interested are you in politics?" with response options ranging from 1 (*not interested at all*) to 5 (*very interested*) and "People have different feelings about politics. What are your feelings?" with a six-item response scale ranging from 1 (*loath*) to 6 (*great fun*). The feeling question was rescaled to a 5-point rating scale and the two items were aggregated.

Internal political efficacy was measured by nine items, all referring to a domain-specific efficacy belief in one's own actions to effect change in society. After the stem "If I really tried, I could manage to . . . ," the participants responded to nine statements, such as "Take on responsibility in a political youth organization," "Be an active member of a political organization," and "Discuss politics with persons with more experience than I have." The response scale ranged from 1 (*I could definitely not manage that*) to 4 (*I could definitely manage that*).

Fear of speaking in front of the class. This was a single item included in an instrument that is a modified version of the Social Phobia Screening Questionnaire (Furmark et al., 1999) designed for adults. The current version has been adapted for children and adolescents up to 18 years of age and is called the Social Phobia Screening Questionnaire for Children. The specific item used was "Indicate how much you are usually afraid of speaking in front of the class." The question was answered on a three-point scale ranging from 1 (*no fear*) to 3 (*a lot of fear*).

Self-perceived activity on political issues in the classroom was a four-item scale with questions such as "Have you ever brought up political issues during class?" and "Has it happened that you have brought up a societal problem for discussion during class?" The response scales ranged from 1 (*has never happened*) to 5 (*very often*).

Two control variables were used. Immigrant status was a dichotomous measure differentiating between students with both parents born outside the Nordic countries (coded 1) and other students (coded 0). Gender was coded 0 = female, 1 = male.

To examine the four explanations for understanding students' political reputation in the classroom—political interest, internal political efficacy, social anxiety, and self-perceived political activity in the classroom—we used two-level random intercept models, also known as multilevel models. These models are appropriate to account for the nested structure of the data (adolescents nested in classes) because they allow us to separate individual-level variation in the dependent variable (in our case, variation in political reputation across adolescents) while controlling for class-level variation (variation in political reputation across classes). After controlling for class-level variation, we estimated the effects of our predictors on political reputation.

The cross-sectional and longitudinal predictions of political reputation in both cohorts are reported in Table 4.1. In the cross-sectional predictions, political interest positively predicted political reputation and social anxiety negatively predicted political reputation in both cohorts ($p < .001$). Perceptions of one's own political activity in the classroom and political efficacy also significantly predicted political reputation in the 16-year-old cohort. Adolescents whose parents were born outside the Nordic countries had lower political reputations than other adolescents. Overall, political interest and social anxiety were the strongest predictors in the 13-year-old cohort, and social anxiety, political interest, and perceived political activity in class were the strongest predictors in the 16-year-old cohort. The R^2 was low in both cohorts, indicating the low predictive power of the independent variables.

The longitudinal predictions reported in Table 4.1 show that social anxiety was a significant predictor (at the .05 level) in both cohorts. In the older cohort, political

TABLE 4.1 Predictions of political reputation in class.

	Cross-sectional: DV Reputation T1								*Longitudinal: DV Reputation T2*							
	Age 13				*Age 16*				*Age 13*				*Age 16*			
	Coeff.	*SE*	*P*	*Std.*[a]	*Coeff.*	*SE*	*P*	*Std.*[a]	*Coeff.*	*SE*	*P*	*Std.*[a]	*Coeff.*	*SE*	*P*	*Std.*[a]
Reputation	–	–	–	–	–	–	–	–	.773	.056	<.001	.716	.806	.085	<.001	.762
Political interest	1.625	.321	<.001	.232	1.975	.386	<.001	.196	.307	.268	.251	.040	.515	.212	.015	.046
Political efficacy	.766	.485	.115	.062	1.876	.624	.003	.104	.678	.365	.063	.051	.457	.567	.421	.023
Own activity in class	−.332	.353	.348	−.032	2.592	.587	<.001	.172	.410	.330	.213	.036	1.181	.359	.001	.073
Social fear	−1.634	.364	<.001	−.146	−2.587	.498	<.001	−.143	−.828	.326	.011	−.066	−1.042	.490	.033	−.054
Gender (1 = male)	1.055	.638	.098	.068	2.111	.859	.014	.084	−.270	.464	.560	−.016	1.101	.802	.170	.042
Immigrant status	−1.525	.679	.025	−.079	−4.097	.855	<.001	−.122	.737	.531	.165	.035	−2.140	.715	.003	−.062
Constant	4.328	.468	<.001		6.093	.650	<.001		4.479	.367	<.001		6.149	.735	<.001	
Level 1—*n*		835				795				734				600		
Level 1—Res. variance	53.335	7.173	<.001		124.88	23.588	<.001		29.840	3.611	<.001		50.775	10.351	<.001	
Level 2—*n*		38				47				38				45		
Level 2—variance	0.165	.762	.828		6.109	7.857	.437		1.043	.619	.092		12.728	3.897	.001	
R^2 level 1	.103	.024	<.001		.203	.022	<.001		.574	.034	<.001		.708	.045	<.001	

Note: [a] Standardized coefficients.

All predictors are measured at T1.

interest was also a significant predictor (at the .05 level), as was perceived political activity in the classroom (at the .001 level). Immigrant status was a negative predictor of change in political reputation from T1 to T2. In both cohorts, the independent variables contributed only 2% of the variance over and above the contribution of political reputation at T1. Apparently, this means that once students' political reputations are established, they are not much affected by the individual characteristics examined here.

Does Political Reputation Affect the Development of Political Interest and Efficacy?

Does political reputation in the classroom affect students' political interest and efficacy? This is a similar question to the one we asked earlier about exposure to political interest triggers and subsequent political interest. We have to few reason to believe that predictions of changes in political efficacy and political interest would be affected by students' social anxiety, but could be affected by students' perceptions of how politically active they perceive themselves to be in the classroom. Therefore, the measure of perceived political activity in the classroom was used as another predictor, along with immigrant status and gender.

We predicted changes in political efficacy and political interest over one year for both cohorts. The results are shown in Table 4.2. Political reputation in the classroom predicted an increase in both students' political efficacy and political interest generally at the .001 level for the 13- and 16-year-old cohorts. Self-perceived political activity in the classroom did not predict political efficacy and political interest in three out of four predictions. It seems as if the outsiders' judgment of the political activity in class is a stronger predictor of political interest and efficacy than the insider's perspective.

Political Reputation as a Mediator

To test whether political reputation may act as a booster of preexisting political predispositions, we applied a mediated model in which political reputation mediates the relationships between political interest at T1 and at T2 and between political efficacy at T1 and at T2 (controlling for gender and immigrant status). The indirect effects of political interest at T1 on political interest at T2 were positive and significant in both cohorts (standardized coefficients: .03, $p < .001$ at age 13, .02, $p = .003$ at age 16), as were the indirect effects of political efficacy at T1 on political efficacy at T2 (standardized coefficients: .02, $p = .02$ at age 13, .02, $p = .003$ at age 16). These analyses show that political reputation in the classroom links students' political interest and political efficacy at T1 to their political interest and political efficacy at T2. The results suggest that political reputation functions in part as a booster of adolescents' initial political dispositions over time. In essence, adolescents who have high political interest and high political efficacy gain in their

TABLE 4.2 Predictions of changes in political efficacy and political interest from T1 to T2.

	Age 13				Age 16			
	Coeff.	*SE*	*p*	*Std.*[a]	*Coeff.*	*SE*	*p*	*Std.*[a]
DV: Political efficacy T2								
Political efficacy T1	.516	.047	<.001	.450	.652	.049	<.001	.581
Political reputation	.014	.003	<.001	.140	.008	.003	.001	.142
Own activity in class	.023	.034	.505	.024	.071	.032	.024	.078
Sex	.065	.052	.214	.045	−.025	.052	.636	−.017
Immigrant background	.007	.064	.914	.004	−.042	.077	.586	−.022
Constant	2.412	.049	<.001		2.683	.049	<.001	
Level 1—*n*			735				599	
Level 1—Res. variance	.382	.021	<.001		.312	.022	<.001	
Level 2—*n*			38				45	
Level 2—variance	.040	.012	<.001		.057	.016	<.001	
R^2 Level 1	.261	.033	<.001		.437	.037	<.001	
DV: Political interest T2								
Political interest T1	.499	.036	<.001	.454	.702	.040	<.001	.658
Political reputation	.027	.005	<.001	.172	.008	.003	.004	.085
Own activity in class	.050	.060	.401	.030	.049	.060	.416	.031
Sex	−.040	.084	.632	−.017	.051	.095	.595	.020
Immigrant background	.225	.093	.015	.073	−.206	.130	.114	.062
Constant	2.870	.080	<.001		3.421	.103	<.001	
Level 1—*n*			738				600	
Level 1—Res. variance	1.034	.057	<.001		0.779	.052	<.001	
Level 2—*n*			38				45	
Level 2—variance	.090	.029	.002		0.296	.071	<.001	
R^2 Level 1	.294	.031	<.001		.500	.031	<.001	

Note: [a] Standardized coefficients.

political interest and political efficacy over time because they have a political reputation in the classroom.

Conclusion So Far

The classroom is an ideal social setting for understanding how an adolescent's political reputation develops and the consequences of having such a reputation. Most obviously, the classroom is a social setting in which students encounter each other on an almost daily basis. These regularly repeated social interactions over time are a hallmark of theoretical ideas about social identity and the development of personal reputation (Emler, 1990, 2013, 2019). This chapter has addressed two fundamental questions about adolescents' political reputation in the classroom: political interest and political self-efficacy as predictors of this social reputation, and the role of political reputation in the further development of political interest and political self-efficacy.

Two key explanations for political reputation in the classroom were students' political interest and internal political efficacy. Cross-sectional analyses showed that political interest predicted political reputation in both age cohorts and that internal political efficacy was a predictor in the older cohort. The longitudinal predictions, on the other hand, showed that only political interest predicted changes in students' political reputations in the older age cohort, but not in the younger. To some extent, these longitudinal findings can be expected. To predict a measure—students' political reputations in their classes—which is very skewed and highly stable over time is challenging. We should not expect many potential predictors to have strong influence.

Students' social fears was proposed as a third explanation for political reputation. We assumed that students who were afraid to speak in front of the class were unlikely to gain a political reputation. Indeed, social fears negatively predicted political reputation concurrently in both age cohorts and social fears was also a significant longitudinal predictor in both cohorts. Perhaps not surprisingly, it takes a social competence to raise political and civic issues in class. The final explanation for political reputation was students' own perceptions of their political activity in the classroom. If some students' social identities are associated with extensive political knowledge and verbal skills, then this self-perception of being politically active in class is something that other classmates will also recognize. This self-perception was a significant concurrent and longitudinal predictor (at the .001 level) in the 16-year-old cohort, but not in the 13-year-olds. We conclude that the hypothesized predictors—political interest, internal political efficacy, social anxiety, and self-perceived classroom political activity—at least concurrently influence classroom political reputation.

We also addressed the question of the role of political reputation in the further development of political interest and political self-efficacy. There was strong evidence that political reputation positively influenced adolescents' political interest and internal political efficacy over time. Being seen by classmates as someone who knows a lot about political issues and who brings this up in class seems to have the effect of increasing these students' political interest and political efficacy over time.

Perhaps the most interesting findings regarding youth agency are the mediation analyses. We were interested in whether students' initial characteristics—high political interest and high internal political efficacy—increased as a function of having a political reputation in the classroom. We found support for the idea that political reputation partly functions as a booster of adolescents' initial political interest and political efficacy over time.

Note that the stability of political reputation in the classroom over a year was high for both the 13-year-olds and the 16-year-olds. This means that political reputations, as perceived by classmates, consolidate very early, at least by age 13. This finding is consistent with findings on other types of social behavior, like aggression, popularity, achievement orientation, and immaturity. They already stabilize in late childhood and early adolescence (Aleva et al., 2017; Bukowski & Newcomb, 1984; Liu et al., 2014).

A sorting process seems to occur in classrooms where some students become known as politically competent. Over time, this reputation fuels these students' political interest and political efficacy. This question of the role of classroom political reputation in adolescent political development has not been addressed in political and educational research earlier. The role of schools is to provide students with knowledge and motivation to engage with information about their society and politics, in many cases by supporting classroom discussions and engagement in civic activities (Schulz et al., 2017). In addition to content knowledge about how political and civic systems are organized, civic education is concerned with democratic values, civic skills, and engagement (Arensmeier, 2018). It is likely that the processes that constitute a political reputation in the classroom depend on the overall climate of discussion in the classroom. If a climate of open discussion does not exist, students will not have the opportunity to engage in multiple exchanges of political and civic information with one another. A communality of opinion about who is politically knowledgeable and vocal in the classroom will not develop. However, an open climate of discussion that allows students to express their opinions seems to be a building block for the emergence of collective judgments about who is politically active in the classroom. The sorting process by which some students gain reputations as politically competent is more likely to occur in classes where teachers encourage their students to express their opinions on various political and civic issues than in classes where students have fewer opportunities to openly present their ideas and opinions. This sorting process has never been addressed in research on open classroom climates.

One notable observation is that students' perceptions of being politically active in the classroom did not predict increases in political interest and political efficacy (with one exception at a low level of significance). But their political reputation as judged by their peers did. Thus, an outsider's perspective on students' political behavior in the classroom is a better explanation for their increases in political interest and efficacy than students' own perceptions of their political behavior in the classroom. We had thought that students would be aware of their political reputations and that this awareness would spur their future political interest and efficacy. However, the correlations between political reputation and students' perceptions of their own political activity in class were unexpectedly low (.07, n.s. at age 13 and .29, p <.001 at age 16).

We were interested in learning more about how adolescents' experiences in different everyday settings might contribute to increased political interest. The school setting is the target of this chapter, and we find that micro-processes in the classroom lead some students to acquire a political reputation that influences and increases their political interest. They also gain greater political efficacy as a result of this reputation. School seems to be a training ground for some students' political sophistication. We do not believe that the processes by which some adolescents develop a political reputation are limited to the classroom. Such reputations should potentially be present in other types of political milieus and civic and political associations. In these other milieus and associations, there will be individuals who are willing to stand up for their ideas perhaps regardless of lack of support from others and/or hostile reactions. We are only scratching the surface of what distinguishes these people from others. They may be people who are different from others in only one milieu, or they may be people who are different from others in different milieus. This is an empirical question that we cannot answer with existing data. However, we believe that we have identified a research question for future studies.

An Afterthought

In this chapter, we have treated political interest and internal political efficacy as two independent predictors. However, it is possible that internal political efficacy acts as a moderator between political interest and political reputation in the classroom. Particularly high political reputations might be expected among politically interested adolescents with high political efficacy. Therefore, we reanalyzed Table 4.1 and included an interaction term between political interest and political efficacy. We did not find a significant interaction term for the 13-year-olds. However, for the 16-year-olds, political efficacy was a significant moderator of political interest (see Figure 4.2).

Politically interested students were more likely to have a high political reputation when their political efficacy was high than when their political efficacy was low. Subsequent simple slope tests indicated that political interest was a good predictor of political reputation in the classroom at high levels of political efficacy (coeff. = 3.582, SE = .712, $p < .001$; 95% CI [2.411, 4.754]), but not at low levels of political efficacy (coeff. = 1.181, SE = .698; $p = .091$, 95% CI [0.033, 2.329]). Apparently, the political efficacy of politically interested adolescents may explain why some of them gain a higher political reputation in class than other politically interested adolescents.

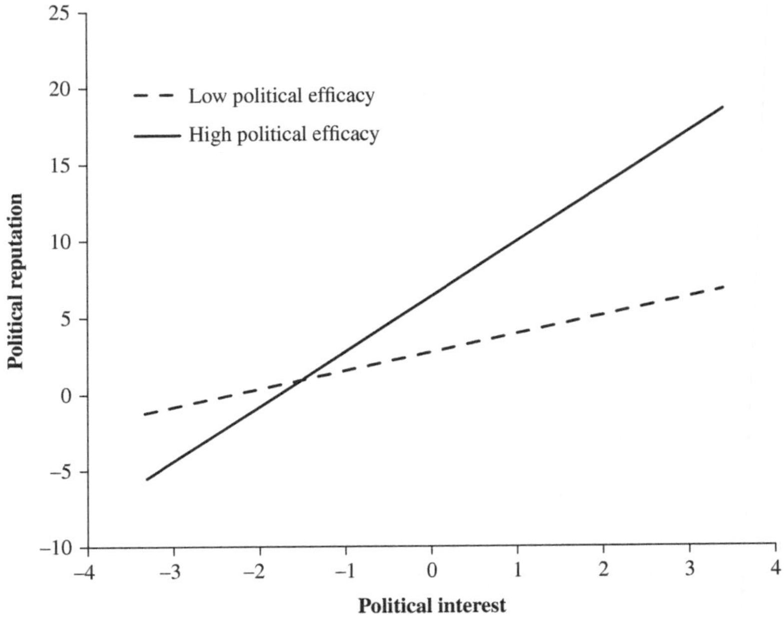

FIGURE 4.2 Interactive effect of political interest and political reputation (age 16 cohort).

The Long-Term Perspective

The increased political interest and internal political efficacy after having a political reputation in class in early and middle adolescence suggests that a political reputation in class may pave the way for a future politically active life. However, this hypothesis needs to be qualified. Two questions need to be addressed: what political activities and what other characteristics of the students are involved?

Future Political Outcomes

A key social skill of students with a political reputation is that they can raise political issues in public and convince others that they have a good knowledge of political, social, and environmental issues. They do not hesitate to engage in political conversations with classmates and to expose their political views to scrutiny and perhaps hostility. Compared to other students, engaging in political activities with others is perhaps where we should expect these students' future political activities to lie. They should be particularly likely to engage in *collective* forms of behaviors (together with others or in front of others), rather than engaging in *solitary* political behaviors, largely unknown to others.

We will focus on the 16-year-olds. Four years later, at age 20, they participated in a new data collection that asked them about engaging in political activities with others and being a member of a political/civic association. We chose this cohort because the year they turned 20 was also a national election year, when they could vote for the first time. The now young adults were asked if they had engaged in two *collective* behaviors during the election: taking a public stand in the election by working on a nonprofit basis for a party and/or supporting a party by wearing their badge or T-shirt. Our hypothesis is that students with a political reputation in the classroom four years later will engage in political activities with others, be members of a political/civic association, and engage in collective forms of taking a public stand for a party more than other students. But they are perhaps no more likely to engage in *solitary* political activities.

What Encourages or Discourages These Students' Future Political Activity?

The role of a political reputation in the classroom for future political activity may depend on how classmates also view other characteristics of these students. Being a student with a political reputation and being seen as popular may increase the student's engagement in political activities that require contact with other people. On the other hand, being a student with a political reputation and at the same time being seen as a person who easily gets angry and causes trouble may discourage them and others from engaging in collective forms of political activities. Here, we decided to examine whether a student's reputation for being popular or angry in class are moderating conditions that increase or decrease the effects of their political reputation on future collective forms of political activity and engagement.

We will follow up the sample of 16-year-olds at age 20. We sought to minimize alternative interpretations of the role of political reputation in the classroom in predicting students' future political activity. First, political interest was included as an independent predictor. This was done to control for the covariation between political reputation and individual differences in political interest in high school. Second, a rival hypothesis is that it is students' own perceptions of their political activity in class, rather than the collective judgment of who is knowledgeable and politically verbal in class, that explains future political activity with others. Accordingly, we controlled for adolescents' own self-perceptions of their political activities in class in high school by including perceptions of their classroom activities as an independent predictor. Third, the two collective forms of political activity at age 20—engaging in collective activities offline and being a member of a civic/political association—were controlled for by the same two political activities measured at age 16.

We measured participants:

Political reputation, political interest, and self-perceived political activity in the classroom. These are the same measures used earlier in this chapter.

Popularity and anger in the classroom. Using the same nomination procedure as for political reputation, all students in each class were asked which classmates were popular (is popular—does things that others follow) and angry (is often angry, disruptive, and causes trouble). The nominations were divided by the total number of students in each class participating on the day of data collection and multiplied by 100.

The age 20 dependent variables were two scales measuring the now young adults' collective political activities and memberships in civic/political organizations. These questions were asked in the age 20 data collection, which took place five months before the election (April/May). Second, a dependent variable was also public participation in the national election, which took place in September.

Participation in offline collective activities. Participants were asked whether they had participated in the following seven activities in the past year, which are thought to be related to participation in collective political activities: "Attended a meeting concerned with political or societal issues," "Collected signatures," "Worked voluntarily for a good cause," "Distributed leaflets with a political content," "Worn a badge or a t-shirt with a political message," "Taken part in a legal demonstration or strike," and "Taken part in a concert or fundraising event with a political message." The response scale ranged from 1 (*never*) to 3 (*several times*).

Membership in a political/civic organization. Participants were asked if they were a member of one of three types of associations: a political association, an environmental association, or a peace or human rights association (peace movement, Amnesty International, etc.). The same two questions were also asked at age 16.

The following questions on electoral behavior were asked in October, after the national elections in September:

Public participation in the national election. Participants were asked whether they had taken an active public stance in the election. Two forms of *collective* participation were measured: "Worked on a nonprofit basis for a party in the parliamentary elections, for example by handing out leaflets for the party" and "Supported a party by wearing their badge or t-shirt." These collective forms of activity were contrasted with two types of *solitary* political activities: "Used the Internet to support the parties I like" and "Followed and 'liked' parties on social networks, such as Twitter and Facebook." Response options were 1 (*no*) and 2 (*yes*).

Control variables were gender (0 = female, 1 = male) and immigrant status, a dichotomous measure distinguishing between students whose two parents were born outside the Nordic countries (=1) and other students (=0).

Attrition analyses showed that the age 20 and post-election data collections were somewhat gender biased. Man were less interested in participating. Nagelkerke's R^2 was .08 for an initial attrition analysis that included the pre-election age-20 data collection, and it was also .08 for the post-election data collection.

Results

First, as seen in the correlation table (Table 4.3) that includes the age 16 measures, the correlations between political reputation and political interest was .32 ($p < .001$), and the correlation between political reputation and self-reported political activity in the classroom was .28 ($p < .001$). The correlation between political interest and self-reported political activity in the classroom was .39 ($p < .001$). In Emler's theory, people's reputations, what others can observe, are likely to reflect their social identities. In the case of political reputation, one would expect that adolescents who are politically interested and perceive themselves as politically active in their classes would be likely candidates for students who gain political reputation. As shown in Table 4.3, the associations between political reputation and these political characteristics are modest at best.

As shown in Table 4.4, political interest and political reputation at age 16 were the two main predictors of offline political activity, political/civic association membership, and the two election-related behaviors at age 20. Political interest significantly predicted all four outcome measures (but did not discriminate between collective and solitary political activities) whereas political reputation, as proposed, significantly predicted the three types of collective activity, but not solitary activities in connection with the election. While political interest was the main predictor of the two measures of election-related political activity, political reputation was the main predictor of engaging in political activity with others and being a member of a civic/political association. Notably, participants' self-perceived classroom activity at age 16 did not significantly predict any of the measures of political activity at age 20.

The main analyses in Table 4.4 predicted changes from age 16 to age 20 for two types of collective political activity: offline political activity with others and membership in a civic/political association. These two types of collective political activity at age 20 were controlled for by the same two measures at age 16. The

TABLE 4.3 Correlations between all measures at T1.

	2	*3*	*4*	*5*	*6*	*7*	*8*	*9*
1. Reputation	.32***	.28***	.11**	.11**	.26***	.11**	.14***	−.08*
2. Political interest	–	.39***	.19***	.20***	.01	−.02	.02	.05
3. Self-perceived activities		–	.26***	.21***	.07*	.00	.03	.08*
4. Political activities			–	.30***	.05	.03	−.04	.12***
5. Member of an association				–	.02	.01	.01	.03
6. Popularity					–	.19***	.07*	−.01
7. Anger						–	.12***	.12***
8. Sex							–	.03
9. Immigrant								–

Note: *** $p < .001$, ** $p < .01$, * $p < .05$.

TABLE 4.4 Prediction of political activity with others and political participation in an election at age 20.

	Political activities with others				*Member of a civic/political association*				*Taking a stand publicly for a party at the election*				*Solitary electoral activities at the election*			
	coeff.	*SE*	*p*	*std.*	*coeff.*	*SE*	*p*	*std.*	*coeff.*	*SE*	*p*	*std.*	*coeff.*	*SE*	*p*	*std.*
Activity at T1	.100	.042	.017	.108	.048	.162	.765	.034	–	–	–	–	–	–	–	–
Political interest	.022	.010	.035	.081	.046	.022	.037	.107	.050	.014	< .001	.141	.100	.037	.007	.154
Self-perceived activity	.018	.022	.429	.045	.049	.054	.362	.081	–.018	.027	.499	–.034	.030	.044	.504	.031
Political reputation	.006	.002	.001	.277	.007	.002	.003	.190	.008	.003	.013	.249	.002	.003	.585	.031
Popularity	.003	.002	.150	.075	.003	.004	.411	.054	.004	.003	.197	.077	–.004	.005	.454	–.039
Anger	.002	.003	.469	.050	–.004	.002	.044	–.078	.005	.004	.257	.090	.015	.004	< .001	.155
Reputation × popularity	.000	.000	.027	.086	.000	< .001	.255	.073	.001	.000	< .001	.273	<.001	.000	.175	.067
Reputation × anger	.000	.000	.015	–.166	.000	<.001	.146	–.055	.000	.000	.005	–.135	< .001	.000	< .001	–.123
Sex	.027	.034	.425	.043	–.029	.048	.541	–.029	.049	.048	.302	.057	–.108	.088	.222	–.069
Immigrant status	.044	.046	.342	.049	.096	.087	.271	.067	–.016	.051	.762	–.013	–.178	.124	.149	–.081
R^2		.181				.107				.250				.072		

table also includes a measure of *collective* political activity related to the election (taking a stand for a party in public by "working on a nonprofit basis for a party in the parliamentary elections, for example by handing out leaflets for the party" and "supporting a party by wearing their badge or t-shirt") and a measure of *solitary* activities in relation to the election ("Use the Internet to support the parties I like" and "follow and 'liked' parties on social networks, such as Twitter and Facebook").

To account for the nested structure of the data (youth nested within classes), we used two-level random intercept models. In this way, we explain individual-level variation in the dependent variables while controlling for variation in mean responses across classes. They are the same type of analyses we used earlier in the chapter.

Being perceived as popular in class at age 16 was not a significant predictor of any of the four measures of political activity at age 20. Being perceived as angry in class by classmates at age 16 negatively predicted being a member of a civic/political association, but positively predicted election-related solitary activities. Neither gender nor immigrant status was a significant predictor of the four outcome measures at age 20. It remains to be seen whether political reputation in the classroom at age 16 is moderated by classmates' nominations of students who were considered popular and angry.

Table 4.4 provides strong evidence that political reputation is moderated by both popularity and anger. Regarding popularity, having a political reputation predicted political activity with others among popular youths (+1SD, coeff. .008, $p < .001$), but less so among unpopular youths (−1SD, coeff. .004, $p = .019$, Figure 4.3a). Having a political reputation predicted engagement in taking a public stand for a party during the election among popular adolescents (+1SD, coeff. .015, $p < .001$), but not among unpopular adolescents (−1SD, coeff. .000, $p = .958$, Figure 4.3b). Regarding anger, participants with a political reputation were less likely to engage in political activities with others and to take a public stand for a party when they were known to be angry in class (+1SD, coefficients for the two outcomes were .005, $p = .002$ and .006, $p = .080$, respectively) than when they were not known to be angry (−1SD, coefficients were .008, $p = .001$ and .010, $p = .001$; Figures 4.3c and d). Finally, we found a significant interactive effect between political reputation and anger in predicting solitary electoral activities, but the two coefficients, +1SD and −1SD, were not significantly different from zero.

We conclude that (i) the unique effects of political interest are significant for three of the four outcome measures, (ii) political reputation in class is more strongly related to future collective political activity than to solitary political activity, and (iii) the role that political reputation has for future political activity depends on other characteristics of these students—their popularity and anger.

Political Reputation as a Mediator

Finally, to test whether political reputation may act as a booster of preexisting political predispositions, we applied a mediation model in which political reputation

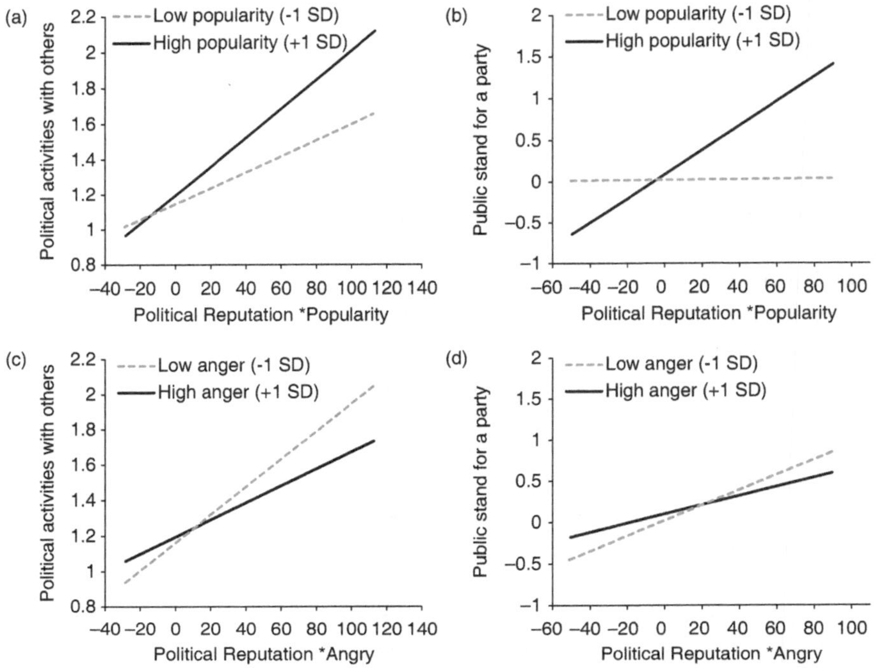

FIGURE 4.3 Interactive effects of political reputation and reputations for being popular and angry.

mediates the relationships between political interest at T1 (age 16) and at T2 (age 20) and between political efficacy at T1 and at T2 (controlling for gender and immigrant status). The indirect effects of political interest at T1 on political interest at T2 were positive and significant in both cohorts (standardized coefficients: .03, $p < .001$ at age 13, .02, $p = .003$ at age 16), as were the indirect effects of political efficacy at T1 on political efficacy at T2 (standardized coefficients: .02, $p = .02$ at age 13, .02, $p = .003$ at age 16). These analyses show that political reputation in the classroom links students' political interest and political efficacy at T1 to their political interest and political efficacy at T2. The results suggest that political reputation partially functions as a booster of adolescents' initial political predispositions over a long time. In essence, adolescents who have high political interest and high political efficacy will gain in their political interest and political efficacy much later because they have a political reputation in the classroom.

Discussion

Having a political reputation in the classroom at age 16 predicted adolescents' political activity four years later, independent of political interest at age 16 and perceptions of one's own political activity in the classroom. Consistent with our hypothesis, political reputation predicted future *collective* political activity, but not *solitary* political activity. Apparently, when some students gain a reputation for knowing a lot about what is going on in the world and do not hesitate to bring it up in class, this has long-term consequences for them with respect to their collective political activities.

Political interest was also an important predictor at age 16. It was a stronger predictor of election-related political activity at age 20 than it was of off-time political activity and membership in civic/political associations. That political interest is a strong long-term predictor is consistent with many previous studies in the literature. Preferably, young people's political interest should be included by default in all predictions of people's political opinions, attitudes, behaviors, and political interactions with others. It is easy to draw erroneous conclusions about the role of a particular predictor if interest in politics is not included.

Political interest is typically based on self-reporting. Political reputation, on the other hand, is based on peer nominations. The correlation between the two measures was modest, $r = .32, p < .001$, suggesting that both self-reported and external information are independent sources of knowledge about adolescents' future political activities.

In terms of what enhances or discourages the future political involvement of students with a political reputation in the classroom, we hypothesized that their reputations for being popular and for being angry and disruptive in the classroom should also be considered. Popularity might enhance the future collective political activities of politically interested students, while being angry and disruptive might discourage these activities. A person who is angry and disruptive would discourage others from engaging them in joint political activities. We found ample evidence that popularity and anger moderated the associations between political reputation and the types of political activities we measured at age 20. Having a political reputation predicted political activities with others and engagement in taking a public stand for a party during the election among popular adolescents, but less so among unpopular adolescents. Regarding anger, participants with a political reputation were less likely to engage in political activities with others and to take a public stand for a party when they were known to be angry in class than when they were not known to be angry. Hypothesized interaction terms in regression analysis are difficult to confirm. But here, five of them were significant in eight separate analyses.

Emler's reputation enhancement theory differs from assumptions in identity theory (McCall & Simmons, 1978; Stryker & Burke, 2000) in that it emphasizes the collective judgment of others' social identity rather than one's own identification of one's social identity. This difference in perspective between peer reputation for political activity in the classroom and an individual student's identification as someone who is politically active in the classroom allowed us to ask whether it is one's own view of being politically active in the classroom or one's reputation for being politically active in the classroom that influences future political activity and involvement. We found that students' perceptions of their political behavior in the classroom were not strongly related to their future political engagement. The main predictor was their political reputation in the classroom as judged by their peers. Information about classroom political interactions from the outside rather than the inside perspective is more important for understanding future political activity in other settings.

We have argued that if teachers encourage discussions about political and civic activities in class, then students in that class will have many opportunities to observe their classmates' interest in civic and political issues, and over time they are likely to develop similar opinions of the students who keep track of what is going on in their society and the world, and who often initiate discussions about societal issues in class. In classes with less open discussion climates, there will be fewer opportunities to observe political interactions in class, and there will be less communality of opinion about who is politically competent. In classes where teachers encourage political discussion, micro-processes will begin to operate, and these group processes will result in some students gaining reputations for being politically competent. Until now, these dynamic group processes in the classroom have been largely unknown. Over time, as we have seen in this chapter, political reputation increases the political interest and political efficacy of these students. Some students have fewer opportunities to acquire such reputations. Students with social anxiety are one example. Fear of speaking in public makes them reluctant to express their opinions. Schools have an obligation to try to involve all students in these discussions, including those who do not have the social skills to bring these issues to public attention.

Finally, participation in collective political activities at age 20 is predicted by political reputation in the classroom at age 16 in upper secondary school. These predictions are independent of students' political interest at age 16. But side by side, political interest, independent of political reputation, is also an important predictor of these political activities at age 20.

Finally, what is the evidence in schools that young people are active agents in their own political development?

Some students acquire political reputations from their classmates. Political interest and internal political efficacy appear to be key student characteristics that at least cross-sectionally explain this political reputation in class.

When they gain a political reputation in class, this reputation has consequences.

The short-term perspective:

- Political reputation partially functions as a booster of students' initial political interest and political efficacy. Students who initially have high political interest and efficacy gain in political interest and efficacy over time as a result of having a political reputation in class.

The long-term perspective:

- By predicting future political activity and behavior in the context of a national election, political reputation functions as a booster of adolescents' initial political predispositions over time—political interest and political efficacy.

PART III

Political Interactions With Parents

5

POLITICAL INTERACTIONS WITH PARENTS IN EARLY AND MID-ADOLESCENCE

Highlights

- *Most young people perceive their parents as politically interested and knowledgeable.*
- *Most young people are open to their parents' political communication: their parents' views are important to them and are perceived as similar to their own views, and their parents' conversations about society and the news evoke positive feelings in them. Most adolescents perceive that their parents respond positively to their political communication.*
- *Parents report that discussions about politics and society take place at home significantly more often than their adolescents report. This is not limited to political discussions. Parents also perceive that discussions about everyday life—about common family activities and school—take place more often than their adolescents report.*
- *On the list of different types of everyday conversations that adolescents have with parents and peers, conversations about politics and society are reported as the least frequent topic. On a similar list, parents are also the least likely to report discussing politics and society with their children.*
- *Adolescents know more about their parents' views than about their friends' views, parents are seen as more knowledgeable than friends, and parents' attempts to make adolescents more aware of what is going on in the world and of environmental issues occur more frequently than friends' attempts.*
- *Early adolescence is potentially the most formative time for young people, according to parents. Parents are more likely to try to influence their 13-year-olds than their 16-year-olds.*

The family is the most fundamental place and group of people for understanding young people's perceptions, knowledge, and interest in politics, their society, and the world. Insights into how political interactions between adolescents and their parents affect adolescents' political development must begin with the similarities and differences in how adolescents and their parents perceive these interactions. Do adolescents perceive their parents as politically knowledgeable? How often do adolescents perceive that their parents' political views are important to them and similar to their own? According to adolescents and parents, how often do political

DOI: 10.4324/9781003371731-8

discussions take place between them? Are adolescents aware that their parents are trying to influence them politically, and are they receptive to their parents' attempts to influence them? Similar questions can be asked of their parents. In this chapter, we will provide an overview of how adolescents perceive their parents' views on politics and society and their political interactions with their parents, as well as how parents perceive their political interactions with their children. We will use the two youngest age cohorts, 13 and 16 years old.

Differences between the two age cohorts and between adolescents and their parents are best described by measures of effect size, reported as Cohen's *d* (small = up to .20; medium = up to .50, large = at least .80). Because the differences between the two youngest age cohorts are small (and do not alter the conclusions we draw), we decided to report the results for both cohorts together and for both genders together. In the running text, we report separately all cases where there are significant differences at the .001 level between the two cohorts and between boys and girls.

Adolescents' Perceptions of Their Parents' Political Sophistication

Are Adolescent Aware of Their Parents' Political Views and Knowledge?

What do adolescents know about their parents' views on political and social issues? We asked two questions. The first was, "How much do you know about your parents' views on and ways of looking at societal issues?" As shown in Figure 5.1, the majority of adolescents, 54%, felt they knew quite well or most of what their parents thought about social issues. Only 17% of adolescents said they did not know anything or not much about their parents' views. A follow-up question was asked: "Are your parents knowledgeable regarding what is going on in Sweden and the rest of the world?" (Figure 5.2). Seventeen percent were unsure of their parents' knowledge. Few reported that their parents were not knowledgeable. But more than 8 out of 10 young people said that their parents had quite good or very good knowledge of what was going on in Sweden and the world. Apparently, most young people perceive that they are aware of their parents' views on societal issues, and most of them perceive that their parents are knowledgeable about what is going on in society.

Next, adolescents responded to two statements about their parents' political interest. The first was, "My parents are interested in what is going on in the world" (Figure 5.3). More than 8 in 10 adolescents said this applied quite well or perfectly. Second, they responded to the statement, "My parents keep themselves in touch with the news," with about 9 in 10 adolescents saying it applied quite well or perfectly. In summary, most adolescents in both cohorts reported that they have good insight into their parents' thinking about social issues, that their parents have good knowledge of what is happening in the world, and that their parents keep up with the news.

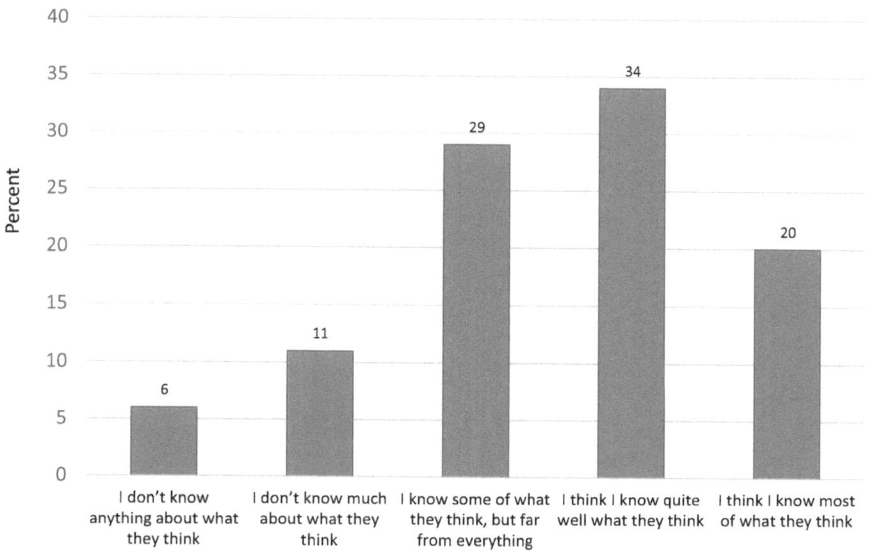

FIGURE 5.1 Adolescents' responses to the question "How much do you know about your parents' views on and ways of looking at societal issues?"

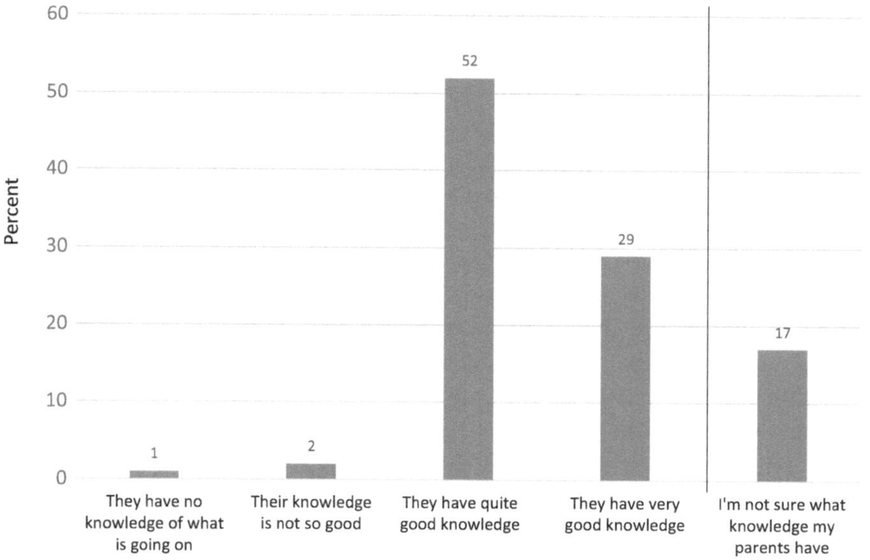

FIGURE 5.2 Adolescents' responses to the question "Are your parents knowledgeable regarding what is going on in Sweden and the rest of the world?"

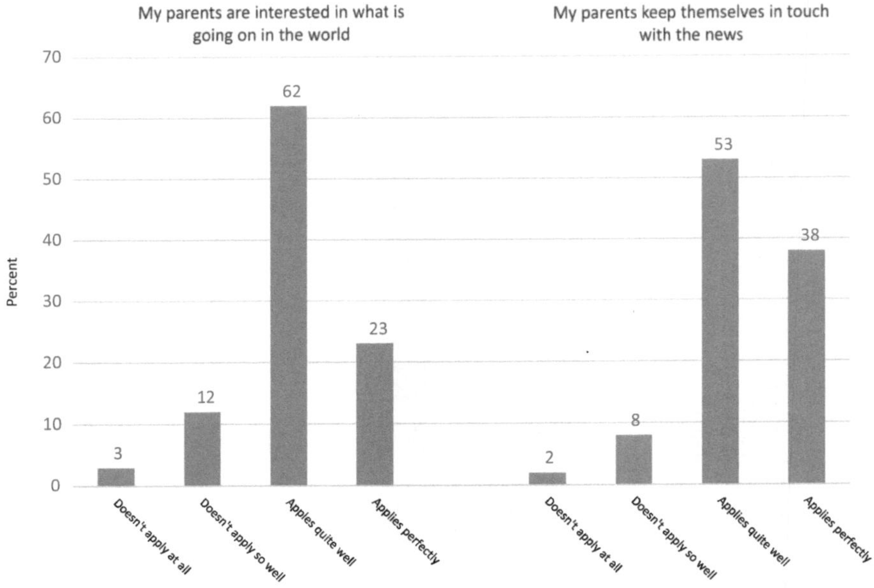

FIGURE 5.3 Adolescents' responses to two statements about parents' political interest and keeping up with the news.

Are Parents' Political Views Important to Adolescents, and Are Their Views Similar to or Different From Their Own?

We asked the direct question, "Are your parents' political views and their ways of looking at societal issues important to you?" As shown in Figure 5.4, 6 in 10 youths responded in the affirmative (in part or very much). Only 8% said their parents' views were not important to them at all. Thus, for most adolescents, their parents' political views are important to them.

We asked the adolescents, "Do you and your parents hold the same or different views on and ways of looking at societal issues?" (Figure 5.5). Twenty-three percent of adolescents could not answer this question. Fifty-five percent said their parents' views were much or quite like their own, 18% said their parents' views were different from their own, while only 3% said their parents' views were almost opposite their own. The overall message is that adolescents typically experience their parents' political views as about the same as their own.

Political Discussions in the Family

How Often Do Political Discussions Take Place?

Against this background of how young people perceive their parents' knowledge of what is going on in society, how important their parents' views are and whether

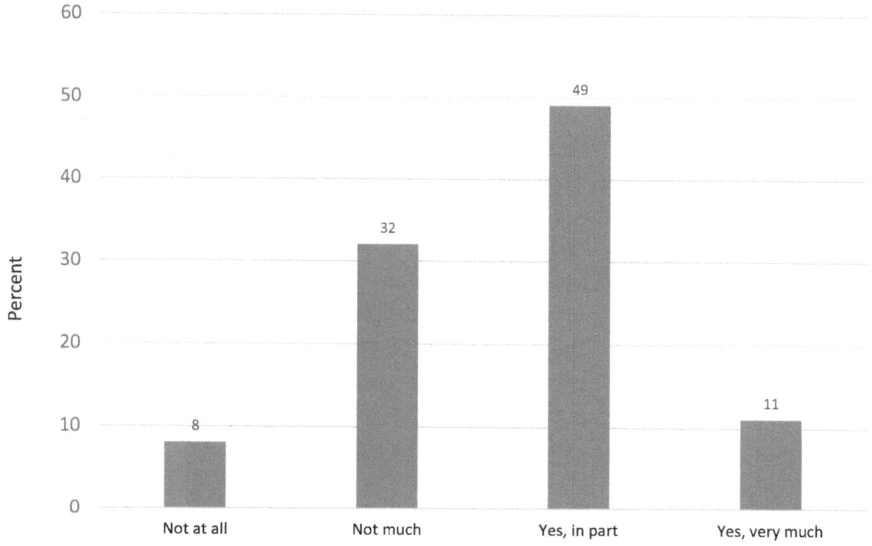

FIGURE 5.4 Adolescents' responses to the question "Are your parents' political views and their ways of looking at societal issues important to you?"

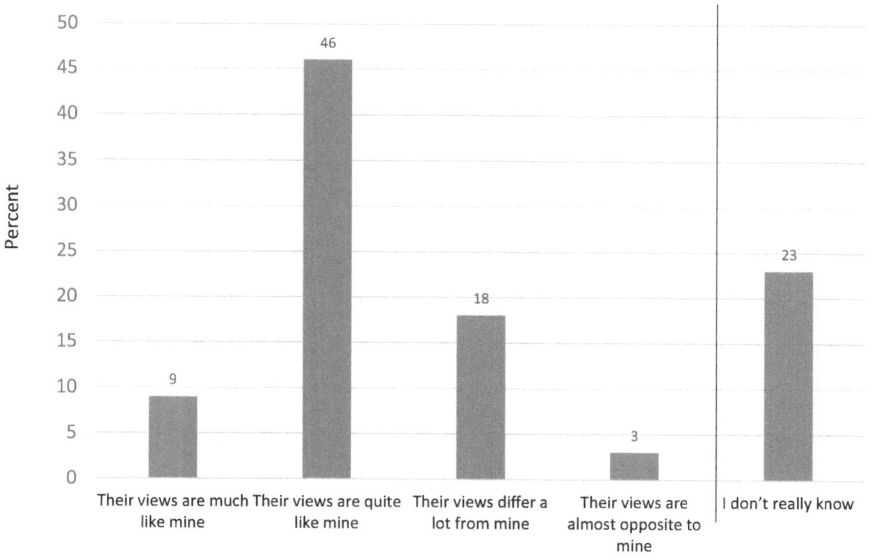

FIGURE 5.5 Adolescents' responses to the question "Do you and your parents hold the same or different views on and ways of looking at societal issues?"

their parents have similar views to their own, we need to know more about how often political discussions take place in families. We also need to know how their parents perceive the frequency of these political discussions.

We asked the adolescents the following question: "How often does it happen that you and your parents talk about what you have heard on the news about what is going on in Sweden and around the world?" According to the adolescents, more than 60% said this type of discussion happens now and then or very much (see Figure 5.6). Eight percent said it never happened. When parents responded, they perceived the frequency of political discussions differently. More than 90% said it happened now and then or very often, and no parent said they never talked about these issues. The mean scores differed significantly between the adolescents' and their parents' reports, with a large effect size (0.88). Thus, although the majority of adolescents perceive that political conversations occur now and then or very often, parents perceive that these political conversations occur significantly more often than their children report.

We also asked the adolescents, "How often does it happen that you and your parents talk about politics or societal issues?" According to the adolescents, most of them perceived that these discussions with parents about political and social issues seldom or never took place (Figure 5.7). In contrast, the most common response from parents was that this type of discussion occurred now and then. It should be noted that one in five adolescents reported that these discussions never took

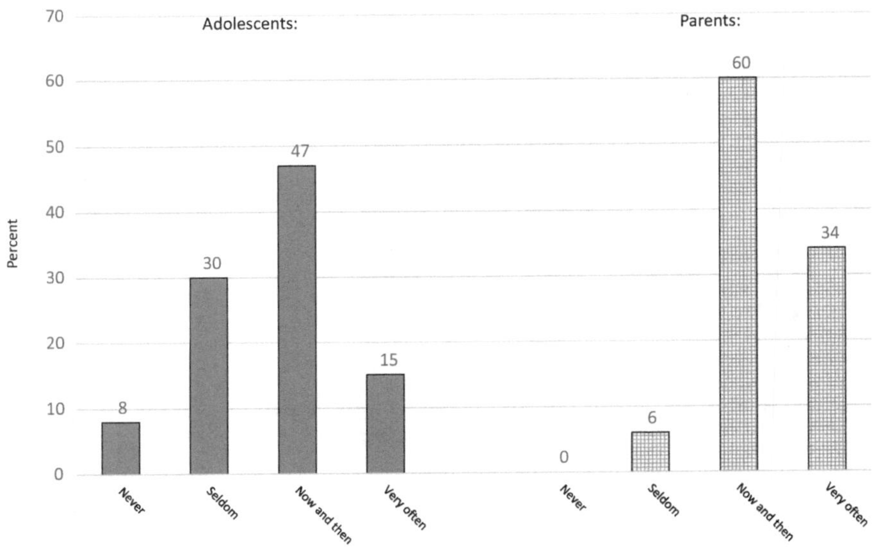

FIGURE 5.6 Responses to the question "How often does it happen that you and your parents talk about what you have heard on the news about what is going on in Sweden and around the world?"

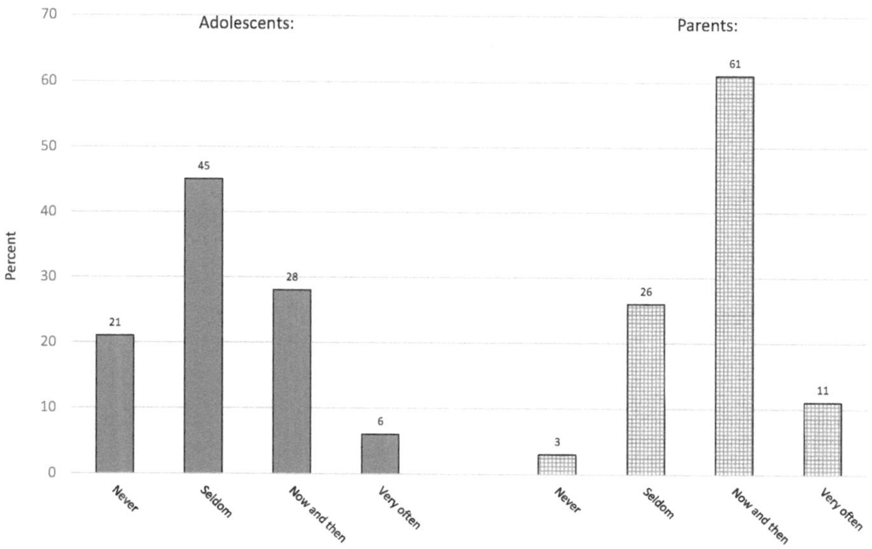

FIGURE 5.7 Responses to the question "How often does it happen that you and your parents talk about politics or societal issues?"

place, while the alternative "never" was reported by very few parents. Overall, parents reported more discussions about political or social issues than did their adolescents. The effect size was large (.85). The most obvious conclusion from these results is that parents perceive that they have political discussions with their adolescents considerably more often than their adolescents perceive that they do.

Do Parents Try to Influence Their Adolescents Politically?

We asked both adolescents and their parents whether parents try to influence their children to be interested in politics and society. On the question "Do your parents try to get you to become more aware of environmental issues?" 60% of adolescents reported that this happened sometimes, often, or almost always (Figure 5.8). Parents' responses to the same question showed that more of them, about 90%, reported that this happened sometimes, often, or always. The difference between parents' and adolescents' responses yielded a medium effect size (0.65).

A follow-up question to the adolescent was "Do your parents try to encourage you to become more aware of what is going on in the world?" Here, more than 80% of adolescents reported that this happened sometimes, often, or almost always (Figure 5.9). With few exceptions, most parents reported that this happened sometimes, often, or almost always. Again, parents were more likely to perceive that they were trying to influence their children politically than adolescents were likely to perceive that their parents were doing so. The effect size for the differences between parents and adolescents was close to medium (0.48).

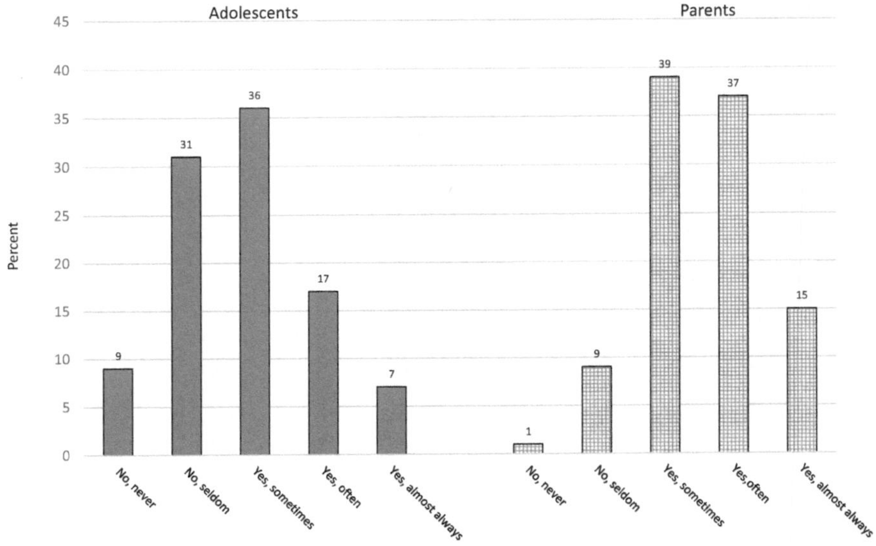

FIGURE 5.8 Adolescents' and parents' responses to the question whether parents try to make the adolescent more aware of environmental issues.

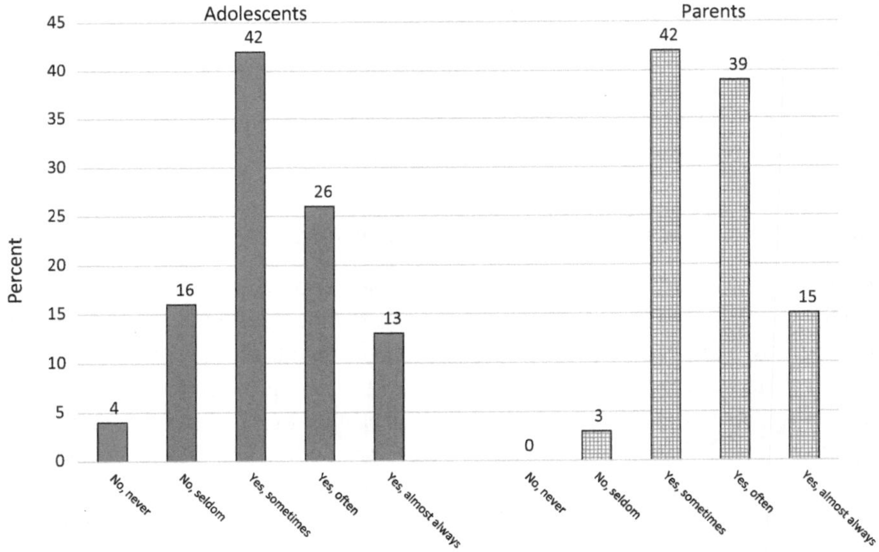

FIGURE 5.9 Adolescents' and parents' responses to whether parents try to encourage the adolescent to be more aware of what is going on in the world.

We also asked both adolescents and parents about the different ways in which parents can politically socialize their children. These included suggesting newspapers, books, or websites where the child can read about politics or social issues (Figure 5.10a), providing information about activities or organizations the child can contact or get involved with (Figure 5.10b), and asking the child to sit down and watch the news on television with the parent (Figure 5.10c). Between 47% and 61% of parents reported that these examples of their children's political socialization kind of applied, applied quite well, or applied very well to what was going on at home. The same percentages were lower for adolescents, ranging from 34%

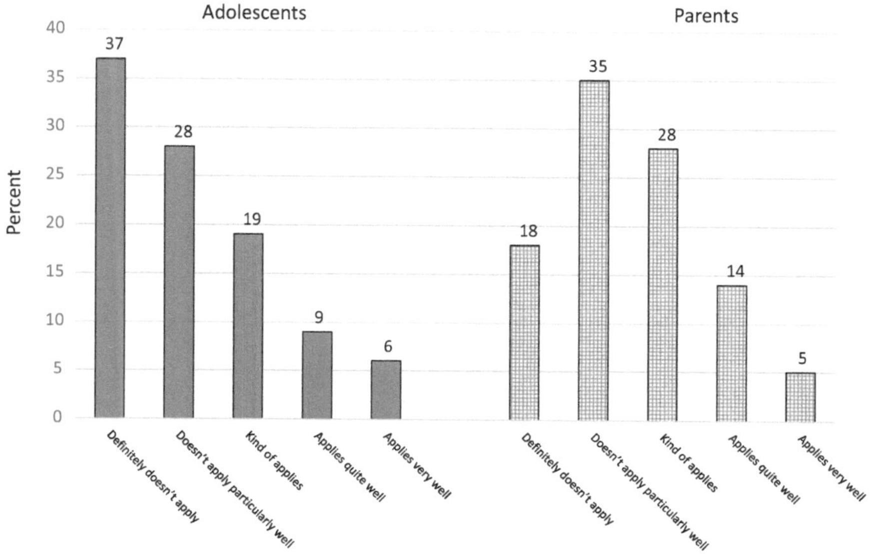

FIGURE 5.10A Adolescents' and parents' responses to whether parents suggest newspapers, books, or websites where one can read about politics or societal issues.

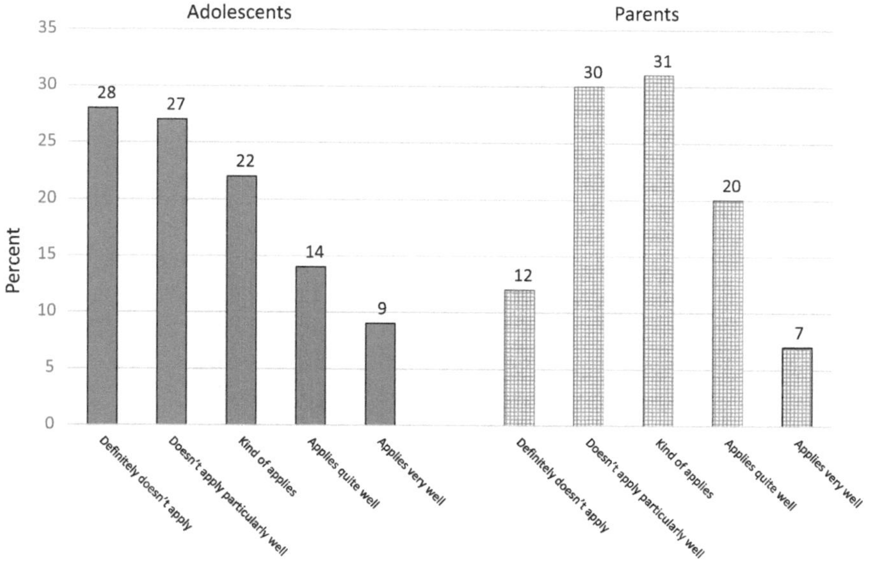

FIGURE 5.10B Adolescents' and parents' responses to whether parents give information about activities or organizations to contact or get involved with.

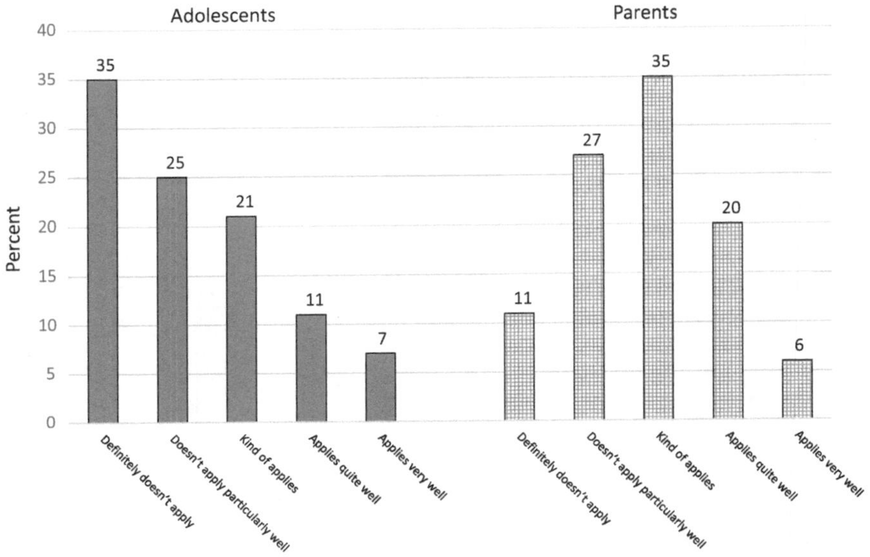

FIGURE 5.10C Adolescents' and parents' responses to the question of whether parents usually want the adolescent to sit down and watch the news on TV with them.

to 45%. It is noteworthy that the percentage of adolescents who said that these attempts by their parents to politically socialize them never happened was more than two to three times higher than what their parents reported. The differences between parents and youth for the three examples of political socialization attempts yielded effect sizes of 0.30, 0.25, and 0.44, respectively. We conclude that a substantial minority of adolescents are aware of the different ways their parents' attempts to influence them politically. Most parents are aware of these different ways to influence their adolescents' political and social views.

How Do Adolescents Perceive Their Parents' Reactions to Their Political Initiatives?

If parents are interested in promoting their children's political development, they would be happy if their adolescents spontaneously discussed political and social issues at home. We asked the adolescents two questions. The first was "You may have tried to start a discussion on some societal or political issue with your parents. How then have they usually reacted?" As shown in Figure 5.11, 45% of adolescents said they had never initiated such discussions at home. Of those who had, most reported that their parents reacted positively (happy and interested or fairly positive). It can be added that a cross-tabulation of this question and cohort shows that there was a significantly higher proportion in the younger cohort than in the older cohort who had never initiated a discussion about political or social issues with their parents.

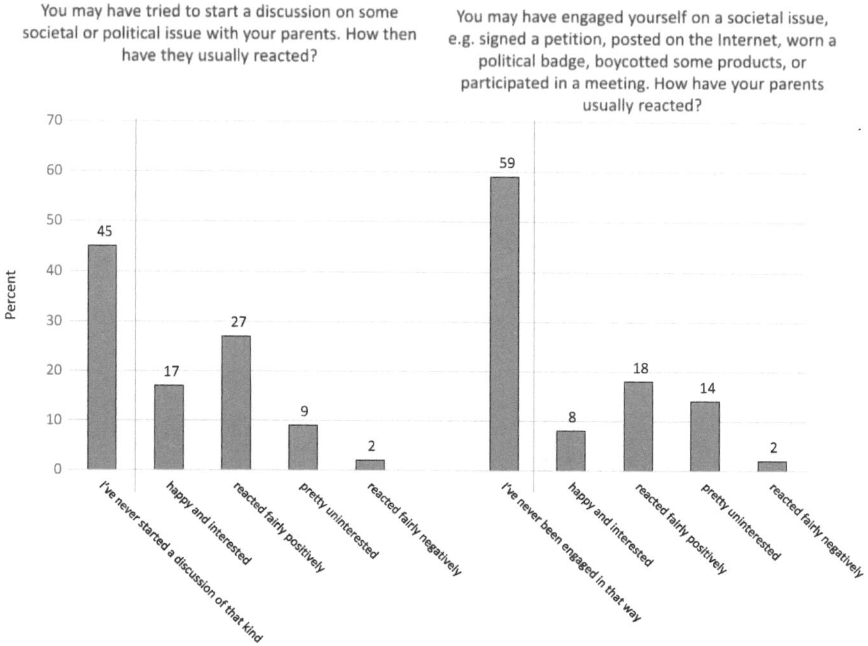

FIGURE 5.11 Adolescents' answers to the question of how parents react to adolescents' political initiatives.

A follow-up question was, "You may have engaged yourself on a societal issue, e.g., signed a petition, posted on the Internet, worn a political badge, boycotted some product, or participated in a meeting. How have your parents usually reacted?" As shown in Figure 5.11, the majority of youths (59%) had never been involved in these types of issues, but of those who had, the majority reported positive parental reactions.

Our conclusion is that young people's attempts to discuss their political views or activism with their parents are generally met with a positive response.

Are Adolescents' Open to Their Parents' Political Socialization?

How do young people perceive their parents' political communication? Are they open to the way their parents talk about political and social issues? We asked two questions about this openness. The first was whether adolescents agreed with the statement "My parents talk about things that happen in the world and in society in such a way that I become curious and want to know more" (Figure 5.12). Here, more than 7 of 10 of the adolescents responded that this statement applied kind of, quite well, or applied very well.

The second question was, "My parents tell me about the news they have heard on TV or read about in a way that evokes strong feelings in me." More than 7 in

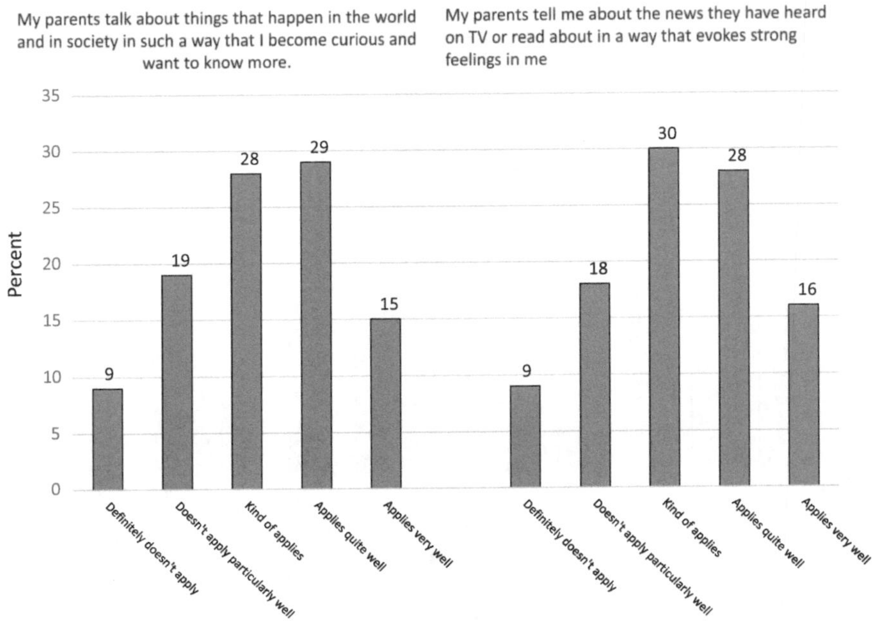

FIGURE 5.12 Adolescents' susceptibility to parents' political communication.

10 adolescents in both cohorts felt that parents' attempts to provide information evoked strong feelings (kind of, quite well, or very well). Overall, it seems that when parents talk about the world, society, and the news, it evokes positive feelings in the majority of adolescents.

How Often Do Adolescents Try to Influence Their Parents Politically?

Parents may try to influence their children's political and social interests, but adolescents may also initiate discussions about these issues with their parents. We asked parents the following general question: "How often does your child try to get you into discussions of politics or societal issues?" As shown in Figure 5.13, only 10% of parents reported that this happened quite often or very often. At the same time, although it didn't happen often, it did happen now and then (44%). Note that 47% of parents said it happened very rarely.

Subsequently, we posed the same question to both adolescents and parents: "Do you try to get your parents more aware of what is going on in the world?" and "Do your children try to get you more aware of what is going on in the world?" (Figure 5.14). Here, a minority of both youth (18%) and parents (14%) reported that this happened often or very often. The most common response from adolescents was that it seldom happened, and the most common response from parents

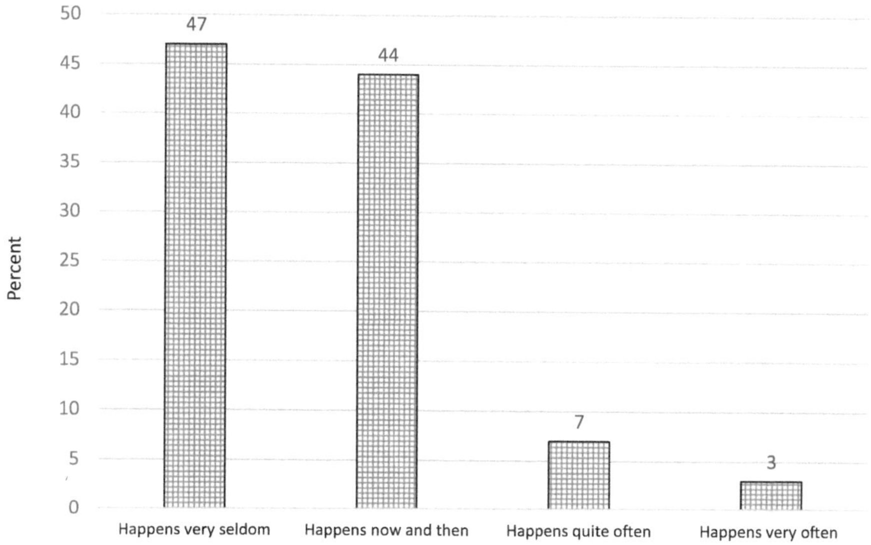

FIGURE 5.13 Parents' answers to the question "How often does your child try to get you into discussions of politics or societal issues?"

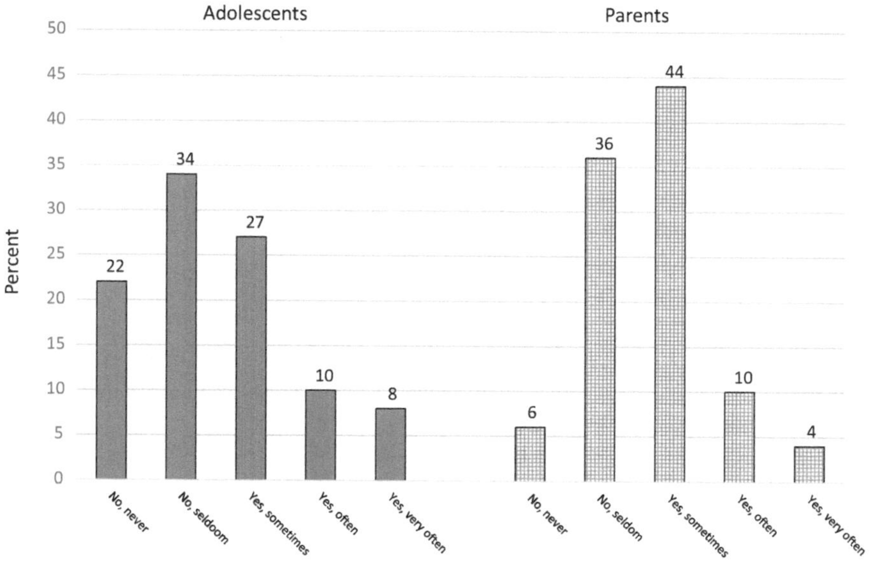

FIGURE 5.14 Adolescents' and parents' responses to the question of whether adolescents encourage parents to be more aware of what is going on in the world.

was that it happened sometimes. The difference between parent and adolescent reports yielded a small effect size (0.19).

Sex Differences

We repeated all analyses up to this point, looking for sex differences ($p < .001$) in both cohorts. We found none. We conclude that there is a general lack of sex differences at the .001 level.

Cohort Differences

In general, there were few significant differences between the responses of the 13-year-olds and the 16-year-olds ($p < .001$). One difference, however, was how often the adolescents and their parents talked about what was going on in Sweden and the world. Older adolescents perceived that this kind of discussion took place more often than younger adolescents. We found a similar difference when we asked how often the adolescents and their parents talked about politics and society. In addition, parents of the older adolescents reported that their adolescents tried to involve them in discussions about politics and society more often than did parents of the younger adolescents. Effect sizes ranged from 0.19 to 0.43.

There seems to be another kind of cohort difference. Parents seem to try to politically socialize their younger adolescents more than their older adolescents. A significant difference with a small effect size (0.33) is that parents are more likely to give their younger adolescents information about activities or organizations to contact or get involved with than their older adolescents. Although the differences were not significant at the .001 level, it also appears that younger adolescents were more likely than older adolescents to report that their parents tried to influence them politically by suggesting newspapers, books, or websites. Younger adolescents were also more likely than older adolescents to report that their parents tried to make them aware of environmental issues and tried to make them aware of what was going on in the world.

Summary

The findings presented so far in this chapter can be summarized as follows:

Parents are seen as politically competent and their views are considered important by most adolescents.

- Most adolescents perceive their parents as knowledgeable about political and social issues.
- Most adolescents perceive their parents as interested in politics.
- Most adolescents say their parents' views are important to them.
- For the majority, their parents' political views are perceived to be about the same as their own. In very few cases, parents' views are perceived to be the opposite of adolescents' views.

Adolescents are open to their parents' political communication and aware of their parents' attempts to influence them.

- Parents' conversations about society and the news evoke positive feelings in the majority of adolescents.
- The majority of adolescents report that their parents encourage them to be more aware of environmental issues and what is going on in the world.
- Parents may use a variety of ways to influence their adolescents politically: suggesting newspapers, books, or websites to read about politics or social issues; providing information about activities or organizations the child can contact or get involved with; or suggesting that their child sit down with them and watch the news together. A substantial minority of adolescents recognize these socialization attempts.

Parents are perceived as open to youth influence.

- When young people have had discussions with their parents or have become involved in a social issue, most of these young people perceive that their parents have responded positively to their communication attempts.

Parents perceive that their joint political interactions occur more often than adolescents experience them.

- There are significant differences between parents and adolescents in how often they perceive political discussions take place in the family. Parents say they occur more often than their adolescents report.
- The vast majority of parents report that they try to influence their adolescents to be more aware of environmental issues and what is going on in the world. Significantly fewer adolescents report this.
- The majority of parents report that they try to provide their adolescents with political information (suggesting newspapers or books; providing information about organizations; watching the news on TV with them). Fewer adolescents recognize that this is the case.
- Parents perceive that their adolescents try to influence their political views more often than adolescents say they do.

There is evidence that older adolescents are more politically active at home than younger adolescents.

- Older adolescents report discussing politics or social issues with their parents more often than younger adolescents.
- Parents report that their adolescents in the older cohort have initiated discussions about politics or social issues more often than parents of adolescents in the younger cohort.

There is evidence that parents are more likely to politically socialize their younger adolescents than their older adolescents.

- Parents are more likely to provide their younger adolescents than their older adolescents with information about activities or organizations to contact or join.

- Younger adolescents are more likely to report that their parents try to influence them politically (suggesting newspapers, books, or websites).

- Adolescents in the younger cohort are more likely to report that their parents try to make them aware of environmental issues and try to make them aware of what is going on in the world.

These are important findings. One could argue that parents would avoid influencing their young people's political beliefs because they assume that their children won't understand or will be upset or that it's irrelevant to them at this age (Patterson et al., 2019). However, the opposite seems to be true. Parents are more interested in making their early adolescents aware of what is happening in the world and trying to influence them politically than they are in trying to influence their middle adolescent children. Early adolescence is perhaps the time when parents think young people are most formative.

On Openness to Parents' Political Socialization

The traditional assumption in political socialization research is that parents transmit their political attitudes and values to their offspring. Their views become the views of their children. Successful socialization means that the child adopts the values and behaviors transmitted by the parents. But children must be open to their parents' socialization attempts if "normal socialization" is to work as it should. This is the basic view of socialization presented in value socialization theory (Grusec & Goodnow, 1994; Grusec & Kuczynski, 1997; Knafo & Schwartz, 2003, 2009).

There is strong evidence that young people are indeed receptive to their parents' political socialization: Parents are perceived as knowledgeable and youth are receptive:

- *Knowledge of parents' political views.* The vast majority of adolescents, more than 8 in 10, believe they have at least some knowledge of their parents' political views.
- *Susceptibility.* A majority of adolescents say their parents' views on social issues are important to them. A majority also report that their parents' conversations about the world, politics, and society evoke positive feelings in them—they become curious and want to know more, or they find it fun and interesting.

Overall, the information on the political socialization of young people that we have brought up in this chapter seems to indicate that young people are open and receptive to their parents' political messages.

Notably, among those who were able to compare whether they and their parents had the same or different views and perspectives on social issues, more than 60% said that their parents' views were very similar or very similar to their own. More than 80% said their parents had a fair or very good knowledge of what was going on in Sweden and the rest of the world. The same percentage said that their parents were interested in what was going on in the world and that they kept up with the news. Furthermore, among the young people who said that they had started a discussion at home about a social or political issue, again about 80% said that their parents had responded positively. Moreover, parents' attempts to politically socialize their adolescents were often met with positive feelings on the part of the adolescents. When asked, "My parents talk about social issues in a way that makes them fun and interesting" and "My parents talk about things going on in the world and society in a way that makes me curious and want to know more," 70% to 80% of adolescents said this kind of applied, applied quite well, or very well. There seems to be massive evidence that at this age parents are politically important discussion partners about politics for adolescents: They are seen as politically competent, open, and positive, and in these discussions they evoke positive feelings in most adolescents.

Extending the Questions

How Often Do Political Talks Take Place Relative to Other Talks?

One finding in this chapter that appears to be well founded is that parents report that political discussions occur more often than adolescents report. In and of itself, not much can be said about the frequency with which adolescents and parents report discussing political and social issues unless that frequency can be compared to other types of topics that are also discussed in families. Here we compare the frequency with which political and social topics are discussed ("Politics and social issues" and "What you have heard in the news about what is going on in Sweden and around the world") with other conversations that take place in families—conversations about "Family activities (doing things together)" and about "School, school work and homework." The two young age cohorts were again paired.

Parents' reports on how often political and everyday topics are discussed in the family are shown in Figure 5.15. As can be seen in this figure, discussions about school, schoolwork, and homework were most common in families, and discussions about politics and society were least common. The effect size for the mean difference between talking about politics and society and talking about school was very large (2.20). The effect size was also large (1.13) when comparing discussions

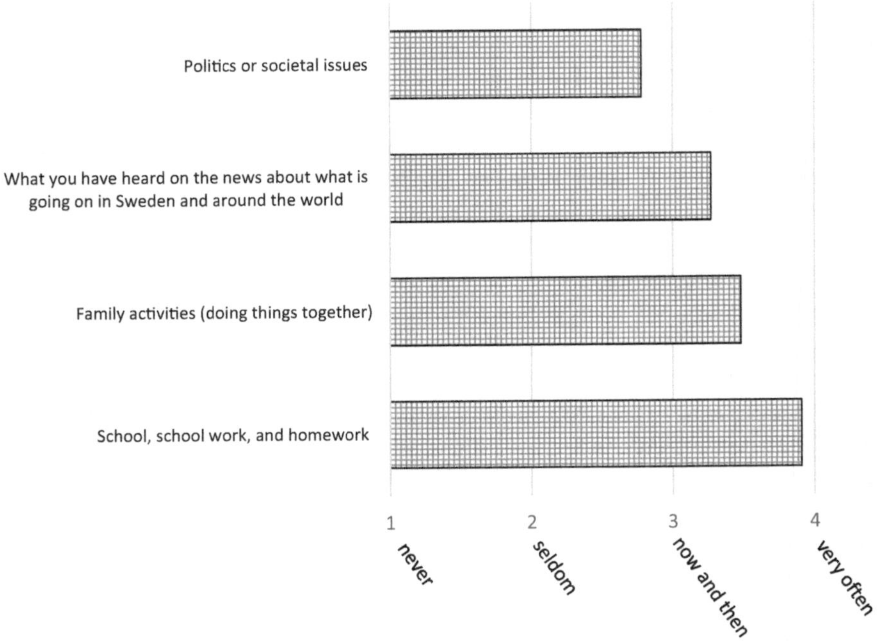

FIGURE 5.15 Parents' responses to the question "How often does it happen that you and your son/daughter talk about the following?"

about politics and society with discussions about family matters. Finally, discussions about what they had heard in the news were more common in families than discussions about politics and society (effect size is 0.80). To provide more detail on these comparisons, in Figure 5.16 we report how often parents perceived that discussions with their adolescents about politics and society took place relative to discussions about school, schoolwork, and homework. Nine out of 10 parents reported that discussions with their adolescents about school took place very often. In contrast, only 1 in 10 parents reported that discussions about politics and society took place very often.

Admittedly, conversations about family activities and school are likely to be more frequent than family discussions about politics and the news. Therefore, we need to include more diverse types of family conversations. This kind of comparison was not possible with the parents because we had to limit the number of questions in the mail questionnaire, but it is possible with the adolescents' reports.

We asked adolescents about the frequency of conversations with their parents on seven different topics (again measured on 4-point scales), *Never, Seldom, Now and then, Very often*):

- School, schoolwork, and homework
- Relatives and friends of the family

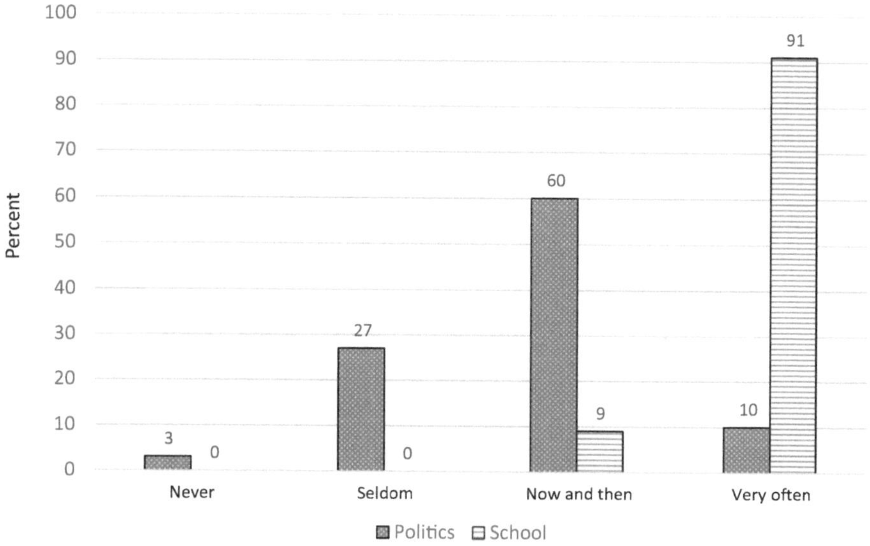

FIGURE 5.16 Parents' answers to the questions "How often does it happen that you and your son/daughter talk about Politics or societal issues and School, school work, and homework?"

- Family activities (doing things together)
- Your friends (what you do in free time)
- Films, music, and TV series
- What you have heard on the news about what is going on in Sweden and around the world
- Politics or societal issues

The last two types of family discussions concern political, environmental, and social issues. As shown in Figure 5.17, these types of family discussions (and especially political or social issues) were not particularly common in the families compared to the other five. Comparing the last five "everyday" discussions with the first two "political" discussions, there is a significant difference with a large effect size (1.16). In short, according to the adolescents, discussions about politics, society, and the environment are not high on the agenda compared to other types of conversations in the family.

To elaborate on these comparisons, Figure 5.18 shows how often adolescents perceived that discussions about politics and society took place compared to discussions about school, schoolwork, and homework. The differences between these two types of family discussions are large. Nine out of 10 adolescents reported that family discussions about school took place now and then or very often. In contrast, only 3 in 10 adolescents said that discussions about politics and society took place that often. Note that both parents and adolescents considered school and family

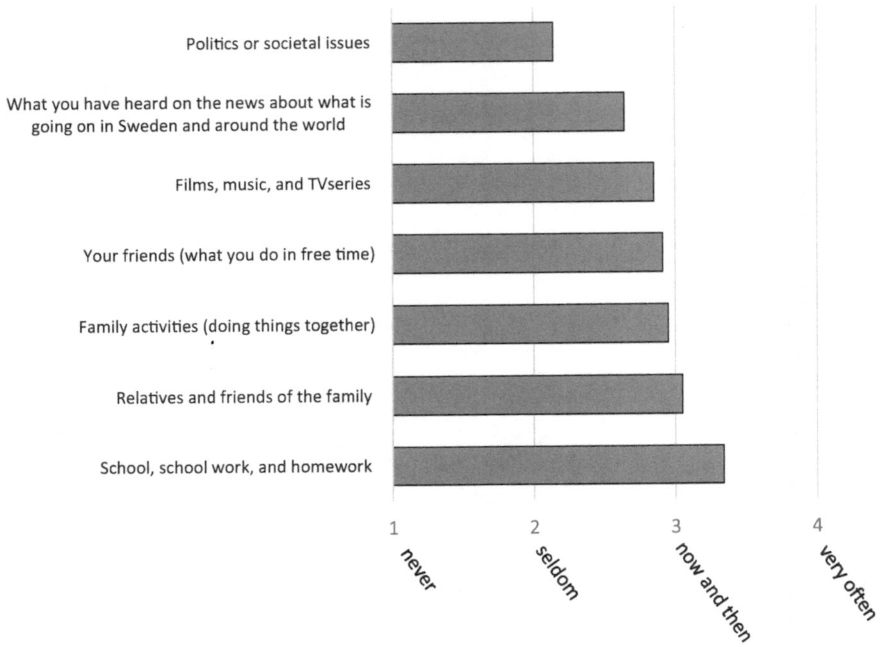

FIGURE 5.17 Adolescents' responses to the question "How often does it happen that you and your parents talk about the following?"

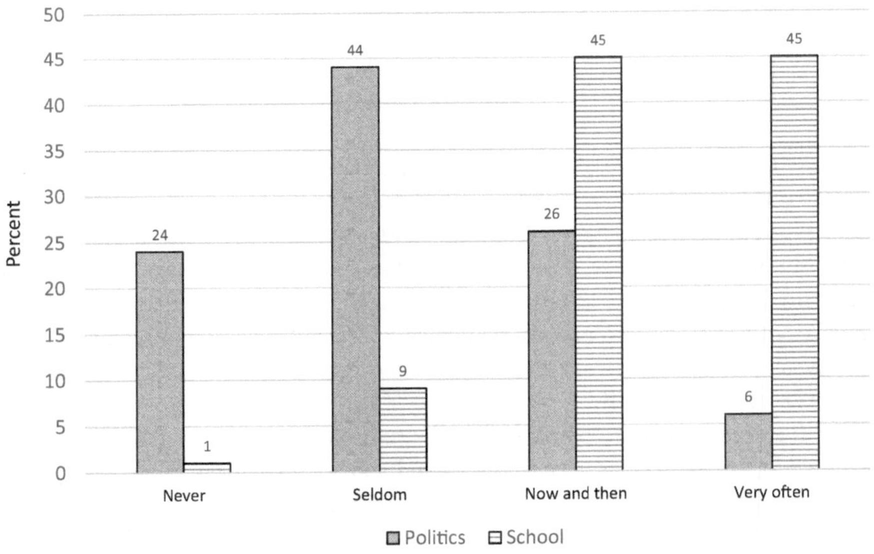

FIGURE 5.18 Adolescents' answers to the questions "How often does it happen that you and your parents talk about Politics or societal issues and School, school work, and homework?"

activities to be among the most frequent types of conversations they had together and discussions about politics or social issues to be among the least frequent.

We conclude that political discussions between parents at home are not regular in most families and are less frequent than discussions about many kinds of everyday issues. Parents perceive that political discussions take place more often than adolescents do. If parents over-report discussing political and social issues with their adolescents, one explanation is social desirability, Consider Figure 5.19. In this figure, which is an extension of Figure 5.16, we have included both parents' and adolescents' reports of how often they talk about the four topics they were both asked about.

As shown in Figure 5.19, parents report more conversations about *all four topics* examined—politics, news, family activities, and school. The differences between parents' and adolescents' reports are substantial with effect sizes that are medium for the first three and large for the last. It appears that parents' reports of how often different topics are discussed in the family—both everyday topics and political topics—are significantly higher than the frequency with which adolescents report discussing these topics. Thus, the parent-adolescent differences we found for political topics do not seem to be unique to these topics. One explanation is that parents are more sensitive to the topics they discuss with their adolescents than their adolescents are. However, it cannot be ruled out that when parents are asked issues connected to their responsibilities as parents, they respond in ways that would

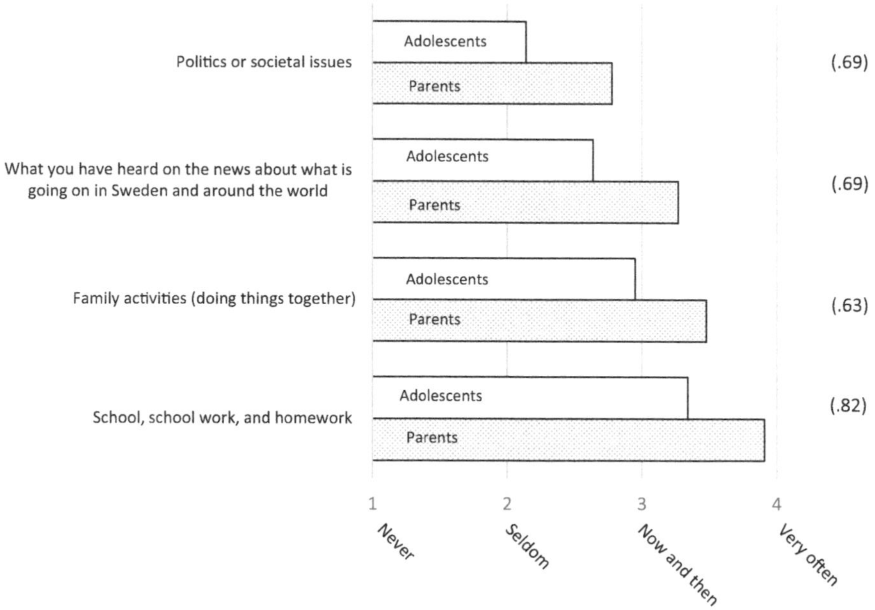

FIGURE 5.19 Parents' and adolescents' responses to the question "How often does it happen that you talk about these things?" Cohen's *d* is shown in parentheses.

be expected of a responsible parent (cf. Kapetanovic & Boson, 2022; Koolstra & Lucassen, 2004). Actually, meta-studies have shown that parents in general tend to report their own behavior in a more positive light compared to what their adolescents report (Hou et al., 2020; Korelitz & Garber, 2016).

Note that adolescents and parents report on what is talked about in *the same setting*—the family setting. Thus, it is not about issues that take place in different settings that are unknown to either of them. This should maximize convergence between adolescents' and parents' perceptions (Kraemer et al., 2003). Correlations between adolescent and parent reports of the four topics in Figure 5.15 are as follows:

- Family activities (doing things together), $r = .22$
- What you have heard on the news about what is going on in Sweden and around the world, $r = .15$
- School, school work, and homework, $r = .16$
- Politics or societal issues, $r = .24$.

These correlations (although significant at the $p < .001$ level) show low agreement between how often adolescents and parents perceive that they talk about different topics at home. They do not differ between the two political topics and the other two everyday life topics. This is the first encounter with how adolescents and parents view their common political and non-political interactions. *Their perceptions are far from similar*. These findings are not unique to this study. Meta-studies in developmental psychology typically show that there are only small to modest associations between parents' and adolescents' reports of parenting behaviors and their joint affective and behavioral interactions (Hou et al., 2020; Korelitz & Garber, 2016) and adolescents' mental health (De Los Reyes et al., 2015). The lack of convergence will be a central research topic in this book. Korelitz and Garber's study of more than 400 comparisons of parenting behaviors and joint interactions also showed, as we found above, that adolescents' and parents' perceptions often show substantial differences in mean levels.

Finally, we need to understand whether adolescents and parents distinguish between talking about *everyday topics* and talking about *political topics*. For validation, adolescents were asked how often they talked with their parents about "Films, music, and TV shows," "Family activities," "School, school work, and homework," "Friends (what you do, etc.)," and "Relatives and friends of the family." This is what we call everyday topics. They also answered how often they talked with their parents about "What you have heard in the news about what is going on in Sweden and the world" and "Politics or social issues." This is what we call political discussions. Principal components analysis of the two political discussion items with the other five everyday life items yielded two factors that separated the political discussion items from the other items. The cross-loadings were small. Parents also reported how often they discussed "Family activities (doing things

TABLE 5.1 Principal component analyses of different types of conversations in the family, assuming a distinction between "everyday" and "political" conversations.

	Adolescent reports		*Parent reports*	
Conversations:	*Everyday*	*Political*	*Everyday*	*Political*
Films, music, and TV series	.57	.07	–	–
Your friends	.69	.10	–	–
Relatives and friends of the family	.71	.17	–	–
Family activities	.66	.26	.79	.12
School, school work, and homework	.65	.18	.81	.05
What you have heard on the news	.26	.82	.19	.83
Politics or society	.12	.88	−.01	.87

together)" and "School, schoolwork, and homework" using the same response scale. They also reported how often they talked about "What you have heard in the news about what is going on in Sweden and the world" and "Politics or social issues." Factor analysis revealed the same two distinguishing factors. The cross-loadings were small (see Table 5.1). It seems that both adolescents and parents make a clear distinction between political conversations and conversations about everyday life.

Are the Political Socialization Attempts of Parents More Important Than the Same Attempts of Other Important Persons?

We have examined various aspects of parents' and adolescents' joint political interactions. It is difficult to draw strong conclusions about the specific role of parents as political socializers of their adolescents from this information alone. We need to go beyond the information and ask the question, Is the role of parents as socializers similar to or different from the role of other people?

Two key questions we asked adolescents were, "My parents talk about things that happen in the world and in society in such a way that I become curious and want to know more" and "My parents tell me about the news they have heard on TV or read about in a way that evokes strong feelings in me." In the questionnaire, we used these two questions and replaced "parents" with "friends" and "teachers." For each of them, we aggregated the two questions. Now we have the opportunity to examine whether adolescents' susceptibility to political information from their parents is higher or lower than their susceptibility to political information from their friends and teachers.

Consider Figure 5.20. Adolescents reported being as susceptible to teachers as they were to parents. This susceptibility to political communication from teachers and parents was higher than for political communication from friends, with moderate effects (.52 and .59). It is interesting to note that susceptibility to significant

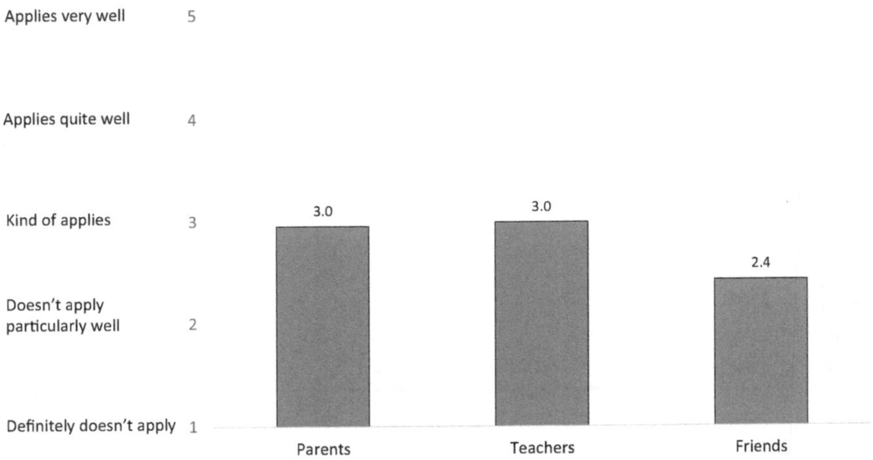

FIGURE 5.20 Adolescents' answers to questions about their receptiveness to political communication from parents, teachers, and friends.

adults was higher than susceptibility to friends. We will have more to say about this in a later chapter.

Comparing Political Interactions Between Parents and Friends

We will extend these analyses and systematically compare political interactions with parents and friends. In the questionnaire, we asked similar questions about friends as we did about parents. In Figure 5.21, we report the differences between parents and friends for six questions: about adolescents' knowledge of parents/friends' social views, whether parents/friends know a lot about what is going on in the world, and whether parents/friends try to make them more aware of what is going on in the world and of environmental issues. We also asked adolescents if they had encouraged their parents and friends to be more aware of environmental issues and what is going on in the world. All of the differences in Figure 5.21 are significant at the .001 level and in the same direction. Adolescents know more about their parents' views than about their friends' views, parents are seen as more knowledgeable than friends, and parents try to make adolescents more aware of what is going on in the world and of environmental issues than friends. The effect sizes are medium and large. Significant differences in the same direction, but with small effect sizes, also appear for the last two questions about whether adolescents try to influence their parents and friends. Overall, whether adolescents perceive their parents' and friends' knowledge and political influence, or their own attempts to make parents and peers more aware, these political interactions are stronger for their political interactions with parents than for these interactions with friends.

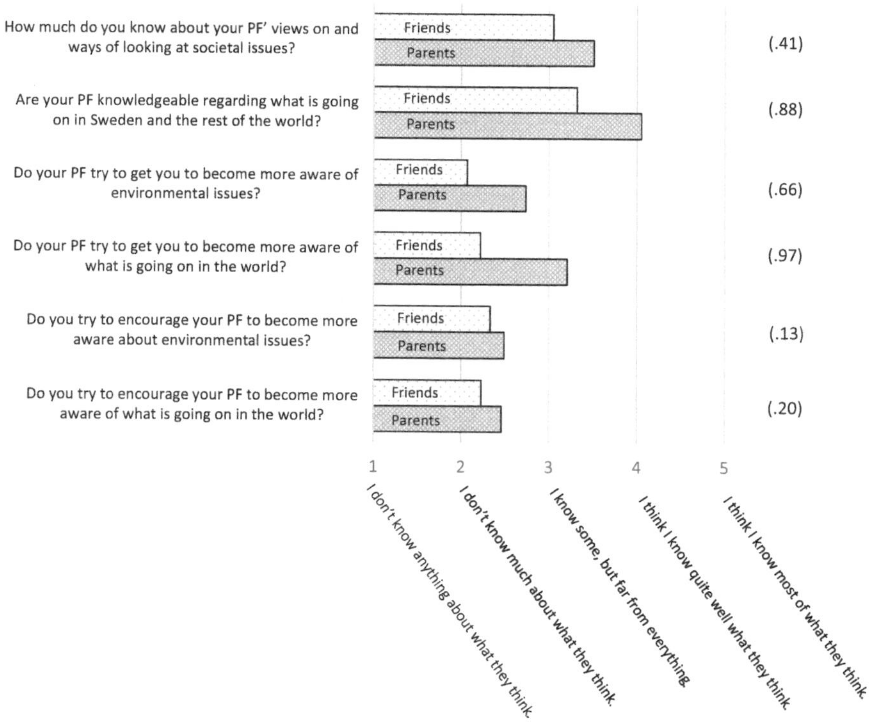

FIGURE 5.21 Comparing political interactions with parents and friends. Cohen's *d* is shown in parentheses.

In Figure 5.22 we use three of the 4-point scales that we have previously reported. We show differences in how interested and knowledgeable the adolescents' parents and friends are perceived to be, and whether the views of their parents and friends are important to them. Again, parents are perceived as more politically interested and knowledgeable than friends. The effect sizes for these two questions are large. Parents' views are also perceived as significantly more important than friends' views, but the effect size is small.

There is one exception to the general trend where there are no differences in what young people say about their parents and friends (Figure 5.23). This is the response to the question whether the young people and their parents (friends) have the same or different views and perspectives on social issues. About the same percentage of participants didn't know what their parents' and peers' views were, and among those who did know, there were no differences in the responses of having similar or different views. This suggests that adolescents perceive that both their parents and their friends have about the same political views as they do.

What do adolescents talk about with their friends that is different from what they talk about with their parents? Examples of topics that the young people talk about

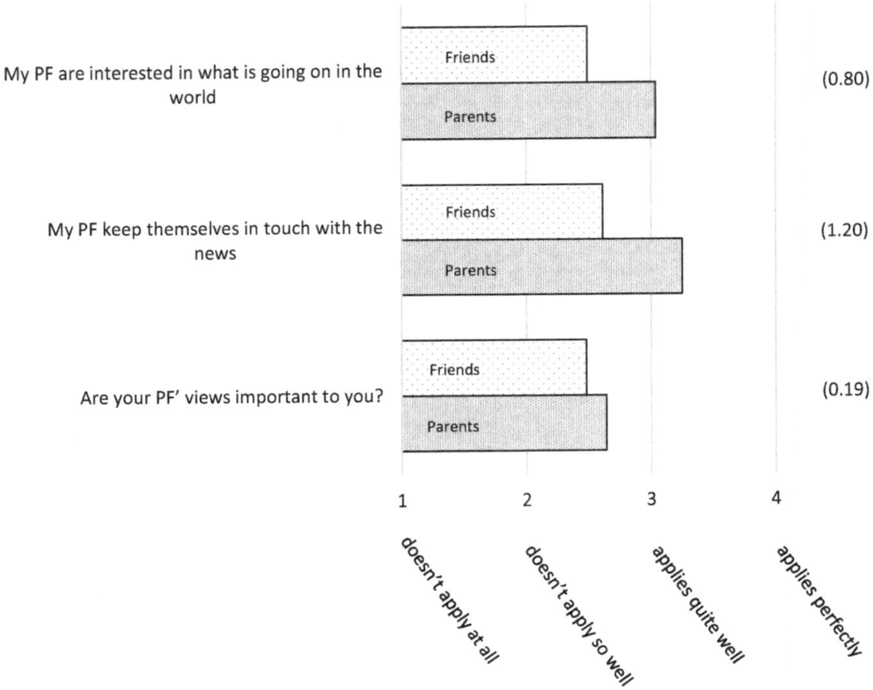

FIGURE 5.22 Comparing attention to news and perceived importance of views of parents and friends. Cohen's *d* is shown in parentheses.

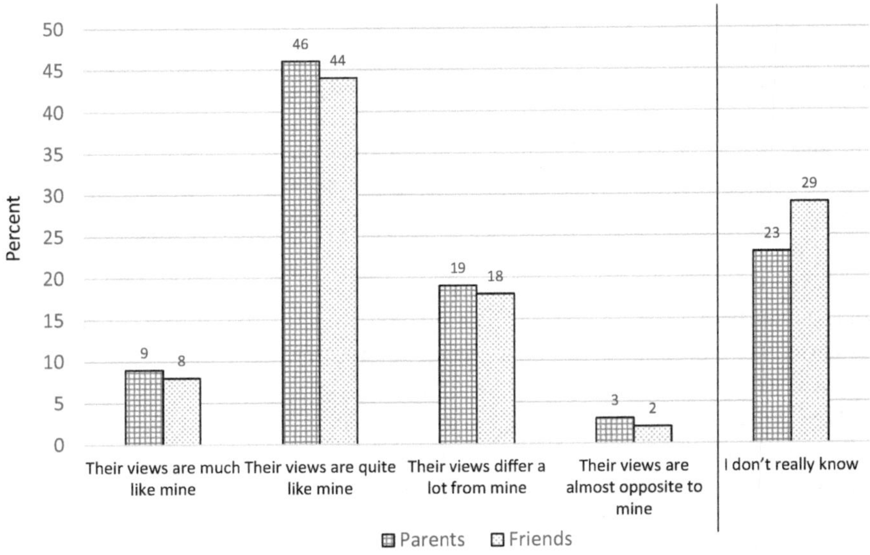

FIGURE 5.23 Adolescents' responses to the question "Do you and your parents (friends) hold the same or different views on and ways of looking at societal issues?"

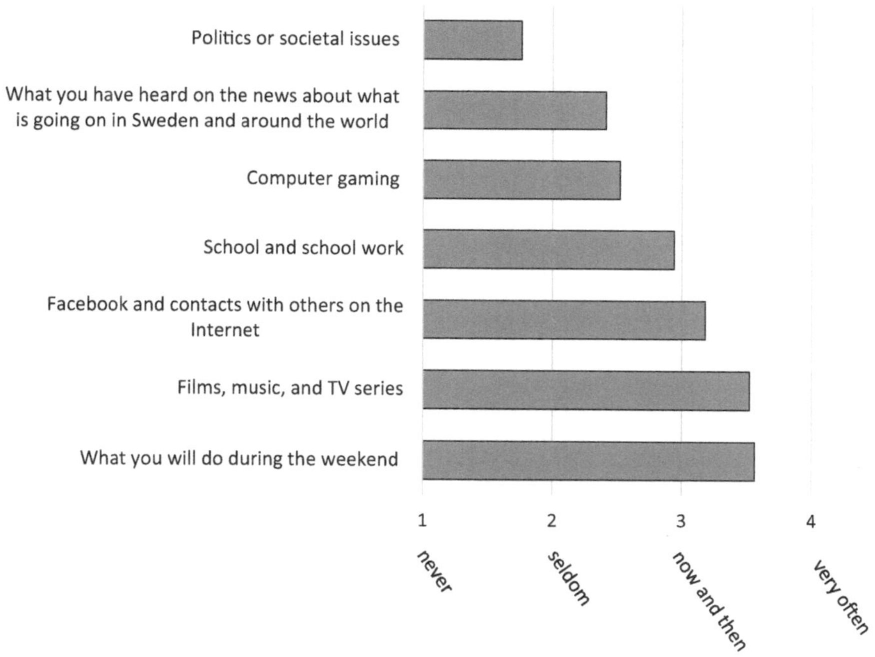

FIGURE 5.24 Adolescents' answers to the question "How often does it happen that you and your friends talk about these things?"

with their friends are shown in Figure 5.24. As can be seen in this figure, talking to friends about 'Politics and social issues' and 'What you have heard in the news about what is going on in Sweden and in the world' was not high on the agenda for the young people. These were the least reported topics discussed with peers in this figure. Talking about what one is going to do on the weekend, movies, music and TV series, and Facebook and contacts with others on the Internet were high on the list.

In Figure 5.25 we have compared the frequency of talking with friends about politics or social issues with the frequency of talking about what to do on the weekend. The distributions are almost opposite. A total of 19% of the young people stated that they sometimes or very often talk to their friends about politics or social issues, while 97% of the young people sometimes or very often talk to their friends about what they are going to do on the weekend.

Five of the topics can be compared between parents and friends. These are the three questions about social issues, the topic of school and schoolwork, and discussions about films, music, and TV series (see Figure 5.26). There are significant differences for all of these topics. Of the five topics, adolescents discussed films, music, and TV series more often with their friends than with their parents. The effect size was large. For the other topics, adolescents talked more with their parents than with their friends. The effect sizes were small, but medium for talking

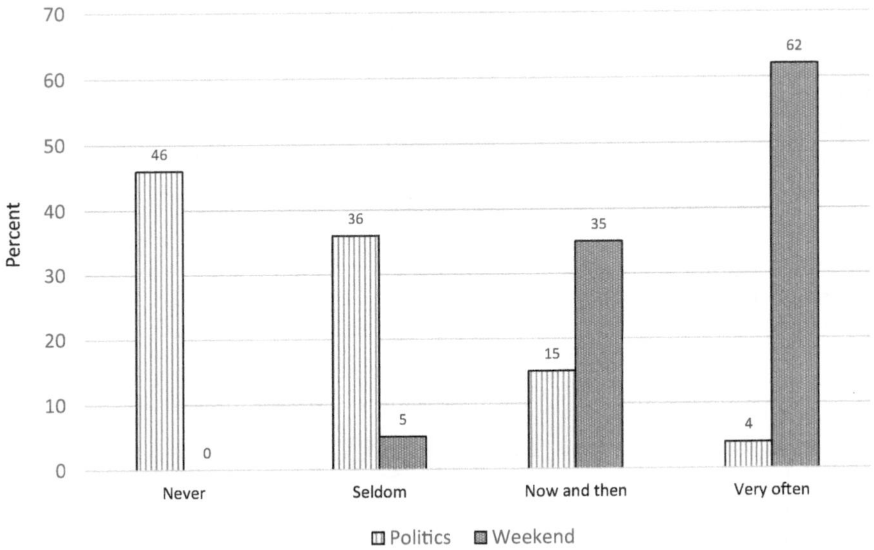

FIGURE 5.25 Adolescents' answers to the questions about how often it happens that you and your friends talk about *Politics or societal issues* and *What you will do during the weekend.*

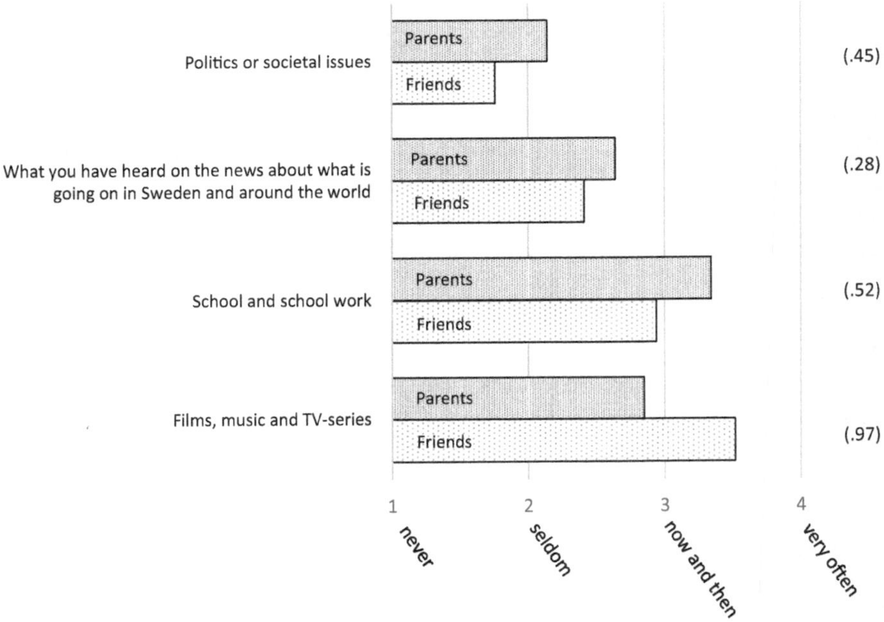

FIGURE 5.26 Adolescents' answers to the question "How often does it happen that you and your parents (friends) talk about these things?" Cohen's *d* is shown in parentheses.

about what they heard in the news. Four of the topics can be compared between parents and friends. These are the two questions about politicaö issues, the topic of school and schoolwork, and discussions about films, music, and TV series (see Figure 5.26). There are significant differences for all of these topics. Of the four topics, adolescents discussed films, music, and TV series more often with their friends than with their parents. The effect size was large. For the other topics, adolescents talked more with their parents than with their friends. The effect sizes were medium, but small for talking about what they heard in the news.

Conclusion

The take-home message is that although the frequency of conversations with parents about societal issues is not comparable in magnitude to conversations about everyday life issues, they are on the agenda in most adolescents' homes. It is therefore not surprising that adolescents report knowing their parents' political views.

From the descriptive findings reported in this chapter, we conclude that parents are the most important people for adolescents to talk to about politics, society, and the news. This does not mean that adolescents readily adopt their parents' political values and views. It appears that the family is seen as a safe training ground for political conversations (McDevitt, 2006).

Outside the family, adolescents show a susceptibility to political communication from their teachers—higher than the susceptibility to political communication from friends. When comparing the political interactions that adolescents have with parents and friends, the results show that parents are the most important political communication partners.

6

POLITICAL INTERACTIONS WITH PARENTS IN EARLY ADULTHOOD

Highlights

It has been commonly assumed that young adults have fewer political discussions with their parents than adolescents because young adults no longer live with their parents, transitional events in young adulthood (marriage and children) interfere with such discussions, and the emergence of new age-appropriate socializing agents, such as work colleagues, college peers, and romantic partners, replace parents as discussion partners. We propose a contrasting view that young adults' political interest is unaffected by these transitional events and changes in socializing agents, and that they have political discussions with parents as often as with alternative socializing agents in early adulthood.

- *In early adulthood, participants discussed political issues with their parents as frequently as with their friends, college peers, and colleagues, but less frequently than with their romantic partner.*
- *Cross-lagged models showed that political discussions with parents positively influenced political discussions with friends from early adolescence to early adulthood, and with colleagues and college peers in early adulthood. The opposite was true for romantic partners. Political discussions with romantic partners and friends in early adulthood fueled political discussions with parents.*
- *Transitional events in early adulthood, such as moving away from home, getting married, and having children, did not affect the frequency of political discussions with parents.*

Quite many studies have suggested that the role of parents as political socialization agents is particularly strong during adolescence, but declines thereafter (Pancer, 2015). Some of the arguments in the literature are as follows:

- During adolescence, parents and children live under the same roof. They have frequent interactions, and parents are the adults with whom children interact most on a daily basis. From a learning perspective, parents can engage their children in political learning through discussion and modeling during these years (Jennings & Niemi, 1974). Things change when children leave the family. There are fewer opportunities for daily political discussion: "[M]ost of these pre-adults are approaching the point at which they will leave the immediate

DOI: 10.4324/9781003371731-9

family. Further political training from the parents will be minimal" (Jennings & Niemi, 1968, p. 171).

- In addition to leaving home, other transitional events typically occur during young adulthood that can shift young people's attention away from discussing political issues with parents and toward more immediate experiences in their lives (e.g., Converse & Niemi, 1971; Jennings & Niemi, 1968; Stoker & Jennings, 1995), such as
    - getting married
    - having children
- Over time, the romantic partner, college peers, and work colleagues may be the people with whom young adults have the most regular political conversations (Dostie-Goulet, 2009; Lee et al., 2013; Vollebergh et al., 2001). They are the people with whom young adults are most likely to interact—not their parents.

In sum, by early adulthood, parents should no longer be considered the primary people young adults turn to for political discussion.

There are three observations that challenge this belief and instead suggest that young adults may discuss political issues with their parents more often than adolescents. First, this should be due to the increase in young people's own political interest from adolescence to young adulthood. Increased political interest is likely to be associated with more political discussions with others, including parents. Indeed, parents may be seen as "safe" partners with whom to discuss political issues during adolescence (Kiousis et al., 2005; McDevitt, 2006), and they may also be the right people for many young adults to discuss political issues with.

Few empirical studies have compared the frequency with which adolescents and young adults discuss politics with their parents. One (Hunter, 1985) examined samples of adolescents of different ages and also a group between the ages of 18 and 20 and reported that the group of young adults had more frequent political discussions with their parents than did the adolescents. Another study, by Rill and McKinney (2011), examined how often college students had political discussions with different socializing agents—parents, close friends, classmates, coworkers, and others—around the time of the 2008 U.S. presidential election. The young adults, ages 18 to 23, had discussions with their parents more often than with close friends, siblings, classmates, coworkers, and people in other relationships. These two studies suggest that parents remain one of the most important sources of political information for young adults.

Second, there is little empirical evidence that transitional events, such as moving away from home, getting married, and having children, substantially change the levels of political attitudes and behaviors of young adults. With one exception (Stoker & Jennings, 1995), studies of the effects of transitional events on young adults' political and civic attitudes and behaviors suggest that these transitional effects are small (Highton & Wolfinger, 2001; Neundorf et al., 2013; Voorpostel & Coffé, 2010).

Third, there is compelling evidence in the developmental literature that parents do not lose their role as communication partners in their children's early adulthood. Cross-sectional and longitudinal studies show that parents continue to play an important role in the lives of young adults (for reviews, see Collins et al., 2011; Galambos & Kotylak, 2011; Lefkowitz, 2005). The majority of young adults report having positive, harmonious, and supportive relationships with their parents (Aquilino, 1997; Masche, 2008; Rice & Mulkeen, 1995; Thornton et al., 1995). In fact, affective relationships between parents and young adults tend to improve rather than deteriorate as a result of adolescents leaving home or cohabiting/marrying (Galambos & Kotylak, 2011; Thornton et al., 1995). Leaving home, marrying, or cohabiting and entering the workforce appear to be associated with experiencing more, not less, parental support (Aquilino, 1997) and less conflict (Aseltine & Gore, 1993; Dubas & Petersen, 1996; Smetana et al., 2004). Taken together, these studies suggest that affective relationships between young adults and their parents should facilitate rather than hinder discussions with parents about society and the world. Still, we need to ask a specific question.

Do Parents Lose Their Role as Political Role Models in Early Adulthood?

In the previous chapter, two key features characterized adolescents' political interactions with their parents during adolescence:

- For most adolescents, parents were seen as knowledgeable, they were perceived as keeping up with the news, their political views were seen as important to adolescents, and parents' political views were seen as close to adolescents' views.
- Adolescents were open to their parents' attempts at political socialization. They were aware of their parents' attempts to influence them, and they were receptive to their parents' political communication.

Here, we will strategically select a few questions for the young adults that tap into parents as communication partners and their openness to parents' political socialization and compare them with the adolescents' reports.

Results

Do Other People Take Over Parents' Role?

In these early adulthood analyses, we will compare the frequency of political discussions with parents relative to political discussions with coworkers, college peers, and romantic partners. We used the first two data collections for each of the three early adulthood cohorts (ages 20, 24 and 26). We also included information on the frequency of political discussions with their friends from age 13 to age 28. The frequency of political discussions was measured by two items asking how often the participants and their conversation partners (parents, friends, college peers, work colleagues, romantic partner) discussed politics: "What you have heard on the news about what is going on in Sweden and around the world" and "Politics or societal issues." The response options ranged from 1 (*never*) to 4 (*very often*). An analysis of the overall developmental trends from early adolescence to early adulthood based on data for each individual age is presented in Figure 6.1.

As can be seen in this figure, participants discussed more with their parents than with their friends throughout adolescence. The largest differences occurred in early adolescence.

Young adults discussed politics most often with their romantic partners ($M = 3.08$, SD = 0.62). The difference compared to talking with parents ($M = 2.83$, SD = 0.67) yielded a Cohen's d of 0.36. The romantic partner is typically the person with whom young adults spend the most time and will be a conversation partner for many of them for a long time, and it is perhaps not surprising that the romantic partner was the most preferred person to discuss political and social issues with. In addition, participants talked with their friends ($M = 2.82$, SD = 0.66) and work colleagues ($M = 2.89$; SD = 0.67) as often as with their parents. Finally, they talked significantly less often with their college peers ($M = 2.32$, SD = 0.34) than with their parents. Cohen's d was 0.96. In short, at this early age of adulthood, parents are still one of the most important discussion partners on political issues. The

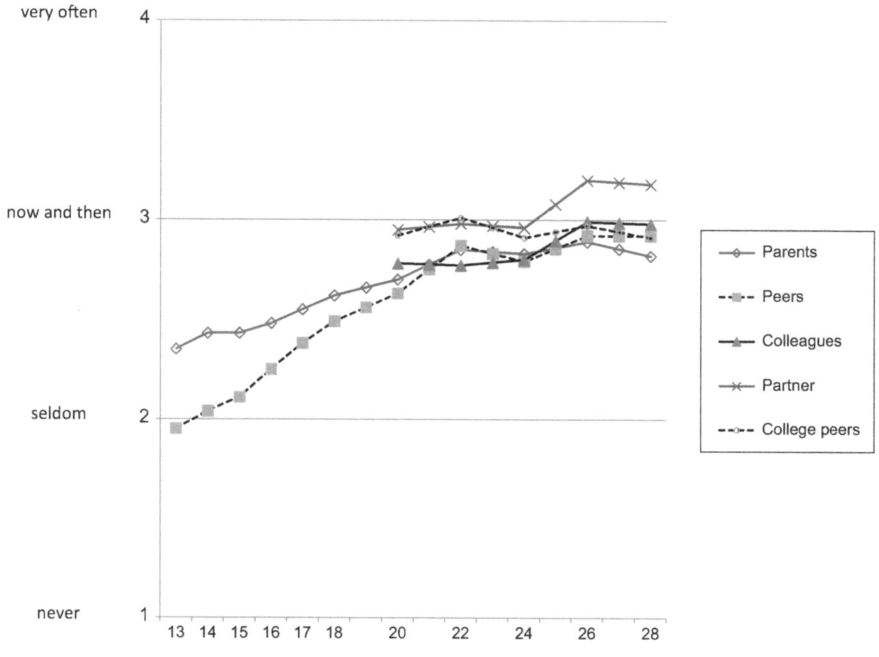

FIGURE 6.1 Trends in political discussion with different socializing agents.

frequency of political discussions with parents among our samples of adolescents and young adults did not decline over time. Thus, there is little support for the argument that young adults are having fewer political discussions with their parents and more with other people they see regularly.

If the political discussions that participants have with their friends, college peers, work colleagues, and romantic partners spur participants to discuss political issues with their parents, then we would observe a change over time in political discussions between adolescents and parents as a result of frequent political discussions with these alternative socialization agents. To examine this, a series of autoregressive cross-lagged (ARCL) models was tested for each discussion partner. These ARCL models provide two types of estimates: first, stability over time for a given discussion partner, and second, estimates of whether political discussions with alternative socializing agents predict future political discussions with parents, and vice versa. In these analyses, we used three control variables: immigrant status—parents born outside the Nordic countries (1) versus other parents (0), gender (0 = male, 1 = female), and feelings of belonging to society (after the question "How well do the following statements describe you?" Participants reported whether they felt at home with "Sweden as a country," "the municipality where I live," and "the neighborhood where I live." The response scale ranged from 1 (*doesn't apply at all*) to 4 (*applies perfectly*).

Spillover Effects of Political Discussions

Figure 6.2 shows this ARCL model for the association between political discussion with parents and friends over time. In this analysis, we examined changes over 2 years, using waves 1 and 3 from the two younger cohorts, and waves 1 and 2 from the three older cohorts.

Do political discussions with friends spill over into political discussions with parents, or is it the other way around? First, as shown in Figure 6.2, the stability of political discussions over 2 years for the five cohorts was higher for discussions with parents than for discussions with friends. This should not come as a surprise, as we can expect the people that participants consider their friends to change over time. Next, for all five two-year intervals, having political discussions with parents positively influenced having political discussions with friends. Having political discussions with friends, on the other hand, showed a more substantial effect on having political discussions with parents only for the three oldest age cohorts. For the second cohort, ages 16 to 18, the path from political discussions with parents at T1 to political discussions with friends at T2 was significantly larger than the opposite path. In short, participants' experiences from their political discussions with parents spill over into their political discussions with friends, but not much in the opposite direction, except in early adulthood. This is consistent with the suggestion in the literature that political discussions in the family lay the groundwork for such discussions in contexts outside the family (Kiousis et al., 2005; McDevitt, 2006).

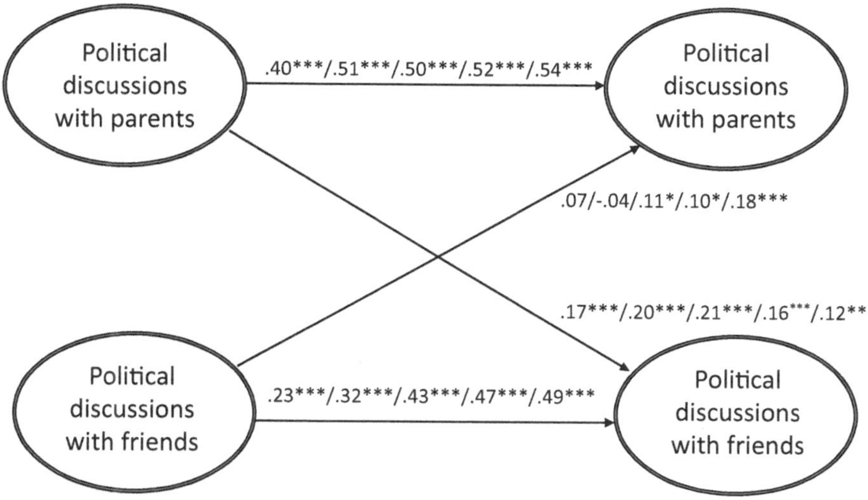

FIGURE 6.2 Longitudinal relationships between political discussion with parents and friends. For each estimate, results are reported using waves 1 and 3 from the two younger cohorts, and waves 1 and 2 from the three older cohorts (ages 13 to 15; ages 16 to 18; ages 20 to 22; ages 22 to 24; ages 26 to 28).

Note that all estimates in Figure 6.2 are positive, indicating that the more participants discussed politics with their parents, the more they discussed politics with their friends. In short, political discussions with parents spill over into political discussions with friends. They help rather than hinder the participants' discussions with their friends. The opposite is also true. Political discussions with friends, especially in early adulthood, are positive for political discussions with parents.

Little, if anything, is known about the spillover effects between political discussions with parents in early adulthood and political discussions with college peers, work colleagues, and romantic partners. We used information from the first and second waves in the three oldest cohorts (ages 20 to 22; ages 22 to 24; ages 26 to 28). The ARCL models are shown in Figure 6.3.

As can be seen in this figure, the more often young adults discussed politics with their parents, generally the more often they discussed political issues with their work colleagues and college peers. With one exception (discussions with college peers between the ages of 22 and 24), the frequency of political discussions with work colleagues and college peers did not lead to more frequent political discussions with parents. The findings suggest that discussions with parents spill over into more frequent political discussions with work colleagues and college peers.

There is one exception. As shown in Figure 6.3(c), political discussions with parents did little to facilitate political discussions with young adults' romantic partners. In fact, the opposite seems to be true. The more 20- and 22-year-olds

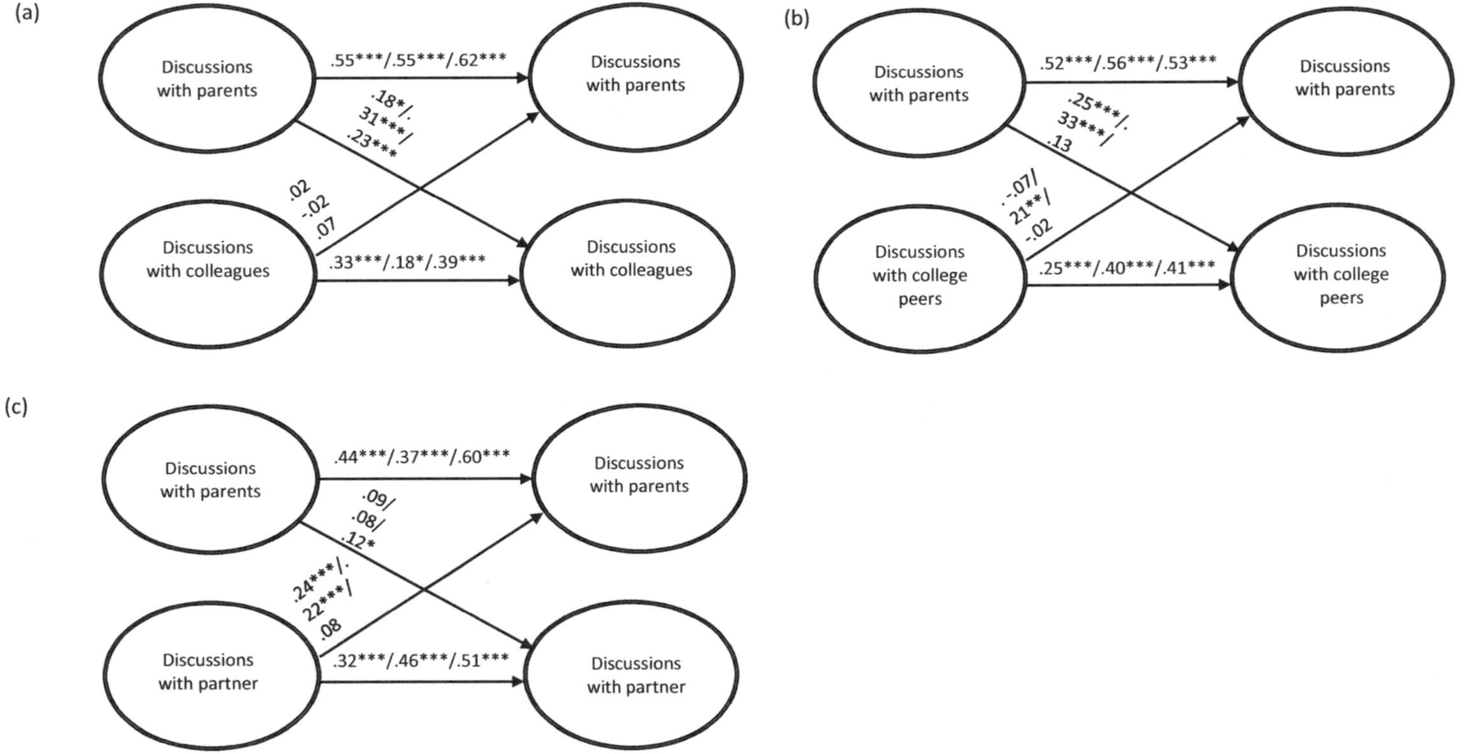

FIGURE 6.3 Longitudinal relationships between political discussion with parents and (a) coworkers, (b) college peers and (c) the romantic partner in early adulthood. For each estimate, results are reported sequentially from waves 1 and 2 for each of cohorts 3 through 5 (20 to 22; 22 to 24; 26 to 28).

discussed political issues with their romantic partners, the more often they discussed politics with their parents. Recall above that of all the socialization agents in early adulthood, young adults discussed political issues most often with their romantic partners. This is the first strong evidence that another socialization agent influences political discussions with parents. It should also be noted that the stability of political discussions over time was generally somewhat higher for romantic partners than for work colleagues and college peers.

The Role of Transitional Events

Do transitional events in young adulthood destabilize political discussions with parents? We looked at three types of transition experiences:

- Move away from home—Have you moved away from home? 1 (*no*), 2 (*yes*)
- Relational status—1 (*married/cohabitating*), 2 (*have a partner in a separate residence*), 3 (*single*)
- Having own children—Do you have children of your own? 1 (*no*), 2 (*yes*)

We examined all possible combinations of *moving from home* for each of the three early adult cohorts (Home to Home, Home to Away, Away to Away, Away to Home), *having a child* (None to None, None to Child, Child to Child), and *marriage* (Single to Single, Single to Marriage, Marriage to Marriage, Marriage to Single). A mixed ANOVA showed that the interaction between time and group membership was not significant for two of the three transition measures: leaving home and having a child (see Table 6.1). However, the interaction was significant for marriage. For this reason, paired sample tests were conducted for each subgroup. An increase over two years in political discussions with parents was significant for continuously married participants. Overall, transitional events such as moving away from home, having a child, and getting married do not seem to change the frequency of political discussions with parents. Perhaps this is to be expected. Parents have experiences in these areas that are now increasingly relevant to young people.

Do Adolescents and Young Adults Perceive Political Interactions With Their Parents Differently?

Do young adults perceive political interactions with their parents as similar to or different from those of adolescents? We asked the young adults a few core questions about their experience of these political interactions. These were questions that the adolescents had also reported on.

The adolescent sample was the 13- and 16-year-olds in cohorts 1 and 2. The young adult sample was the 20- and 26-year-olds in cohorts 3 and 5 (about 1,750 adolescents and 1,200 young adults). No significant differences were found between the two young adult cohorts on any of the study variables reported here.

TABLE 6.1 Results from mixed ANOVAs.

Experience type	*Group membership*	*M(SD)* at T_1	*M(SD)* at T_2	*Mixed ANOVA*[a]	*Post-hoc*[b]
Moving away	Home and Home ($n = 128$)	2.77 (.74)	2.79 (.76)		–
	Home and Away ($n = 162$)	2.87 (.67)	2.80 (.67)	$F(3, 1723) = 1.60$	
	Away and Away ($n = 1405$)	2.86 (.66)	2.89 (.66)	$p = .19, = .00$	
	Away and Home ($n = 32$)	2.88 (.71)	3.00 (.62)		
Having a child	None and None ($n = 1433$)	2.87 (.67)	2.88 (.67)		–
	None and Child ($n = 147$)	2.77 (.65)	2.85 (.61)	$F(2, 1727) = 1.46$	
	Child and Child ($n = 150$)	2.75 (.70)	2.82 (.73)	$p = .23, \eta_p^2 = .00$	
Marriage	Single and Single ($n = 720$)	2.89 (.70)	2.91 (.71)		$t(719) = -0.87, p = .39, d = .03$
	Single and Marriage ($n = 308$)	2.88 (.66)	2.82 (.62)	$F(3, 1734) = 2.88$	$t(307) = 1.88, p = .06, d = .10$
	Marriage and Marriage ($n = 588$)	2.81 (.64)	2.86 (.63)	$p < .05, \eta_p^2 = .01$	$t(587) = -1.99, p < .05, d = .08$
	Marriage and Single ($n = 122$)	2.76 (.64)	2.84 (.67)		$t(121) = -1.26, p = .33, d = .12$

Note: In the analyses, data from waves 1 and 2 were entered as T1 and T2 among cohorts 3 to 5. Regarding cohort 4, data from waves 2 and 3 were also entered as T1 and T2.

[a] The presented results concern the interaction between group membership and political discussion with parents over time.

[b] Dependent *t*-test.

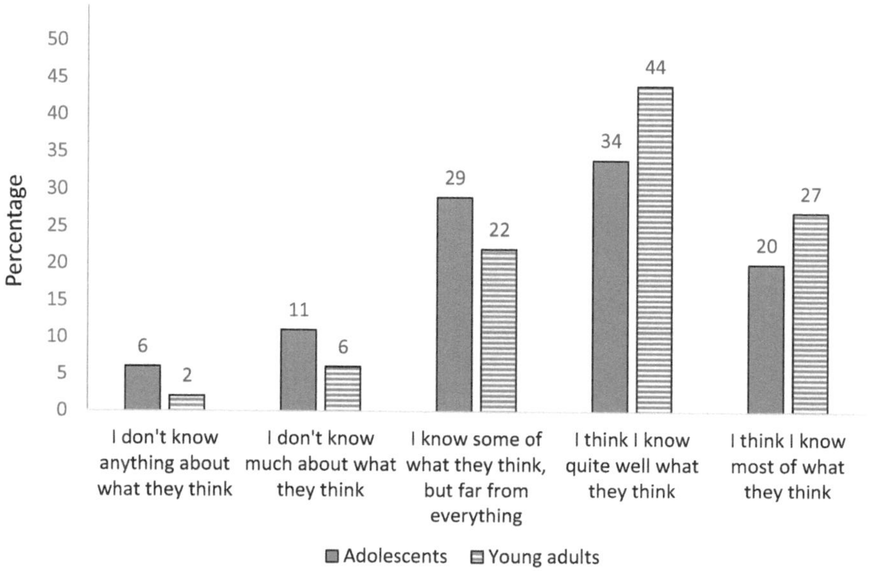

FIGURE 6.4 Adolescents' and young adults' responses to the question "How much do you know about your parents' views on and ways of looking at societal issues?" Cohen's *d* is 0.34.

When asked how much they knew about their parents' views on and ways of looking at societal issues (Figure 6.4), significantly more young adults thought they knew than adolescents. More than 50% of adolescents and more than 70% of young adults said they knew quite well or very well what their parents thought about social issues. The Cohen's *d* for this difference was high, 1.04. When asked whether their parents knew what was going on in Sweden and the rest of the world (Figure 6.5), there were no significant differences between the adolescent and young adult samples. About 8 out of 10 reported that their parents had quite or very good knowledge. Participants were asked whether their parents' views and perspectives on social issues were important to them (Figure 6.6). Slightly more young adults than adolescents reported that their parents' views were important to them. Cohen's *d* was 0.13. Approximately 6 out of 10 participants answered yes, in part, or yes, very much to this question.

Participants were asked whether they and their parents had similar or different views and perspectives on social issues (Figure 6.7). Twenty-three percent of adolescents but only 11% of young adults said they did not know whether they and their parents had similar or different views (a Cohen's *d* of 0.13 for the dichotomy between not knowing and knowing). Slightly more young adults perceived their parents' views as similar to their own than did adolescents (71 vs. 55%). The Cohen's *d* for this difference was 0.13. Finally, young adults were more likely

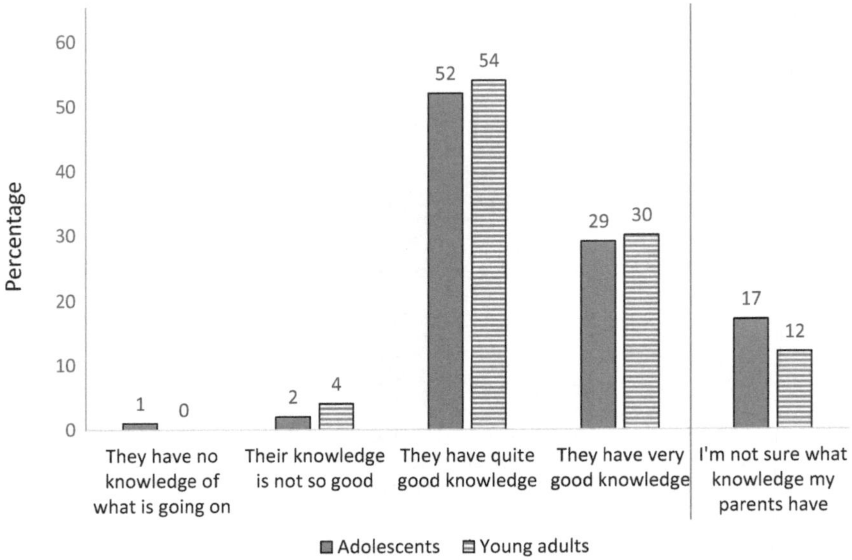

FIGURE 6.5 Adolescents' and young adults' answer to the question "Are your parents knowledgeable regarding what is going on in Sweden and the rest of the world?" Cohen's *d* is 0.05.

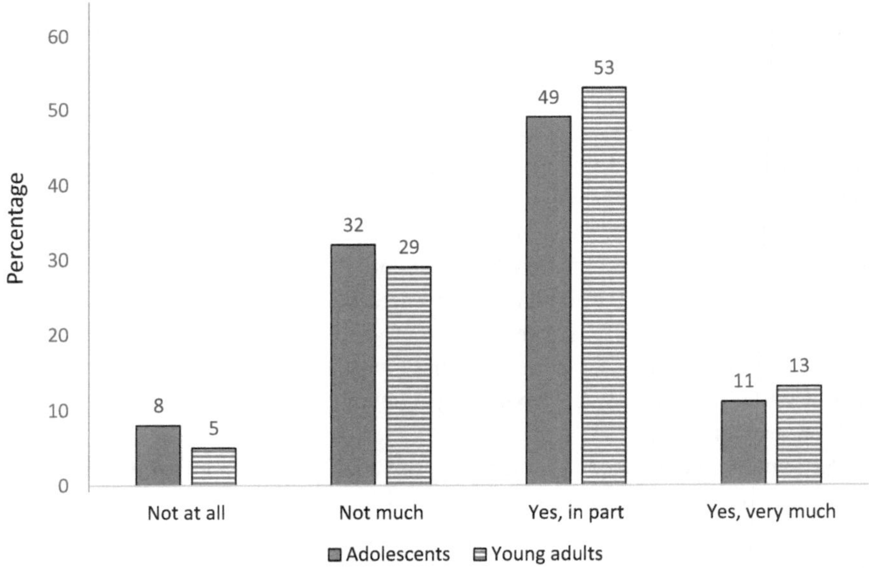

FIGURE 6.6 Adolescents' and young adults' answer to the question "Are your parents' views on and ways of looking at societal issues important to you?" Cohen's *d* is 0.13.

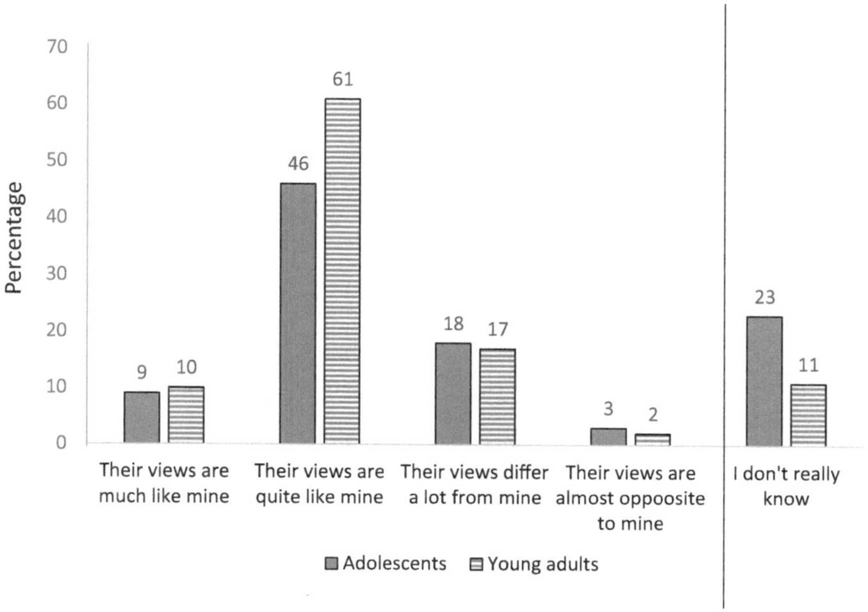

FIGURE 6.7 Adolescents' and young adults' response to the question "Do you and your parents have similar or different views and perspectives on social issues?

than adolescents to say that they and their parents often talked about what was going on in Sweden and the world (Figure 6.8) and about politics and social issues (Figure 6.9). The Cohen's *d*s for these two questions were high, 0.91 and 1.02, respectively.

To summarize these comparisons, it appears that both adolescents and young adults have positive views of their political interactions with their parents. Most know what their parents think about social issues, most see their parents as knowledgeable, most perceive that their parents' views are important to them, and most perceive that they and their parents have similar views (subsequently, few adolescents and young adults think they have different views from their parents). Young adults report slightly higher levels of agreement than adolescents on these issues. More than 8 in 10 young adults talk with their parents now and then or very often about what is going on in the world. The same is true for 6 in 10 adolescents. When asked if they talk about politics or society, 68% of young adults and 43% of adolescents say they talk about these topics now and then or very often. Overall, if we can consider parents as role models for adolescents, this characterization seems even more true for young adults.

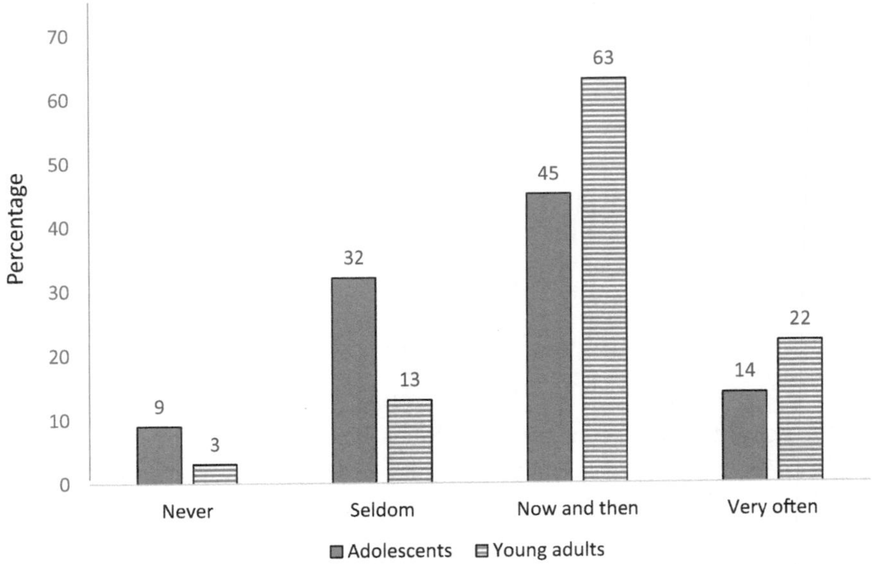

FIGURE 6.8 Adolescents' and young adults' responses to the question, "How often does it happen that you and your parents talk about what you have heard on the news about what is going on in Sweden and around the world?" Cohen's *d* is 0.91.

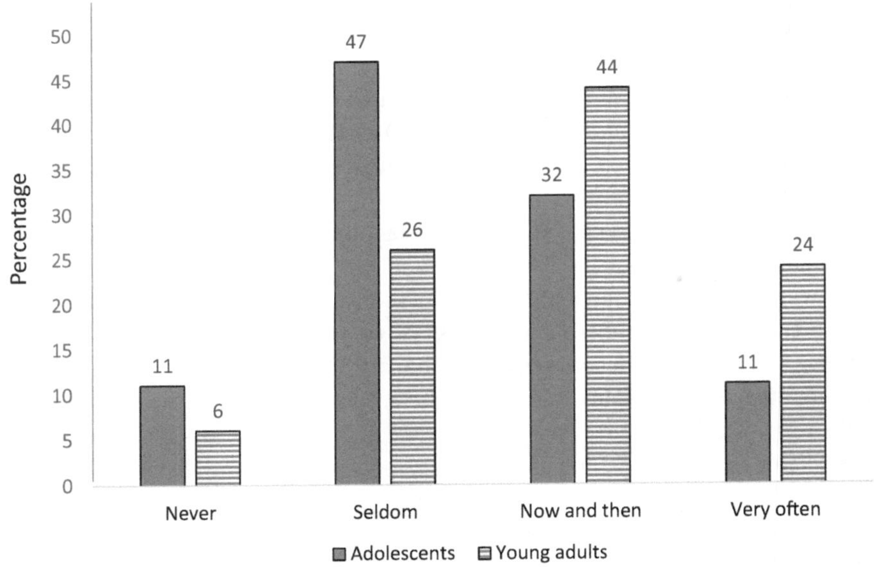

FIGURE 6.9 Adolescents' and young adults' responses to the question "How often does it happen that you and your parents talk about politics or societal issues?" Cohen's *d* is 1.02.

Discussion

Contrary to the popular belief that young people discuss political issues with their parents less after adolescence, this chapter provides empirical evidence that they discuss politics with their parents more often in young adulthood than in adolescence. If social learning is at work, it is difficult to explain why young adults who have moved away from home and do not have daily interactions have more political interactions with their parents than adolescents. This is likely due to the fact that young people's own political interest increases from adolescence to young adulthood. Moreover, they discuss politics with their parents significantly more often than with their friends in adolescence. In early adulthood, they are just as likely to discuss politics with their parents as with their friends.

Physical proximity is not necessary to have political discussions with parents. We draw this conclusion both from finding an increasing trend from early adolescence to early adulthood in the frequency of political discussions between parents and young people and from a more rigorous examination of the differences between young adults who were still living in their parents' homes and those who had moved out. Other potential threats to the increase in political discussion with parents are changes in relationship status and having children. We did not find much evidence that these transitional experiences had an impact on political discussion with parents.

College peers or coworkers do not take over as the primary discussion partners for political issues in early adulthood. But the romantic partner is the person with whom young adults prefer to have the most political discussions.

Our findings suggest that young adults engage in political discussions with all socializing agents over time, rather than substituting one agent for another. If young adults were replacing their parents as political discussion partners with their coworkers, college peers, and romantic partners, then we would expect the ARCL models to yield negative coefficients, indicating that engaging in political discussions with coworkers, college classmates, and romantic partners over time lead to a decrease in such discussions with their parents. This was not found. Young adults do not substitute other people for political discussions with parents in early adulthood. In general, political discussions with parents positively spill over into political discussions with friends, and in early adulthood there is also an effect in the opposite direction. Political discussions also spill over into political discussions with college peers and coworkers. But—and this is a key finding—political discussions with parents do not spill over into political discussions with romantic partners. The opposite is true.

The brief conclusion of the findings reported in this chapter is that transition events or newcomers to daily life do not prevent young adults from having political discussions with their parents. The findings are consistent with those of the few studies of political discussions with parents among adolescents of different ages and among young adults (Hunter, 1985; Rill & McKinney, 2011). The frequency of political discussions between young adults and their parents appears to depend more on the perception of the family as a safe zone for sharing political experiences than on their physical distance or other transitional events.

Finally, comparisons of key measures of family political communication between adolescents and early adults show that similar proportions of adolescents and early adults believe that their parents have a good knowledge of what is going on, that their parents' views are important, and that they have similar political views. More early adults than adolescents consider themselves knowledgeable about their parents' political views.

7

DIRECTION OF EFFECTS AND CONGRUENCE BETWEEN ADOLESCENTS' AND PARENTS' VIEWS

Highlights

- *A common assumption in political socialization research is that parents transmit their political attitudes and values to their offspring. Their views become the views of their children. This is a shaky assumption unless it can be shown that parents' political values and attitudes are closely linked to the same attitudes and values in their children. Reliance on cross-sectional surveys is of little help in confirming this assumption. This study finds bidirectional, not unidirectional, relationships from ages 13 to 28.*
- *Consistent with research from the 1960s and 1970s, we show that parents' political attitudes and values and perceptions of political interactions with their adolescents do not match adolescents' attitudes and values and perceptions of joint political interactions with their parents.*
- *There is a need to understand the mechanisms that govern adolescents' perceptions of their political interactions with others and the mechanisms that govern parents' perceptions of the same interactions. This is because adolescents and parents seem to live in different perceptual worlds when it comes to their views of political attitudes, values, and joint political interactions.*

A common assumption in the field of political socialization is that parents shape the political development of their adolescents. They transmit their political ideas, attitudes, and values to their offspring, and these views become the views of their children. This one-sided view of parent-adolescent political interactions is found in most journal articles, books, and textbooks in the field of political socialization. With few exceptions, the reader of this literature will encounter study after study claiming that there is ample support for a strong intergenerational transfer of worldviews, attitudes, and values from parents to children. Consistent with this view, the previous chapter suggested that adolescents—as well as young adults—are receptive to their parents' views in discussions of political issues at home. It is time to examine the evidence that parents shape their children's political development.

DOI: 10.4324/9781003371731-10

Three Influential Studies

Let us look at three studies in the literature that have examined the role that parent-adolescent discussions about politics plays in adolescent political development. We have chosen these studies because they are fairly representative of the research designs that have been used, and because these studies are highly cited and, as such, have had a strong influence on how researchers have tended to view the consequences of political discussions with parents for adolescents' political attitudes and values.

The first study is based on a national sample of 1,500 young people between the ages of 15 and 25 who, in the aftermath of September 11, reported on many different aspects of their political attitudes and involvement, ranging from local civic participation to national politics (Lake Snell Perry and Associates, 2002). Of particular strength were the findings that frequent political discussions with parents were associated with a range of political attitudes and behaviors—that is, higher levels of political activity, knowledge of and attention to political news, stronger beliefs that political leaders pay attention to young people's concerns, higher levels of trust in government, higher levels of importance placed on voting and volunteering, and higher levels of internal political self-efficacy. In this study, parent-adolescent political discussion was considered a parenting behavior: "This data, like so many studies before, point to the significance of parents' political behaviors is shaping the attitudes and engagement level of young adults" (p. 7). This is a cross-sectional study. The authors cannot say much about how parents shape the political attitudes and behaviors of their youth.

There are other, equally well-cited studies that have provided information about the importance of parents as political role models through discussions with their adolescents, particularly for voting behavior. One study by Andolina et al. (2003) was a retrospective study of two samples of more than 1,000 adolescents and young adults, ages 15 to 25, who were representative of the national population in several ways. The young adults were asked to report retrospectively on their high school experiences. Compared to participants who reported low frequency of political discussion at home, those who reported high frequency were significantly more likely to report voting and to vote regularly. There are two problems with this study. The first is that it mainly reports results that are consistent with the authors' predictions. Second, a retrospective design is rarely a researcher's first choice because it is extremely difficult to interpret. Among other things, people tend to believe that how they think, feel, act, and relate to other people in the present is what they perceive they did in the past. The opposite is also true. The activities people believe they will engage in in the future tend to be among the activities they already engage in or aspire to engage in. Ignoring these limitations, in this study, as in the first, political discussions at home were seen as a training ground for the young people's parents: "By talking about politics, families teach their children that it is important to pay attention to the world around them—and to take the next step of doing something"—voting (p. 277).

The third is a study by McIntosh et al. (2007). This is a study of what parental characteristics influence their political discussions with their adolescents so that the adolescents become more politically knowledgeable and civically competent (e.g., news monitoring, political knowledge, engagement in public communication, and community service). This is a two-step idea. First, it assumes that parental characteristics (most importantly, parents' civic experiences) influence the frequency with which parents engage in political discussions with their adolescents. Second, it assumes that these discussions make adolescents more politically and civically active. The authors are upfront about the direction of causality. It is stated in the title—"The influence of family political discussion on youth civic development: Which parent qualities matter?" Despite the clear idea that causality runs from parents to their children, this study had a cross-sectional design and has little to say about how parents influence adolescents' civic development over time. The authors used a 1996 National Household Education Survey. This survey cannot say much about causality, nor can it say much about the consequences for adolescents' civic development over time.

What is unique about the McIntosh et al. (2007) study is that the authors also used parental reports. Parents did not report how often they discussed political issues with their adolescents (this was based on adolescents' reports), but they did report on a number of other issues, such as socioeconomic conditions (ethnicity, income, education) and a number of measures of their civic behavior as well as civic skills, knowledge, and attitudes. Did parents' civic experiences affect the frequency of political discussions they had with their adolescents? This is the first of two questions that should have been asked in the proposed two-stage model. It was not reported. Therefore, we do not know the extent to which parents' civic experiences and demographic characteristics affect the frequency of political discussions as perceived by adolescents.

Next, when the authors controlled for how often adolescents perceived that discussions about political issues occur with their parents in predicting adolescents' news monitoring, public communication, and community service, information about parents' reports of sociodemographic conditions and civic behavior did not add much predictive power. Adolescents' reports of family political discussions were the best explanation for three of the four dependent measures. The authors concluded that the act of discussing politics with their parents influenced adolescents' news monitoring, public communication, and community service: "parents who take the time to talk with their adolescent children about the public affairs of the day may have a positive influence on the civic development of these adolescents" (p. 498). Note that parents' reports of their civic experiences did not add much information in predicting adolescents' reports of their political knowledge and civic experiences after controlling for adolescents' reports of their political discussions with their parents—so no new information was provided about how family discussions are related to parents' civic experiences.

In sum, these three studies share the same assumption: Parents shape their adolescents' political development. This may be true, but these three studies share two fundamental limitations.

Reliance on Cross-Sectional Designs

Perhaps the strongest evidence that parents are successful in shaping their children's political development through political discussions at home concerns young people's political interest. Correlations between adolescents' perceptions of the frequency of political discussions with their parents and their own political interest are sometimes in the range of 0.40 to 0.50 in different studies, which can be considered substantial (Koskimaa & Rapeli, 2015; Oswald & Schmid, 1998; Schmid, 2012; Warner & Warner Colander, 2016). Although these studies were cross-sectional, the authors interpreted the strong associations as solid evidence that when parents initiate political discussions in the home, it influences adolescents' political interest.

It is possible to change the dependent variable and come to the exact opposite conclusion. This is what Levinsen and Yndigegn (2015) did when they wanted to understand whether having different opinions from one's parents negatively affected the likelihood of having political discussions with one's parents. They found that adolescents who reported that their mothers and fathers held attitudes different from their own were less likely than other adolescents to discuss political issues with their parents. Their regression analyses included a measure of adolescents' political interest among many other potential predictors. Of all the variables measured, adolescents' political interest was by far the most important predictor of having political discussions with their fathers and mothers. Here, adolescents' political interest predicted their perceptions of how often they had political discussions with their parents.

A problem with the socialization perspective in political socialization research is that many findings are based on cross-sectional designs. Different developmental conditions have been hypothesized to produce high levels of political interest. Abstracts, introductions, and discussions of these studies contain words like "impact," "influence," "determine," and "increase," even though cross-sectional designs cannot establish causality. Sometimes causality is found in the titles of these studies: "Habits from Home, Lessons from School: Influences on Youth Civic Engagement" and "Democracy Begins at Home: Democratic Parenting and Youth Support for Democratic Values." It may seem odd to assume causality in cross-sectional designs, and odd that reviewers did not raise doubts about it. Historically, however, social learning models have dominated political socialization theory (Jennings & Niemi, 1974; Niemi & Hepburn, 1995; Jennings et al., 2009). These learning models provide explanations for how external conditions are transformed into young people's political interest and engagement.

Longitudinal studies are needed to answer the question of what affects what over time. Unfortunately, such longitudinal studies are rare. Two of them built the hypothesized direction of causality into their studies by using adolescents' political interest as the dependent variable (Dostie-Goulet, 2009; Shehata & Amnå, 2017). Both studies confirmed that parents influence their adolescents' political interest through political discussions at home. Shehata and Amnå's (2017) study examined both political conversations with parents and peers in a model that also included adolescents' news media use. The study found a significant association between political conversations with parents at age 14 and adolescents' political interest two years later. The model overestimated the effect of political discussion, though, because the researchers controlled for political interest one year earlier, at age 13, at a time when political interest has not yet crystallized. To predict adolescents' political interest, Dostie-Goulet (2009) compared political discussions with parents and friends, and the study also included discussions with teachers about political issues. Analyses over one year that predicted changes in political interest over one year—from ages 14 and 15 to 15 and 16 and from ages 15 and 16 to 16 and 17—showed that discussions with parents in particular were significant predictors of changes in political interest over time at the .05 level.

So there are at least two studies in the literature that have confirmed longitudinally that having political discussions with parents affects changes in adolescents' political interest. But this is a one-sided view. What is needed are studies that simultaneously examine how the two are related over time.

Are joint political discussions and adolescents' political interest unidirectionally linked? In the previous chapter, we found that young people's perceptions of having political discussions with their parents increased with age—from age 13 to early adulthood. Because of the increasing political interest of adolescents and young adults as they age, which we reported in Chapter 1, we might expect that young people's increasing political interest would facilitate their engagement in political discussions with their parents. Alternatively, in line with the intergenerational transmission view, we would expect that the political discussions young people have with their parents would spur their political interest, perhaps over the entire age span covered in our study, from ages 13 to 28. We tested these predictions.

Political interest was measured using two items: "How interested are you in what is going on in society?" and "How interested are you in politics?" The response options for both items ranged from 1 (*totally uninterested*) to 5 (*very interested*).

Political discussion with parents was measured by two questions asking adolescents how often they and their parents discussed politics: "What you have heard on the news about what is going on in Sweden and around the world" and "Politics or societal issues." The response options ranged from 1 (*never*) to 4 (*very often*). The adolescents' sex, immigrant background, and feelings of belonging to the society were control variables.

We used an autoregressive cross-lagged (ARCL) model to test how much one variable—interest or discussion—contributed to the change in the other over time, and vice versa. At the first assessment, participants in the five age cohorts were 13, 16, 20, 22, 24, and 26 years old. We included a two-year window for each cohort to cover ages 13–28 (C1: ages 13–15; C2: ages 16–18; C3: ages 20–22; C4: ages 24–26; C5: ages 26–28). As shown in Figure 7.1, there is evidence that political interest and political discussion are bidirectionally related. Political discussion produced significant changes in political interest, especially in the early age cohorts (ages 13–15, 16–18, but also 20–22). In contrast, political interest produced significant changes in political discussion in early adulthood (ages 20–22, 24–26, 26–28), but also in early to middle adolescence (ages 13–15). The bidirectional effects in the ARCL models were positive and significant in 7 out of 10 cases. Political discussions with parents and political interest are mutually reinforcing. The magnitudes of the bidirectional effects were compared. None were significantly different. The results suggest that political discussion and political interest are bidirectionally related. Preliminarily, the results seem to indicate that political discussions with parents affect young people's political interest primarily in adolescence, while young people's political interest affects political discussions with parents primarily in early adulthood when their relationships are more egalitarian.

The longitudinal links between political interest and political discussion do not appear to be solely parent-to-youth driven. They cannot be interpreted exclusively as consequences of intergenerational transmission or as an effect of parents' actions on adolescents and young adults. Political interest and political discussion shape each other over time. The finding of bidirectional relations between political discussion in the family and young people's political interest in this longitudinal design show that correlations in a cross-sectional study between political interest

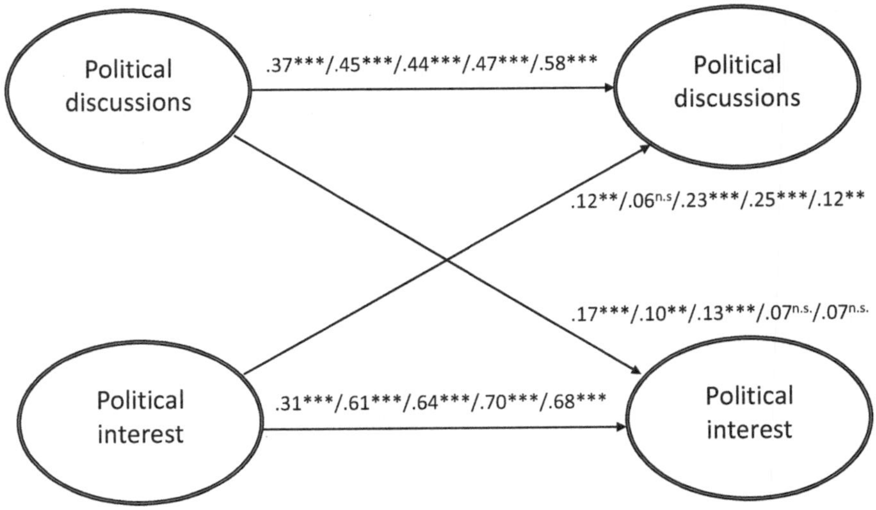

FIGURE 7.1 Longitudinal relationships between political discussions with parents and political interest among adolescents (ages 13–15, 16–18, 20–22, 24–26, and 26–28).

and political discussion at home cannot automatically be translated into an effect of parents' political socialization attempts on political interest.

We do not disagree with the notion that parents can contribute to the development of adolescents' political opinions by acknowledging, encouraging, and challenging their ideas and sharpening their arguments. Parents can be attentive listeners and responders to adolescents' political initiatives. In fact, as shown in the previous two chapters, parents appear to be the most important discussion partners for adolescents and remain important discussion partners into early adulthood, providing young people with opportunities for political experience.

All of the studies that we have mentioned in this chapter - including the ARCL model just reported - relied on adolescent reports of both the independent and dependent variables. The study by McIntosh et al., (2007) added parental reports as another independent variable. Adolescents reported both their own political interests and their political discussions with their parents. This selection of adolescents as sole reporters is common in research.

What was not considered was the extent to which adolescents' reports of the frequency of political discussions match their parents' reports of the frequency of political discussions at home. Nor was it considered whether other political aspects they reported about their parents match what their parents themselves report. This is an issue we will address here.

Lack of Similarity Between the Reports of Adolescents and Parents Not Taken Into Account

This brings us to the second limitation of the three well-cited studies in this area of research. They did not mention in their studies that parents' reports of their political views, attitudes, and values and their perceptions of their political interactions with their adolescents typically show little correspondence with adolescents' views, attitudes, and values and with adolescents' perceptions of their political interactions with their parents.

All of the studies that we are aware of that have compared parents' and adolescents' reports of various sociopolitical measures have found low to modest associations at best, with one exception—party identification. However, even this exception can be criticized (Ojeda & Hatemi, 2015). These low correlations between what parents report and what adolescents report were known very early, as early as the 1960s and 1970s (Connell, 1972). Social attitudes and values were found to be consistently low between adolescents and parents (Jennings & Niemi, 1968, 1974). When adolescents' reports of their parents' political attitudes and values do not match their parents' reports of their attitudes and values, it is difficult to infer an intergenerational transfer of political attitudes and values from parents to adolescents. As early as 1968, Jennings and Niemi examined the concordance of various sociopolitical values between parents and adolescents, found low concordance, and concluded that "any model of socialization that rests on the assumption of pervasive streams of parent-child value transmission of the types examined here is in serious need of modification" (Jennings & Niemi, 1968, p. 183). This study is a good example of the lack of strong agreement between adolescents' and their parents' sociopolitical values and attitudes that has been reported later in the literature (Acock & Bengtson, 1980; Geißler, 1996; Gniewosz & Noack, 2006; Noack, 2001; Oswald & Schmid, 2006; Patterson et al., 2019; Ter Bogt et al., 2001; Vollebergh et al., 2001). Even when children and parents appear to share the same opinions, parent-child convergence is low. For example, Patterson and coworkers (2019) interviewed children between the ages of 5 and 11 prior to the 2016 U.S. presidential election. Most of the children, 62%, reported that their parents were very interested in the upcoming election. Most of the children themselves, 58%, were also very interested in the election. Children's preferences for presidential candidates were significantly related to their parents' preferences. However, children's interest in the election was not significantly related to their parents' political interest or to their parents' political communication. The studies that based their findings on adolescents' reports and confirmed that parents politically socialized their adolescents through political discussions at home rarely referred to all the studies that examined the actual congruence between parents' and adolescents' reports. Research has consistently failed to document strong causal relationships between parent and child behavior (McDevitt, 2006). How is is possible that these studies are forgotten?

Comparing Adolescent and Parent Reports

To cross-validate previous research on the concordance between adolescents' and parents' political views, we asked adolescents and their parents the same questions about various aspects of their political interactions with each other and their attitudes toward specific sociopolitical issues in the youngest cohort at ages 13 and 17:

- *Parents' political interest*
- *Parents' political knowledge*
- *Frequency of joint political discussions*
- *Parents' political influence attempts*
- *Parents' political support*
- *Adolescents' political influence attempts*
- *Everyday environmental protection*
- *Concern for other people's welfare*
- *Concern for nature*
- *Achievement values*
- *To be active as a norm for citizenship*
- *Trust in people*
- *Positive/negative attitudes toward immigrants*

The specific items/scales behind these measures are shown in Table 7.1.

TABLE 7.1 Scales and items used in the chapter.

Concept	*Items*	*Response scale*
Parents' political interest		
A: "My parents are interested in what is going on in the world"	1	1 (*doesn't apply at all*) 5 (*applies very well*)
P: How interested are you in politics or societal issues? (for mother and father separately). The correlation between the two items was .37, $p < .001$ at age 13 and .54, $p < .001$, at age 17.	1 & 1	1 (*totally uninterested*) 5 (*very interested*)
Parents' political knowledge		
A: "My parents keep themselves in touch with the news"	1	1 (*doesn't apply at all*) 4 (applies perfectly)
P: "Can be described as a person who tries to keep informed about what is going on in the world"; "Follows the news daily to know what other people are talking about." Separately for father and mother. The reliability for the four items was .77 both at age 13 and at age 17.	2 & 2	1 (*doesn't apply at all*) 3 (*applies perfectly*)
Joint political discussions		
A: How often does it happen that you and your parents talk about these things? "What you have heard on the news about what is going on in Sweden and around the world"; "Politics or society"? The correlation between the two items was .56, $p < .001$ at age 13 and .62, $p < .001$ at age 17.	2	1 (*never*) 4 (*very often*)
P: How often does it happen that you talk with your son/daughter about these matters? "What you have heard on the news about what is going on in Sweden and around the world"; "Politics or society"? The correlation between the two items was .44, $p < .001$ at age 13 and .56, $p <.001$ at age 17.	2	1 (*never*) 4 (*very often*)
Parents' influence attempts		
A: "Do your parents try to get you to become more aware of environmental issues?"; "Do your parents try to get you to become more aware of what is going on in the world?" The correlation between the two items was .66, $p <$ .001 at age 13 and .64, $p < .001$ at age 17.	2	1 (*no, never*) 5 (*yes, almost always*)
P: "Do you try to get your son/daughter to become more aware of environmental issues?"; "Do you try to get your son/daughter to become more aware of what is going on in the world?" The correlation between the two items was .48, $p < .001$ at age 13 and .55, $p < .001$ at age 17.	2	1 (*no, never*) 5 (*yes, almost always*)

(*Continued*)

TABLE 7.1 (Continued)

Concept	*Items*	*Response scale*
Parents' political support		
A: My parents: "Suggest newspapers, books or websites where you can read about politics or societal issues"; "Give me information about activities or organizations that you can contact or get engaged in (they talk about what these organizations do and how you get in contact with them)"; "Want me to sit down and watch the news on television with them" The reliability for the three items was .68 at age 13 and .64 at age 17.	3	1 (*definitely doesn't apply*) 5 (*applies very well*)
P: "We parents use to suggest newspapers, books or websites where our child can read about politics or societal issues"; "We parents use to give information about activities or organizations that you can contact or get engaged in"; "We parents use to suggest that the children sit down with us and that we watch the news together." The reliability for the three items was .82 at age 13 and .66 at age 17.	3	1 (*definitely doesn't apply*) 5 (*applies very well*)
Adolescents' influence attempts		
A: "Do you try to encourage your parents to become more aware about environmental issues?"; "Do you try to encourage your parents to become more aware of what is going on in the world?" The correlation between the two items was .66, $p < .001$ at age 13 and .67, $p < .001$ at age 17.	2	1 (*no, never*) 4 (*yes, almost always*)
P: "Does your child try to get you more aware of environmental issues?"; "Do your children try to get you more aware of what is going on in the world?" The correlation between the two items was .57, $p < .001$ at age 13 and .63, $p < .001$ at age 17.	2	1 (*no, never*) 4 (*yes, almost always*)
Everyday environmental protection		
A: How often do you do the following things for environmental reasons? "Choose environmentally friendly products"; "Choose to use public transport rather than being taken by/driving a car"; "Turn off the TV and computer completely when I'm not using them (by using the power switch, not just the stand-by button)." The reliability for the three items was low (0.53) at age 13 (inter-item correlation was .48) and it was low (0.63) also at age 17 (inter-item correlation was .59).	3	1 (*almost never*) 5 (*always*)

Concept	Items	Response scale
P: How often do you do the following things for environmental reasons? "Choose environmentally friendly products"; "Take public transport, cycle or walk rather than traveling by car"; "Turn off the TV and the computer completely when they are not being used (by using the power switch not just the stand-by button)" The reliability for the three items was low, .48 at age 13 (inter-item correlation was .35), and it was low, .48, also at age 17 (inter-item correlation was .25).	3	1 (*almost never*) 5 (*always*)
Concern for other people's welfare		
A and P: "Equality, equal opportunities for all people"; "A peaceful world free from war and conflicts"; "Helping other people"; "Social justice, fighting injustice, and caring about the less fortunate in society"; "Working together with others for a better society." Reliability for adolescents was .80 at age 13 and .84 at age 17. Reliability for parents was .80 at age 13 and .78 at age 17.	5 & 5	1 (*not at all important*) 5 (*very important*)
Concern for nature		
A and P: "Respecting nature and thinking ecologically," "Protecting the environment and preserving nature," "Preventing pollution of the environment and not wasting resources." Reliability for adolescents was .89 at age 13 and .93 at age 17. Reliability for parents was .90 at age 13 and .88 at age 17.	3 & 3	1 (*not at all important*) 5 (*very important*)
Achievement values		
A: "Always doing my best"; "Working hard on school work"; "Studying so that I get good grades"; "Learning new things"	4	1 (*not at all important*) 5 (*very important*)
P: "Always doing our best," "Working hard to achieve the goals we have set," "Getting better at what we do," "Learning new things"	4	1 (*not at all important*) 5 (*very important*)
Reliability for adolescents was .78 at age 13 and .85 at age 17. Reliability for parents was .78 both at age 13 and at age 17.		

(*Continued*)

TABLE 7.1 (Continued)

Concept	*Items*	*Response scale*
Norms of citizenship: Active		
A: How active should people be on political issues? What do you think? For me it is important to "Join political parties and organizations to bring up the issues that are important to me"; "Be involved so that politicians get to know what people think"; "Actively try to influence societal issues"; "Make my voice heard on societal issues"	4	1 (*not important at all*) 4 (*very important*)
P: "Be involved so that politicians get to know what people think"; "Actively try to exert influence on societal matters"; "Constantly make my voice heard on societal issues"	3	1 (*not important at all*) 4 (*very important*)
Reliability for adolescents was .83 at age 13 and .81 at age 17. Reliability for parents was .73 at age 13 and .75 at age 17.		
Social trust		
A and P: "Most people can be trusted," "Most people are fair, and don't try to exploit you." The correlation between the two items for adolescents was .64, $p < .001$ at age 13 and .66, $p < .001$ at age 17. The correlation between the two items for parents was .80, $p < .001$ at age 13 and .86, $p < .001$ at age 17.	2 & 2	1 (*doesn't apply at all*) 5 (*applies perfectly*)
Positive attitudes toward immigrants		
A and P: "Our culture gets enriched when people from other countries move here," "In the future, Sweden will be a country where there are exciting encounters and meetings between people from different parts of the world," "That people move to Sweden is good for the Swedish economy," "We should welcome people who have fled from problems in their own countries." Reliability for adolescents was .77 at age 13 and age 17. Reliability for parents was .77 at age 13 and .88 at age 17.	4	1 (*doesn't apply at all*) 4 (*applies very well*)
Negative attitudes toward immigrants		
A and P: "It happens only too often that immigrants have customs and traditions that do not fit in into Swedish society"; "Immigrants often come here just to take advantage of the welfare in Sweden"; "Immigrants often take jobs from people who are born in Sweden." Reliability for adolescents was .75 at age 13 and .76 at age 17. Reliability for parents was .67 at age 13 and .80 at age 17.	3	1 (*doesn't apply at all*) 4 (*applies very well*)

A, adolescent reports; and P, parent reports.

We use the youngest cohort. The same questions asked at age 13 were also asked of them and their parents four years later at age 17.

We calculated correlations between the adolescents' and parents' reports. These are summarized in Table 7.2. The correlations in Table 7.2 range from a low of .02 to a high of .24 at age 13. They were higher at age 17, ranging from .09 to .40. The average correlation at age 13 was .15 and it was .23 at age 17. Significantly higher correlations at age 17 than at age 13 were found for joint political discussions, adolescents' attempts to influence others, trust in others, and attitudes toward immigrants. Similar age-related differences have been reported previously (Westholm, 1999). We conclude that adolescents' and parents' reports on various aspects of their political interactions and sociopolitical issues are not very similar—similarity is somewhat higher for measures of their joint political interactions than for measures of attitudes and values.

The findings in Table 7.2—a general lack of agreement between adolescents' and parents' reports——are similar to what has been reported previously in the literature. These findings have implications for our understanding of the role of parents in adolescent political development. We cannot infer from these low correlations a strong intergenerational transfer of political attitudes and values from parents to adolescents. Nor can we assume that adolescents' reports of their political interactions with their parents (frequency of joint political discussions, parental attempts at political influence, parental political support, adolescent attempts at political influence, etc.) match their parents' perceptions of these same political interactions. Thus, there is little evidence that parents' political and civic perceptions translate into similar political and civic perceptions among their adolescents. Small to modest correlations between adolescents' and parents' reports are to be expected.

TABLE 7.2 Agreement between adolescents' and parents' perceptions of various sociopolitical issues at ages 13 and 17 in the youngest cohort. Correlation coefficients.

	13 years		*17 years*			
	r	*p*	*r*	*p*	*Z*	*p*
Parents' political interest	.14	.001	.28	<.001	−1.94	.052
Parents' political knowledge	.16	<.001	.21	.003	−0.67	.503
Joint political discussions	.15	<.001	.38	<.001	−3.22	.001
Parents' influence attempts	.23	<.001	.19	<.001	0.56	.570
Parents' political support	.16	<.001	.20	<.001	−0.57	.583
Adolescents' influence attempts	.24	<.001	.40	<.001	−2.36	.018
Everyday environmental protection	.23	<.001	.18	<.001	0.14	.889
Concern for other people's welfare	.14	.001	.11	.059	−0.07	.946
Concern for nature	.12	.004	.17	.005	−0.51	.606
Achievement values	.14	.002	.15	.014	−0.99	.321
Norms of citizenship: Active	.02	.714	.09	.143	−0.22	.829
Social trust	.05	.217	.31	<.001	−3.50	<.001
Positive attitudes toward immigrants	.19	<.001	.38	<.001	−2.78	.005
Negative attitudes toward immigrants	.17	<.001	.20	.018	−0.54	.580
Average	.15		.23			

A political socialization science suggesting that parents shape young peoples' political attitudes and values is simply not valid given the lack of evidence that parents' political attitudes and values translate into similar political attitudes and values in their young people.

New ideas are needed. The most central is to understand the mechanisms that govern adolescents' perceptions of their political interactions with their parents, and the mechanisms that govern parents' perceptions of the same interactions with their adolescents. We propose that adolescents' and parents' own political interests are the driving force behind their respective perceptions.

Epilogue

Recall that in Chapter 5 we reported that most adolescents perceived their parents' political views as similar to their own, which was taken as one of several indicators of adolescents' openness to their parents. Adolescents' openness to their parents' political communication was evident in many ways. Most adolescents believed their parents' views were important to them and similar to their own, and their parents' conversations about society and the news evoked positive feelings in them. How adolescents' political attitudes, values, and perceptions of their interactions with their parents match their parents' perceptions is the question we have raised here. Does a general openness to parents' views imply a strong convergence of opinions? Apparently not. Parents' and adolescents' views do not converge well.

We begin to discern a different outline of young people's perceptions of political issues, one that is not necessarily shaped by their parents. It is a perception in which politically interested young people's own curiosity about politics, society, and the world strongly influences their political views and behavior. It has long been known that political interest is perhaps the best predictor of the full range of political attitudes, values, and behaviors (Prior, 2019), but theoretical models of *how* adolescents' intrinsic political interest influences their knowledge, views, and political interactions with others are lacking. This is an issue that will occupy much of the remainder of this book.

8

EMOTIONAL RELATIONSHIPS AND TRANSFERS ACROSS CONTEXTS

Highlights

Are everyday and political conversations between adolescents and parents influenced by similar motivational factors?

- *We propose that the conditions that predict everyday and political conversations at home are substantially different. The frequency of everyday conversations between parents and adolescents depends on adolescents' and parents' perceptions of a warm relationship, but political conversations are strongly influenced only by the political interests of both parties.*
- *Results from a one-year longitudinal analysis of 13- and 16-year-olds support this proposition. Adolescents' political interest predicted their perceptions of the frequency of joint political discussions at home, and parents' political interest predicted their perceptions of the frequency of joint political discussions. Emotional relationships between parents and adolescents influenced parents' and adolescents' conversations about everyday topics, but not their conversations about political topics.*

Similarly, we proposed that adolescents' political activity in the classroom would be predicted by their own political interest rather than by their emotional bonding to school or their perception of being receptive to teachers' political communication.

- *We found that neither adolescents' emotional bonding to school nor their perception of and susceptibility to teachers' political communication explained their political activity in class. Only their political interest was a significant predictor.*

Additional longitudinal analyses examined whether perceptions of own political activity in the classroom or political reputation in the classroom spill over to political discussions at home over the course of a year, or whether the direction of influence is the opposite. The results showed that the more political discussions that took place at home, the more politically active the adolescents were in class. The opposite was not found. Surprisingly, having a political reputation at school had a positive effect on the frequency of political discussions with parents. Students with a political reputation seem to be the students who provide input from school to political discussions with parents.

DOI: 10.4324/9781003371731-11

Introduction

Whether it concerns attachment, social-learning or social-construction theory, or parenting styles, *well-functioning and harmonious parent-adolescent relations are considered the foundation upon which the effectiveness of parents' socialization attempts are based* (Grusec & Davidov, 2021). Frequent and open everyday parent-child communication in adolescence is a key marker of a harmonious family climate. Being at ease when talking to parents shows that the adolescent's views are valued and respected, that the adolescent appreciates family relationships and is open to parents' socialization attempts (Kerr & Stattin, 2000). Adolescents and parents can talk about various issues at home. They can talk about things that unite their interests—films, music and TV series, common family activities, and relatives and friends of the family—or about what happens in the adolescents' lives that is vital for parents to know about—school and friends. In addition, they can talk about matters that widen their information circles—about what happens in the world and political and social issues. In this chapter, we propose that parent-adolescent conversations about everyday issues are highly dependent on affective family relationships, whereas emotional family relationships have much less influence on conversations about political and societal issues. It is to be expected that these conversations about political and social issues will depend largely on whether or not young people and their parents are politically interested. Consequently, the foundation upon which the effectiveness of parents' socialization attempts rests, good parent-adolescent relations, is not a necessary condition for the political talks that take place between adolescents and their parents.

Political socialization is commonly defined as the process through which young people acquire their political ideologies, opinions, and attitudes. Parents are one of the agents of this socialization. We will argue that political socialization is primarily an issue for the parents who are politically interested themselves. Likewise, openness to parents' talks about societal and political issues may be expected primarily to apply to adolescents who themselves are politically interested. Indeed, adolescents whose political interest is an intrinsically motivated behavior may not stop them from pursuing their political interactions with their parents even if the parents do not possess high political interest (cf. Deci & Ryan, 1991; Meadowcroft, 1986). In short, behind the political talks that go on in families, there should be politically interested parents and adolescents, although parents' and adolescents' political interests do not necessarily overlap. The different perceptual worlds of parents and adolescents are an indication of a lack of a general intergenerational transmission process regarding political messages.

Value Transmission

Early political socialization studies aimed at explaining the intergenerational transmission of values on the basis of the agreement between adolescents' and parents' self-reported sociopolitical values (e.g., Jennings & Niemi, 1968, 1974). This line of research shifted over time to focus on adolescents' perception of their parents' values. Here, value transmission from parents to children became largely a question of whether adolescents correctly perceive their parents' socialization messages (Grusec & Goodnow, 1994; Tedin, 1980; Westholm, 1999). Good parent-child relations can be expected to play a vital role in general socialization if adolescents are able to accurately perceive their parents' ideologies, values, and opinions (Grusec & Goodnow, 1994; Grusec & Kuczynski, 1997). In one frequently cited study, Knafo and Schwartz (2003) employed the set of values in Schwartz's basic human values model and compared adolescents' perceptions of the values they thought their parents wanted them to have with those their parents reported that they wanted their adolescents to have. Accuracy in reporting parents' values was positively predicted by parents' warmth and receptiveness, and negatively by autocratic and indifferent parenting and love withdrawal. Similar findings, with good relations encouraging young persons' perceptual accuracy of parents' values and poor relations discouraging perceptual accuracy, appeared in other studies of adolescents using the value types in Schwartz's model (Barni et al., 2011; Friedlmeier & Trommsdorff, 2011; Schönpflug, 2001), and also for other types of value orientations (Roest et al., 2009; Taris & Semin, 1997; Tsai et al., 2015; Wu et al., 2018). In the political socialization sphere, Dunkel and Decker (2012) found that the relationship between college students' perceptions of the political orientation of their parents and their own political orientation was stronger for students with high levels of identification with their parents than for students with low levels. Overall, these studies suggest that whether young people accurately perceive their parents' values can be dependent on their affective relations with their parents. Although several studies have reported supportive findings, the moderating effect of affective parent-child relationships has been rather weak in most of these studies. Also, from the earliest studies in political science, conflicting results have been reported. Jennings and Niemi (1968) found no effect of affective parent-child relationships on the congruence between parents' and adolescents' views, but Tedin (1974) found such an effect, contrary to his hypothesis. Importantly for our focus on political interests, the above studies did not consider the political interests of parents and children. For the most part, cross-sectional designs were used.

Potentially, having good relations with parents may impact adolescents' ability to *perceive* their parents' values less than their willingness to *accept* their parents' values. This interpretation was advocated by Ojeda and Hatemi (2015). They suggested a perception and adoption model similar to the value-socialization model of Grusec and Goodnow (1994). In the Ojeda and Hatemi study, parents' social support was included as one measure of affective parent-child relations. Social support did not increase the probability of correctly perceiving parents' party identification but did increase the probability of adopting parents' party identification. Strictly speaking, having the same party preference as parents does not necessarily mean that an adolescent has adopted their parents' party identification. A similar preference might equally well be interpreted as showing that an adolescent's party identification happens to coincide with that of their parents. Nevertheless, the study provides the important information that the role that parent-child relations plays in the transmission of values from parents to adolescents may be more than a question of whether parent-child relations affect adolescents' perceptions of their parents' socialization messages. Again, the political interest of parents and youth was not considered.

Family Communication Patterns

The idea presented here, that political discussions at home are primarily dependent on parents' and adolescents' political interests and not their emotional relations, differs from the most well-known theoretical idea on political communication in families, developed by mass communication researchers in the 1970s (Chaffee et al., 1973; McLeod & Chaffee, 1972; Stone & Chaffee, 1970). In this literature, the critical issue was *how* parents communicate their political messages. Families are categorized according to two communication styles. The parents who communicate political issues less frequently are the ones who strive to maintain conformism, and who are not open to discussions that challenge their belief systems. These are parents with a *socio-oriented* communication pattern. By contrast, parents who communicate political issues more frequently are the ones who are open to opinions that challenge their own beliefs and encourage their children to adopt stances of their own. These are parents with a *concept-oriented* communication pattern. This distinction spurred much research on political communication during the 1980s and 1990s. For example, a highly concept-oriented communicative style was found to be associated with high knowledge, political discussions, and media use on the part of adolescents, whereas the opposite was true of the socio-oriented communication pattern (e.g., Chaffee et al., 1973; Liebes & Ribak, 1992; Meadowcroft, 1986). In the 1990s, these communication patterns were extended to broader behavioral orientations of the parents: to conversation and conformity orientations and their elaborations (Koerner & Fitzpatrick, 2002; Ritchie, 1991; Ritchie & Fitzpatrick, 1990).

The empirical studies in this tradition treat family communication patterns as set up by parents. A problem with this, however, is that adolescents seem to have different conceptions of socio-oriented and concept-oriented communication than their parents have. Low correlations have been found between parents' and adolescents' reports on concept-oriented and socio-oriented measures (Meadowcroft, 1986; Ritchie & Fitzpatrick, 1990; Rauscher et al., 2020; Saphir & Chaffee, 2002; Tims & Masland, 1985). From the perspective of the present chapter, however, the most important limitation of the family communication-pattern approach is that empirical studies did not control for parents' and adolescents' political interest in the first place, introduced political interest as a mediator between family communication patterns and political outcomes, or sought explanations for differences in adolescents' and parents' reports of communication patterns in terms of their different political interests.

Everyday and Political Talk

We will differentiate between everyday and political conversations and this differentiation is similar to Schudson's (1997) distinction between sociable conversations and political talk. Sociable conversations are casual and happen spontaneously in daily life, giving people pleasure in interacting. Political talk, by contrast, is oriented toward exchange of rational arguments and information, problem solving, and goals. Scheufele (2000) operationalized these two dimensions and applied them to an adult sample. In line with Shudson's expectations, attendance to news, political participation, and political knowledge were mainly associated with political talks. Scheufele (2000) could not attend to the direction of effects in his cross-sectional design, or to the spillover between sociable conversations and political talk. This is an issue that will be brought up here.

The Current Chapter

We use a longitudinal design over one year for one age cohort and over two years for another age cohort of adolescents to examine the role that good parent-adolescent relationships and parents' and adolescents' political interest play in conversations about everyday and political matters. If political socialization is similar to "normal" socialization, then emotional parent-adolescent relationships should affect political conversations in families in much the same way as they affect normal everyday conversations. However, we expect the role of affective parent-adolescent relations to be different for everyday family talk and political talk.

Everyday conversations at home will be strongly influenced by affective parent-child relations, with good relations being a key factor in everyday parent-child communication in families. This hypothesis is based on a wealth of research on parent-child relationships in adolescence (Kerr & Stattin, 2000; Grusec & Davidov, 2021). In contrast, in the absence of strong evidence that emotional relationships between adolescents and parents influence political discussions, we hypothesize that political talk at home is primarily predicted by adolescents' and parents' political interests and is not strongly influenced by emotional parent-child relationships. The frequency of political talk between adolescents and their parents is expected to depend primarily on the respective political interests of parents and adolescents. This is consistent with Schudson's (1997) distinction between social and political talk.

First, we predict that the frequency of everyday conversations at home will depend strongly on affective parent-child relationships. Second, we do not expect political conversations to be strongly influenced by affective parent-child relations. Instead, we expect the frequency of political conversations between adolescents and their parents to depend primarily on the political interests of both parents and adolescents. If adolescents report that political discussions occur frequently in the family, this should reflect the adolescents' own, rather than their parents', political interest. Similarly, if parents report that political discussions occur frequently, this should reflect the parents' political interest rather than that of their adolescents. We expect the same reporter specificity for everyday conversations. We also examine whether political conversations spill over into everyday conversations and vice versa. These analyses provide information on whether political conversations promote everyday conversations over time, and whether everyday conversations facilitate political conversations over time. We do not propose specific hypotheses about these spillover effects. Gender, immigrant status, and parental education level are controlled for in all analyses.

Finally, we attend to the reverse direction of effects. Hence, we examine the roles of the frequency of everyday and political talks in parents' and adolescents' reports of political interest and their emotional relations.

Method

Participants

We use the two youngest age cohorts of adolescents. The first cohort is the sample of 13-year-olds followed over two years. According to class lists, this sample comprised 960 students, of which 856 (89.2%) answered questionnaires at school and had complete data on the measures in the study. This is the analytic sample. Parents answered questionnaires at home ($N = 571$; 59.5% of the target sample). Complete responses from parents and adolescents at Time 1 (T1) were available for 528 participants (61.7% of the analytic sample). The participants' ages averaged 13.41 years ($SD = 0.55$). Of the 528 parent-student pairs with complete data at T1, 303 parent-student pairs were followed up two years later (35.4% of the analytic sample at T1 and 57.4% of the parent-student pairs at T1).

The second cohort, cohort 2, was the sample of 16-year-olds. The target sample comprised 1052 students. Of these, 831 (79%) answered questionnaires at school and had complete data on the measures in the study: the analytic sample. Parents answered the questionnaires at home ($N = 577$). Complete responses from parents and adolescents at T1 were available for 498 participants (59.9% of the analytic sample). The participants' ages averaged 16.57 years ($SD = 0.68$). Of the 498 parent-student pairs with complete data at T1, 268 parent-student pairs were followed up one year later (32.2% of the analytic sample at T1 and 53.8% of the parent-student pairs at T1).

Measures

Concerning satisfying parent-adolescent relations from the perspective of the adolescents, we included measures tapping parents' warmth and responsivity to the adolescents (cf. Grusec & Goodnow, 1994) and, in parent reports, parents' perceptions of the adolescents' warmth toward them.

The following measures were used:

Parental warmth, adolescent report
Adolescents' warmth, parent reports
Political interest, adolescent reports
Political interest, parent reports
Everyday and political talks, adolescent and parent reports

Covariates:

Immigrant status
Gender
Parents' level of education

Information about these measures is reported in Table 8.1. As we have reported earlier in Chapter 5 (Table 5.1), items covering the everyday and the political talks made up two distinct factors.

Attrition Analyses

First, we used logistic regression to compare the participants whose parents responded at T1 with the participants whose parents did not respond. This analysis included all adolescent reports at T1 and the covariates. Significant differences were obtained for immigrant status in both cohorts (cohort 1: $OR = 2.28$, $p < .001$; cohort 2; $OR = 2.43$, $p < .001$) Significant results were also found for adolescents' political interest in cohort 2 ($OR = 2.43$, $p = .035$). Participants whose parents responded contained fewer persons of immigrant background, and adolescents' political interest was higher for participants with parent reports. Nagelkerke R^2 was .04 for cohort 1 and .05 for cohort 2.

Second, in the longitudinal analyses, logistic regression comparisons were made between participants with self and parent reports at both T1 and T2 with the participants who had self and parents reports at T1 but not at T2. This analysis included all adolescent and parent reports and the covariates at T1. There was one significant difference in cohort 1. Parents of the student-parent participants with data from both T1 and T2 reported a higher level of political talks ($OR = 1.50$, $p = .05$). There was also one significant difference in the second cohort. Participants with an immigrant background had a lower response rate ($OR = 2.11$, $p = .012$). Nagelkerke R^2 was .05 in cohort 1 and .04 in cohort 2. In view of low Nagelkerke R^2 coefficients, and given that the differences in terms of significance when converted to Cohen's *d* can be regarded as small, bias can be considered low in the two comparisons.

TABLE 8.1 Scales measuring emotional relationships, political interest, and everyday and political conversations.

Content	*Number of items*	*Response scale*
Parental warmth (A)		
Adolescents reported on their mothers' and fathers' warmth separately, "Do small things that make you feel special, for example, winks, smiles?" "Constantly shows how proud she/he is of you?" "Focuses on the positive, but seldom the negative, things you do?" "Shows with words and gestures that she/he likes you?" and "Always shows that she/he likes you—almost regardless of what you do?" Cronbach alpha at T1 was .88 for cohort 1 and .91 for cohort 2.	5	1 (*never)* 3 (*usually*)
Adolescents' warmth toward parents (P)		
"How often does it happen that your child says she/he likes you and is proud of you as parents?" "How often does your child do little things to show tenderness (e.g., hug you, or smile)?" "How often do you think that your child does something nice for you without there being any special reason?" "How often does it happen that your child says appreciative things about what you try to do for her or him?" and "How often does your child show that she/he likes you, almost regardless of what you do?" Cronbach alpha at T1 was .88 for cohort 1 and .89 for cohort 2.	5	1 (*almost never*) to 5 (*extremely often*)
Adolescents' political interest (A)		
"How interested are you in politics?" and "How interested are you in what is going on in society?" They answered on a scale ranging from (1) *totally uninterested* to (5) *very interested*. The correlation between the items was .46 in cohort 1 and .59 in cohort 2.	2	(1) *totally uninterested* to (5) *very interested*
Parents' political interest (P)		
This question was asked separately about fathers' and mothers' political interest: "How interested are you in politics or societal issues?" The response scale ranged from 1 (*totally uninterested*) to 5 (*very interested*). The correlation between fathers' and mothers' political interest was .37 in cohort 1 and .51 in cohort 2.	1 & 1	1 (*totally uninterested*) to 5 (*very interested*)

Everyday and political talk (A and P)		
Concerning everyday talks, adolescents were asked how often they and their parents talked about "Family activities (doing things together)," "School, school work, and homework," "Your friends (what you do in free time)," and "Relatives and friends of the family."	4	1 (*never*) 4 (*very often*)
Parents reported: "Family activities (doing things together)" and "School, school work, and homework." Both adolescents and parents reported on two types of political talk:	2	1 (*never*) 4 (*very often*)
"What you have heard on the news about what is going on in Sweden and around the world" and "Politics or societal issues." We treat the everyday and political talk measures as frequency counts, that is, the number of times these talks take place in the family.	2 & 2	1 (*never*) 4 (*very often*)
Factor analyses of the everyday and political talks yielded two factors, everyday and political talks, as reported in Chapter 5		
Covariates:		
Immigrant status was a dichotomous measure, differentiating between participants whose parents were born outside the Nordic countries (1) and other participants (0). Sex was coded as 0 (*male*) and 1 (*female*). Fathers' and mothers' level of education were aggregated. They were measured on a scale ranging from 1 (*less than 9 years of study*) to 5 (*university college/university education*).	4	

Adolescents' sex, immigration status, and parents' education were regressed on all the measures of talks at both T1 and T2. They are omitted for the purpose of brevity.
A, adolescent reports; P, parent reports.

Results

Descriptive Results

Table 8.2 reports descriptive statistics and correlations between the study variables at T1 and T2. At T1 for both cohorts, the frequency of political talks reported by adolescents was most strongly associated with the adolescents' own political interest, and the frequency of political talks reported by parents was most strongly associated with parents' own political interest. When adolescents in cohort 1 reported a high frequency of political talks at T1 and T2, they also tended to report a high frequency of everyday talks at T1 and T2 ($r = .45, p < .001$; $r = .45, p < .001$). To a somewhat lesser extent, the adolescents in cohort 2 reported the same ($r = .30, p < .001$; $r = .38, p < .001$).

Regarding parents' and adolescents' warmth toward each other, at T1 in both cohorts, adolescents' perceptions of parents' warmth toward them were most strongly associated with their reports of everyday talks. In both cohorts, parents' perceptions of the adolescents' warmth were more strongly associated with their reports of everyday talks than their reports of political talks.

There are some indications, particularly in the younger cohort, that the frequency of political talks in the family are related to the frequency of everyday talks. However, for the most part, political talks, reported by the adolescents and the parents, were related to their own political interests. The lack of agreement between parents and adolescents about how often political and everyday talks take place at home is noteworthy (correlations ranging from .16 to .33).

Main Results

In order to test the effects of political interest and parent-child relations on political and everyday talks, a path model was constructed (see Figure 8.1), which was tested using Mplus 8.8 (Muthén & Muthén, 1998–2017), both cross-sectionally at T1 and longitudinally from T1 to T2. We address two main issues. First, we were interested in the effects of warm relations and political interest respectively on everyday talks and political talks. Second, we were interested in the spillover of effects between everyday talks than their reports of political talks.

The significant results of the path model that was tested cross-sectionally are reported in Figure 8.2. In line with our hypotheses, in both cohorts, adolescents' reports of everyday talks were most strongly associated with their perceptions of parental warmth, and parents' reports of everyday talks were most strongly associated with their perceptions of their adolescents' warmth. Similarly, adolescents' reports of political talks with their parents were most strongly associated with their own political interest, and parents' reports of political talk were most strongly associated with the parents' own political interest. There were several examples of the emotional-relation measures being significantly associated with political talks in the families. For example, in both cohorts, parents' reports of

TABLE 8.2 Descriptive statistics and correlations between the study variables for cohorts 1 ($N = 303$) and 2 ($N = 268$).

	M (SD)	*1*	*2*	*3*	*4*	*5*	*6*	*7*	*8*	*9*	*10*	*11*	*12*
		3.11 (1.02)	*3.69 (0.76)*	*0.08 (1.13)*	*3.37 (0.83)*	*3.01 (0.49)*	*3.63 (0.39)*	*2.49 (0.66)*	*3.12 (0.48)*	*2.99 (0.52)*	*3.55 (0.40)*	*2.63 (0.69)*	*3.07 (0.48)*
1. Political interest at T1 (A)	2.81 (0.89)	–	.13*	.13*	.12	.20***	.07	.57***	.22***	.09	.12	.52***	.22***
2. Political interest at T1 (P)	3.62 (0.67)	.22***	–	.06	.06	−.11	.13*	.15*	.46***	−.01	.09	.23***	.36***
3. Warmth at T1 (A)	0.14 (1.10)	.17**	.13*	–	.29***	.38***	.19***	.18**	.06	.36***	.23***	.20***	.10
4. Warmth at T1 (P)	3.51 (0.86)	.18***	.24***	.21***	–	.21***	.24***	.20***	.14*	.24***	.24***	.17**	.15*
5. Everyday talks at T1 (A)	3.16 (0.47)	.23***	.08	.39***	.13*	–	.25***	.30***	.03	.62***	.29***	.24***	.04
6. Everyday talks at T1 (P)	3.78 (0.31)	.03	.13*	.10	.33***	.01	–	.05	.21***	.31***	.26***	.19***	.20***
7. Political talks at T1 (A)	2.36 (0.70)	.50***	.24***	.32***	.17**	.45***	.02	–	.24***	.20***	.10	.58***	.31***
8. Political talks at T1 (P)	3.01 (0.52)	.16**	.45***	.02	.27***	−.04	.22***	.16***	–	.04	.18**	.29***	.52***
9. Everyday talks at T2 (A)	3.11 (0.48)	.14*	.09	.23***	.16**	.33***	.00	.23***	.03	–	.28***	.38***	.06
10. Everyday talks at T2 (P)	3.69 (0.39)	−.03	.16**	.17**	.28***	.04	.44***	.06	.25***	.03	–	.22***	.26***
11. Political talks at T2 (A)	2.49 (0.68)	.31***	.19***	.23***	.08	.23***	−.09	.47***	15**	.45***	.02	–	.33***
12. Political talks at T2 (P)	2.93 (0.55)	.14*	.42***	.11*	.20***	−.01	.05	.15**	.58***	.06	.29***	.24***	–

Note: Cohort 1 is under the diagonal and cohort 2 above.
A, adolescent reports; P, parent reports.
$^{*}p < .05$ $^{**}p < .01$ $^{***}p < .001$.

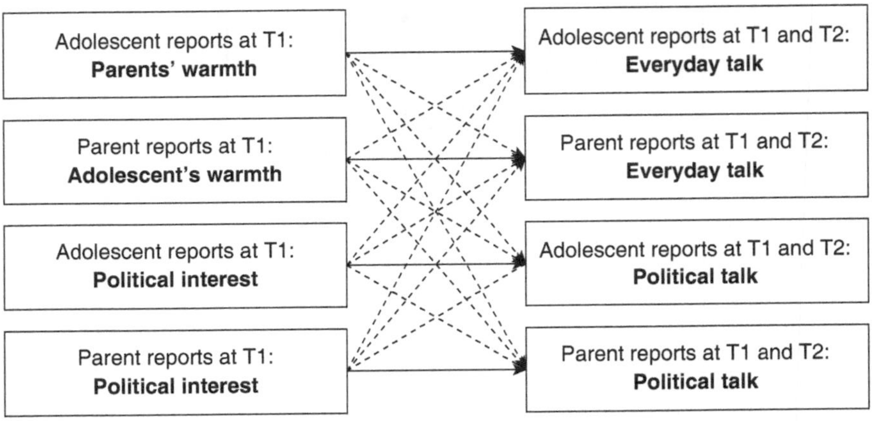

Solid lines represent our expectations of strong associations and dotted lines our expectations of weak associations.

FIGURE 8.1 Conceptual model of the study. Cross-sectionally, warmth and political interest at T1 predict everyday and political talk at T2. Longitudinally, warmth and political interest predict everyday and political talk at T2, after controlling for everyday and political talk at T1.

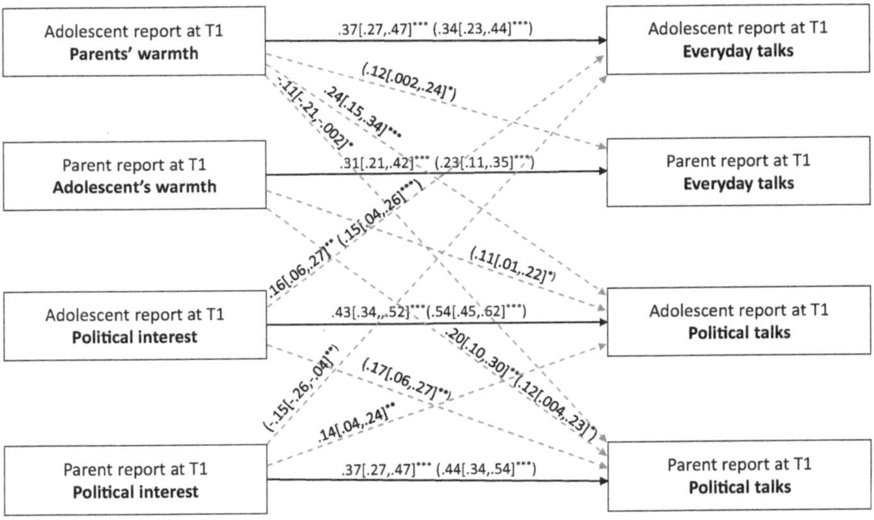

FIGURE 8.2 Cross-sectional predictions of everyday and political talk at T1 from warmth and political interest at T1 (cohort 1: $N = 303$; cohort 2: $N = 268$).

The reported coefficients above are the standardized regression coefficients, followed by their 95% confidence interval. Associations without parentheses are for cohort 1 and associations within parentheses are for cohort 2. Solid lines represent our expectations of strong associations and dotted lines our expectations of weak associations.

* $p < .05$, ** $p < .01$, *** $p < .001$.

their adolescents' warmth were significantly associated with parents' reports of the frequency of political talks, and, in both cohorts, adolescents' reports of their political interest were positively associated with their reports of how frequently everyday talks took place. At the same time, in the older cohort, parents' reports of their political interest were negatively associated with adolescents' reports of everyday talks. Overall, the cross-sectional findings give the first support for the study hypotheses that everyday talks are mainly associated with emotional parent-child relations and political talks are primarily associated with adolescents' and parents' political interest.

The significant results from the longitudinal analyses are reported in Figure 8.3. Here, we were interested in whether warmth and political interest predict changes in everyday and political talks over one year (cohort 2) and two years (cohort 1). For this purpose, we regressed everyday talks and political talks at T2 on warmth and political interest at T1 after controlling for everyday and political talks at T1. As shown in Figure 8.3, in both cohorts, adolescents' reports of their parents'

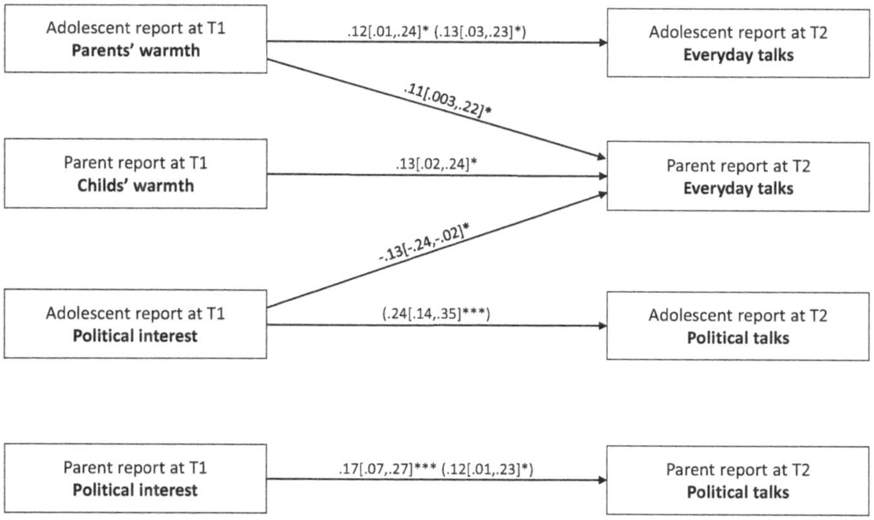

FIGURE 8.3 Longitudinal predictions of everyday and political talk at T2 from warmth and political interest at T1, controlling for everyday and political talk at T1 (cohort 1: $N = 303$; cohort 2: $N = 268$).

The reported coefficients above are the standardized regression coefficients, followed by their 95% confidence interval. Associations without parentheses are for cohort 1 and associations within parentheses are for cohort 2. Solid lines represent our expectations of strong associations and dotted lines our expectations of weak associations.

$^{*}p < .05$, $^{**}p < .01$, $^{***}p < .001$.

warmth positively predicted the frequency of everyday talks as perceived by the adolescents. In both cohorts, parents' reports of their political interest at T1 positively predicted their perceptions of how often political talks took place at T2. Moreover, parents' reports of their adolescents' warmth toward them at T1 positively predicted how frequently they perceived those everyday talks took place at T2 in cohort 1, and adolescents' reports of their political interest at T1 positively predicted their perceptions of how frequently they perceived that political talks took place at T2 in cohort 2. In addition, parents' reports of adolescents' warmth at T1 predicted adolescents' reports of everyday talks at T2 in the younger cohort, and adolescents' reports of their political interest at T1 negatively predicted parents' reports of everyday talks at T2 also in the younger cohort. We conclude that the longitudinal analyses support the study hypotheses that everyday talks are mainly affected by adolescents' and parents' emotional relations with each other and that political talks are affected by adolescents' and parents' own political interests. There is also much to suggest that adolescents' and parents' political interests affect their own, but not the others', perceptions of how frequent political talks take place at home, and the same is true for everyday talks.

Spillover Effects

Do political talks spill over into everyday talks, and/or vice-versa? We regressed political and everyday talks at T1 on political and everyday talks at T2. No spillover effects were found in the older cohort. In the younger cohort, parents' reports of everyday talks negatively predicted both parents' own ($\beta = -.10$, $p = .034$, 95% CI [−.20,−.01]) and adolescents' ($\beta = -.13$, $p = .012$, 95% CI [−.23,−.03]) reports of political talks. However, parents' reports of political talks positively affected their reports of everyday talks two years later ($\beta = .12$, $p = .034$, 95% CI [.01,.24]). The spillover effects were not large, and political and everyday talks seem to affect each other both positively and negatively.

Reverse Direction of Effects

Finally, we tested whether everyday and political talk at T1 predicted adolescents' and parents' political interest and emotional relationships at T2. This analysis was conducted by reversing the order of the variables in Figure 8.1. That is, we regressed teens' and parents' political interest and perceptions of emotional relationships at T2 on everyday and political talk at T1, after controlling for political interest and perceptions of warmth at T1 (see Table 8.3).

First, when looking at predictions of political interest, none of the predictors were significant in cohort 2. However, for cohort 1 participants, their perceptions of the frequency of political talks at T1 positively predicted their own interest at T2 ($\beta = .29$, $p < .001$). Their perceptions of the frequency of everyday conversations negatively predicted their political interest ($\beta = -.15$, $p = .01$). Similarly, parents' perceptions of the frequency of political talks at T1 positively predicted their own political interest at T2 ($\beta = .22$, $p < .001$) in the younger cohort.

TABLE 8.3 Results of reverse causality analyses (cohort 1: $N = 297$; cohort 2: $N = 254$).

	Dependent variable at T2							
	Political interest (A)		*Political interest (P)*		*Warmth (A)*		*Warmth (P)*	
	Cohort 1	*Cohort 2*	*Cohort 1*	*Cohort 2*	*Cohort 1*	*Cohort 2*	*Cohort 1*	*Cohort 2*
Warmth (A)	.10[−.01,.21]	−.03[−.12,.06]	.05[−.05,.15]	.06[−.04,.17]	.45[.35,.55]***	.67[.59,.74]***	.05[−.04,.15]	.10[.01,.20]*
Warmth (P)	−.01[−.11,.10]	−.02[−.11,.07]	−.09[−.19,.01]	−.02[−.13,.08]	.21[.11,.32]***	.04[−.05,.14]	.66[.58,.73]***	.68[.60,.75]***
Political interest (A)	.29[.18,.39]***	.67[.60,.77]***	.07[−.04,.17]	.03[−.09,.14]	.01[−.09,.12]	−.04[−.15,.06]	−.03[−.13,.06]	.06[−.04,.16]
Political interest (P)	.02[−.09,.13]	.03[−.07,.12]	.48[.38,.57]***	.58[.49,.68]***	−.01[−.12,.09]	−.01[−.10,.09]	−.00[−.10,.10]	−.04[−.13,.06]
Everyday talks (A)	−.15[−.26, −.04]**	.03[−.06,.13]	.03[−.07,.14]	−.07[−.18,.04]	−.05[−.16,.06]	.14[.04,.24]**	−.03[−.13,.07]	.03[−.07,.13]
Everyday talks (P)	−.04[−.14,.06]	−.02[−.11,.07]	−.08[−.17,.02]	−.02[−.12,.08]	−.01[−.10,.09]	−.01[−.10,.08]	.00[−.09,.09]	.02[−.08,.11]
Political talks (A)	.29[.17,.41]***	.10[−.01,.20]	−.00[−.12,.11]	.10[−.02,.22]	.12[−.00,.23]	.00[−.11,.11]	−.03[−.13,.08]	−.07[−.18,.04]
Political talks (P)	.10[−.01,.21]	.03[−.06,.13]	.22[.17,.32]***	.03[−.08,.14]	−.08[−.19,.03]	.03[−.07,.13]	.06[−.04,.16]	.02[−.08,.12]

Note: The reported coefficients above are the standardized regression coefficients, followed by their 95% confidence interval.

A, adolescent reports; P, parent reports.

$^{*}p < .05$, $^{**}p < .01$, $^{***}p < .001$.

Second, with regard to predictions of warmth, in the older cohort, adolescents' reports of the frequency of everyday conversations positively predicted perceptions that their parents were warm toward them (β =.14, $p < .01$). In cohort 1, adolescents' perceptions of their parents' warmth at T2 were positively predicted by their parents' perceptions of how warm the adolescents were toward them at T1 (β =.22, $p < .001$). Similarly, parents' perceptions of adolescents' warmth at T2 were predicted by adolescents' reports of parents' warmth at T1 in cohort 2 (β =.10, $p < .05$).

What is striking about these analyses is that the more young people perceived how often political discussions took place with their parents at T1, the more their political interest increased over time, and the more parents perceived how often political discussions took place with their young people at T1, the more their political interest also increased over time. These predictions were found in cohort 1, at a time when parents' attempts to politically socialize their children seem to be most intense (see Chapter 5). They were not found in the older cohort. Second, the analyses do not show that adolescents' emotional relationships with their parents influence political discussions in the families. Third, surprisingly, parents' political interest at T2 was predicted by their perceptions of the political discussions at T1. This is analogous to McDevitt and Chaffee's (2000, 2002) findings that their children's political experiences in school spur parents' news viewing. Third, adolescents' political interest was predicted by their own perceptions of political talk, and parents' political interest was predicted by their own perceptions of political talk. Parents' and adolescents' perceptions of their shared political interactions do not overlap.

Discussion

For parents' socialization attempts to be successful, good parent-adolescent relations are needed (Grusec & Davidov, 2021), and frequent and open parent-adolescent communication about everyday issues is a key marker of such good relations (Kerr & Stattin, 2000). Whether good parent-adolescent relations are required for parent-adolescent communication about political and societal issues has been the research question here. We focused on changes that occurred over one year in everyday and political talks between 16-year-olds and their parents, and over two years for a sample of 13-year-olds. In line with the study hypotheses, good relations, defined as perceiving each other as warm, was the main factor behind everyday talks but political talks were primarily explained by the adolescents' and parents' respective political interests. There was little longitudinal evidence that everyday talks spilled over into political talks, and vice-versa. We conclude that good or bad emotional relations between parents and adolescents have little effect on how frequently parents and adolescents talk with each other about politics and society.

Parents and adolescents seem to live in different perceptual worlds when it comes to how they view their joint political interactions. In this study, the adolescents' political interest primarily affected their own perceptions of the frequency of political talks at home, and parents' political interest primarily affected their own perceptions of the frequency of political talks. Adolescents' reports of political talks at T1 predicted their reports of political talks at T2, and the same was found for parents' reports of political talks. That adolescents' and parents' perceptions are unique to them can also be seen in other ways. Parents and adolescents seem to be poor at recognizing each other's perceptions. For the political-talks and everyday-talks measures that we analyzed in this study, the raw correlations between adolescents' and parents' reports were .33 at the highest ($p < .001$). This is in line with many previous political-socialization studies. Parents' and adolescents' reports of how often they engage in political discussions with each other show low to at most moderate associations (Meadowcroft, 1986; Pacheco, 2008; Ritchie & Fitzpatrick, 1990; Saphir & Chaffee, 2002; Tims & Masland, 1985), and parents' political interest shows only low to moderate associations with their children's political interest (Jennings et al., 2009). Overall, it appears that adolescents' political interest strongly affects their own perceptions of political interactions with parents, and vice-versa for parents, and that adolescents and parents are far from perceiving their political interest and political talks in a similar way. They have their own unique ways of perceiving their common political interactions.

In this chapter, we have shown that the political interactions that take place at home are interpreted differently by parents and adolescents. Parents' perceptions of these political interactions are governed much by parents' own political interest, and adolescents' perceptions of these political interactions are governed much by the adolescents' own political interest. We found a similar pattern for normal, everyday talks between adolescents and parents. Parents' perceptions that their adolescents are warm toward them longitudinally predicts parents' judgments of how often they engage in everyday talks at home. Also, adolescents' perceptions that their parents are warm toward them predict longitudinally their judgments of how often they have everyday talks with their parents. In the first case, the political interactions are determined considerably by parents' and adolescents' respective political interests, while in the second case, concerning their views of how often everyday discussions take place, this type of interactions is more determined by the perceptions of each other's warmth toward them. Apparently, there is a need to try to understand the conditions that make adolescents' and parents' perceptions of their common everyday interactions similar and different from each other.

An understanding of political communication in the family has to include both adolescents' and parents' attentiveness to political issues. That adolescents' and parents' political interests substantially predict how frequently they perceive that they talk about politics and society with each other casts doubt on the family-communication-patterns model (Chaffee et al., 1973; McLeod & Chaffee, 1972; Stone & Chaffee, 1970), and on the validity of research into conversation and conformity orientations (Ritchie, 1991; Ritchie & Fitzpatrick, 1990). These lines of research have focused on how parents communicate their political values and attitudes to their children but have not considered the role that parents' political interest (and adolescents') play in political communication. It might matter a lot for how parents communicate political information to their children if the parents are highly politically interested or if they have little interest in politics. Hence, attending to the political interests of parents and adolescents may pave the way for more theoretically nuanced models of political communication in the family.

Several studies that have examined the intergenerational transmission of values have confirmed the moderating role that emotional parent-adolescent relationships play in such transmission. These studies have been based on the motivational values included in Shalom Schwartz's theory of basic human values (1994, 2016; Schwartz et al., 2012) or have included other more specific types of values, such as work obligation, hedonism, religious commitment, family obligation values, and educational aspirations (Roest et al., 2009; Taris & Semin, 1997; Tsai et al., 2015; Wu et al., 2018). Many of these values are likely to be values that most parents want to instill in their children. However, one can draw a different conclusion about political values and attitudes. Since we found that emotional parent-adolescent relationships were not much associated with political communication in the family, perhaps political values and attitudes should not be considered key topics for all parents to pass on to their children. The transmission of political and social information to their children may only be important for some parents, those who are highly politically interested themselves. One more thing: the previous intergenerational transmission studies were mainly cross-sectional, in contrast to our longitudinal analyses.

We used three covariates in the study: gender, immigrant background, and parents' education. Concerning these covariates, it is noteworthy that parents' educational level was primarily associated with parents' own political interest and parents' perceptions of the frequency of everyday and political talks. The extent to which parents' education was associated with adolescents' reports on the study variables was similar to the other two covariates—sex and immigrant background. This is a first indication that the level of education of the parents does not automatically translate into a political interest on the part of their children.

In the final analyses we examined the reverse direction of effects over one year for the older cohort and over two years for the younger cohort. In the younger cohort, parents' perceptions of the frequency of political talks positively predicted their political interest two years later. The same associations over time were found in the adolescents' reports. These are strong indications that political talks are motivational sources for political interest in early adolescence.

This study has implications for research on parent-child relations more generally. When adolescents report on their everyday and political talks with their parents, their reports are based on their own perceptual experiences. In line with the study hypothesis, adolescents' perceptions of parents' warmth toward them affect their perceptions of how often they have everyday talks, and their own political interest affects how often they perceive that political talks take place. When parents are the reporters, their reports are also based on their own perceptual experiences.

Their perceptions of how warm their adolescents are toward them affect their perceptions of how often they have everyday conversations with their adolescents, and parents' political interest affects their perceptions of the frequency of having political conversations with their adolescents. This also pertains to our findings about the reversed causality of political conversations. In the younger cohort, how often the adolescents perceived that they had political conversations with their parents positively affected their own future political interest, and how often parents perceived that they had political conversations with their adolescents positively affected their own future political interest. The potential problem is that adolescents' and parents' psychological experiences are not well matched, and there is little longitudinal evidence that adolescents' reports of political and everyday talks, warmth, and political interest affect parents' reports on these issues, and vice-versa. The conclusion is that researchers need to realize that adolescents' and their parents' reports about their common interactions—about everyday life and political issues—are perceptual experiences that often do not converge and should not be used as unbiased indicators of family interactions. This is a common problem in research on parent-child relations: attributing what happens in the family to either children's or parents' perceptions. The problem of using one family member's perceptions as valid indicators of what happens in the family not only applies to political science research but extends to the social sciences and beyond (De Los Reyes, 2013).

No prior study has contrasted everyday and political communications in adolescents' families. It is the main strength of the current study that it proposes and confirms that it is adolescents' and parents' political interests that primarily affect their political communication at home, and that emotional parent-child relations have only a limited role to play. By contrast, emotional relations between parents and adolescents affect communications about everyday matters. The findings are robust in that they apply to both parents' and adolescents' reports and that a longitudinal design was used with two age cohorts of adolescents.

Conclusion

Good relations between parents and adolescents, as represented by regular and open communication at home, are regarded as fundamental to parents' successful socialization of their children. We proposed that talks about political and societal issues are highly dependent upon parents' and adolescents' political interests but less so on their good relations. The results also show that the communication that parents and adolescents have about political and societal issues is very much based on their respective political interests, but that emotional parent-adolescent relations do not affect these political talks much. It seems as if the transmission of political and societal information to their children is particularly important for highly politically interested parents. In sum, an understanding of political communication at home needs to attend to the specific motivational source that distinguishes political socialization from general socialization, namely, the political interests of parents and adolescents. We conclude that well-functioning and harmonious parent-adolescent relations are not the particular foundation upon which the effectiveness of parents' political socialization attempts are based (c.f. Grusec & Davidov, 2021).

School

Explaining Adolescent Political Activity in the Classroom

Adolescents may enjoy their time at school. They may like their classmates and teachers and be satisfied with their schoolwork. Some of them may see themselves as politically active in the classroom. Their emotional bonding to school may explain, to some extent, their willingness to be politically active in the classroom. Alternatively, they may be influenced by teachers' attempts to initiate political discussions in class and be receptive to teachers' political communication. Emotional attachment to school and perceptions of teachers' political initiatives are two rival explanations for being politically active in class relative to their own political interest. Also, emotional attachment to school and perceptions of teachers' political initiatives may moderate the relationship between political interest and classroom political activity.

We did not find much evidence that the adolescents' emotional relationship with their parents influenced their political discussions with their parents. Transferred to school, there is little reason to believe that emotional attachment to school plays a role in their political activities in the classroom compared to their general political interest. The perception of having teachers who bring up political issues and being receptive to these attempts by their teachers is, however, potentially a more direct explanation for adolescents' political activities in the classroom. In cohort 1 and cohort 2 we measured emotional bonding to school and perceptions of teachers' political initiatives and examined whether they provided additional explanations for classroom political activity beyond political interest. Four different scales measured emotional attachment or bonding to school and two scales measured perceptions of teachers' political initiatives. These scales are presented in Table 8.4.

Principal component analyses of the measures of emotional attachment to school and teachers' political initiatives yielded two factors for both cohorts (see Table 8.5). All the scales loaded either on the bonding factor or teacher factor for the two age cohorts, with the exception that the Like Teachers scale loaded on both factors for the 13-year-olds. The factor scores were retained and, together with the adolescents' political interest, predicted change in political activity from ages 13 to 14 and from ages 16 to 17. The effects of gender and immigration status were controlled.

TABLE 8.4 Scales measuring emotional attachment to school and perceptions of teachers' political initiatives.

Content	*Number of items*	*Response scale*
Political interest "How interested are you in politics?"	1	1 (*totally uninterested)* 4 (*very interested*)
Political activities in class "Have you brought up things that have to do with the environment (recycling, saving energy, etc.) during class?" "Have you ever brought up political issues during class?" "Has it happened that you have brought up a societal problem for discussion during class?" "Has it happened that you have brought something that has to do with climate change during class?" Cronbach alpha was .90 for cohort 1 and .88 for cohort 2.	4	1 (*has never happened*) 5 (*very often*)
Like class "I feel alone and like a stranger in my class" (rev.), "We help each other in my class," "There are classmates who harass me" (rev.), "We are nice to each other in my class," "There are classmates who bully me" (rev.), "We like to do things together in my class." Cronbach alpha was .75 for cohort 1 and .76 for cohort 2.	6	1 (*absolutely disagree)* 4 (*absolutely agree*)
Like teachers "Most of my teachers treat me fairly," "Most of my teachers listen to what I have to say," "Most teachers are keen that their students feel good." Cronbach alpha was .76 for cohort 1 and .78 for cohort 2.	3	1 (*absolutely disagree)* 4 (*absolutely agree*)
Satisfied with schoolwork "How do you like it in school?" "Do you do the best that you can in school?" "Do you feel like you are forced to go to school?" "How would you describe the relationship between yourself and school?" "Are you satisfied with how it's going for you in school?" Cronbach alpha was .72 for cohort 1 and .76 for cohort 2.	5	1 (*very bad*) to 5 (*very good*) 1 (*almost never*) to 5 (*usually*) 1 (*most often*) to 5 (*almost never*) 1 (*as enemies*) to 5 (as best friends) 1 (*almost never*) to 5 (*usually*)

(*Continued*)

TABLE 8.4 (Continued)

Content	*Number of items*	*Response scale*
Teachers' political initiatives		
"There are teachers at my school who try to involve students in discussions about political issues," "There are teachers at my school who try to encourage students to become more aware of environmental issues," "There are teachers at my school who try to encourage students to become more aware of what is going on in the world?" Cronbach alpha was .86 for cohort 1 and .88 for cohort 2.	3	1 (*doesn't apply at all*) 4 (*applies very well*)
Susceptible to teachers' communication		
I have teachers who "Talk about politics and societal issues in a way that makes them fun and interesting," "Talk about things that happen in the world and in society in such a way that I become curious and want to know more," "Talk about the news they have heard on TV or read about in a way that evokes strong feelings in me." Cronbach alpha was .87 for cohort 1 and .89 for cohort 2.	3	1 (*definitely doesn't apply*) 4 (*applies very well*)

TABLE 8.5 Principal component analysis with varimax rotation for measures of bonding to school and perceptions of teacher political initiatives.

	Age 13		*Age 16*	
	bonding	teacher	bonding	teacher
Like school	.77	−.04	.80	−.01
Like class	.77	−.08	.76	.04
Like teachers	.60	.44	.70	.04
Satisfied with schoolwork	.66	.29	.69	.21
Teachers initiate discussions	−.04	.79	.08	.86
Susceptible to teachers' communication	.14	.75	.15	.86

The results are presented in Figure 8.4. As can be seen in this figure, neither emotional bonding to school nor teachers' political initiatives significantly predicted adolescents' political activity in class for the two cohorts. Only political interest was a significant predictor for both cohorts. We found a significant moderator, but with a negative sign. Among the highly politically interested adolescents,

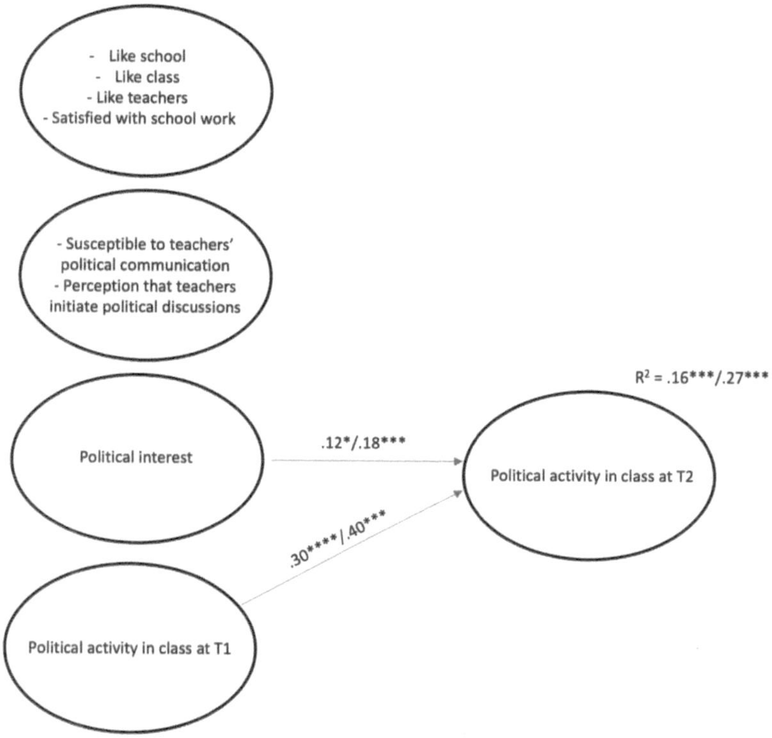

The first figure is for Cohort 1 and the second for Cohort 2. The effects of sex and immigration status were controlled for, but are not presented above for brevity purpose.

FIGURE 8.4 Prediction of adolescents' political activity in the classroom.

those with high emotional bonding to school reported less political activity than the politically interested adolescents with low emotional bonding (high PI group: $B = -.14$, $t = -3.07$, $p < .01$). No differences were found among the low politically interested adolescents (low PI group: $B = .02$, $t = .63$, $p > .05$). We conclude that, as with the home environment, adolescents' emotional bonding to school does not explain how often adolescents bring up political and social issues in class, nor, apparently, do adolescents' perceptions of their teachers' political initiatives in the classroom or their own susceptibility to teachers' political communication.

A sense of belonging in school, feeling accepted and respected in class, and feeling supported by teachers are important interpersonal conditions for students' academic motivation and achievement (Goodenow, 1993; Roeser et al., 1996). However, we did not find much evidence that adolescents' sense of belonging to school influences their initiatives to bring up political discussions in class. It is the political aspect, their political interest, not the affective, that seems to shape adolescents' political discussions in class.

Spillover Effects From Home to School and From School to Home

With the design we have used to find out whether it is the political or the affective, or both aspects, that are effective in understanding adolescents' classroom political activity, we have the opportunity to address another type of research question that has often been raised in political socialization research: the spillover effects of political discussion from one milieu to another.

In a series of seminal studies, McDevitt, Chaffee, and colleagues challenged the conventional parent-adolescent view of family discussions. They proposed that a newly awakened political interest in school could change young persons' political interactions with their parents (McDevitt & Chaffee, 2000, 2002; Saphir & Chaffee, 2002). Specifically, school-induced political interest in a particular issue may motivate adolescents to bring up these experiences in the family context and spur parents to acquire more information. These studies, based on quasi-experimental designs and election-related classroom exposure, confirmed that students' political experiences in school spill over into adolescent-initiated discussions at home, and that these discussions change the family communication patterns.

Civic education in school may change some adolescents' interest in politics, but a powerful event such as an upcoming election, when discussed in class, can increase many students' political interest and encourage them to discuss this event with their parents at home. McDevitt and coauthors have argued that it takes a more dramatic event, such as an upcoming political election, for political experiences at school to transfer to the home because the majority of adolescents are not interested in politics (McDevitt & Chaffee, 2000; Kiousis et al., 2005).

This raises the question of whether, under normal circumstances, adolescents' political discussions in their classrooms tend to influence their political discussions with their parents, or whether the reverse is to be expected. To our knowledge, there is no empirical information on these spillover effects from school to home and from home to school. But there are reasons to believe that spillovers of political discussions from home to school are to be expected. First, the school experiences triggered by a campaign may be situational and may not have lasting effects on students' intrinsic political interest. Thus, what happens at home in the short term may not persist over time. Second, as Devitt and colleagues have repeatedly emphasized, the uniqueness of the home is that the family environment is a safe training ground for political discussion (McDevitt, 2006). Most youths should feel free to express their views and experiences, should experience social and political support, and should not feel embarrassed for expressing their opinions at home.

As we showed in Chapter 5, when the 13- and 16-year-olds were asked "Have you ever tried to start a discussion with your parents about a social or political issue? How did they usually react?" the majority of those who had initiated such discussions at home reported that their parents responded positively. At home, in a supportive and emotionally safe environment, young people can receive good feedback on their political and social views, be encouraged to think critically, and develop a sense of what is central and what is peripheral. They will have time to ask questions, develop counter-arguments to their parents' views, and build an argumentative competence. In short, adolescents should feel ready to express their views in other everyday settings now that their arguments have passed those of their parents. The views and attitudes that adolescents develop under safe conditions at home are likely to be different from the school environment, where conflicts between viewpoints may arise and criticism from classmates, and the risk of ridicule, and public embarrassment may silence students (Hess, 2002; Hess & McAvoy, 2014) (see Chapter 4 for characteristics of students who developed political reputations in the classroom). Overall, *under normal conditions*, we would expect that argumentative competence on a variety of issues developed at home should spill over into raising these issues in classroom discussions, rather than that adolescents' experiences of their political activity in the classroom are transferred to the home.

Analyses

Here, both adolescents' own reports of political activity in the classroom and their political reputations as judged by their peers are two critical features of adolescents' political activity in the classroom. We conducted a model to estimate the spillover effects over 1 year between adolescents' political activities in class and their political reputation and the frequency of political discussions at home. In an autoregressive cross-lagged (ARCL) model, the three study variables at T2 were regressed on the same variables at T1, estimating both stability coefficients of each variable over one year and change coefficients representing the aforementioned spillover effects from one study variable to another over one year. We looked separately at the 13-year-olds and the 16-year-olds. The ARCL model included students' gender and immigration status as control variables and was tested using multilevel modeling with students nested within their classroom membership at T2. The results of these analyses are presented in Figure 8.5.

First, in line with our hypothesis, adolescents' political discussions with their parents influenced their political activities in the classroom in both cohorts. Adolescents' perceptions of being politically active in the classroom did not spill over to political discussions with parents at home. This was the case in both cohorts. What we did not expect was the role of having a political reputation in the classroom. This political reputation, based on classmates' perceptions of particular students' political knowledge and ability to express that knowledge in class, positively influenced political discussions at home between adolescents and parents. This was found for both 13- and 16-year-olds. In addition, for 13-year-olds, political reputation in class positively predicted perceptions of students' own political activity in class, and for 16-year-olds, perceptions of students' political activity in class positively predicted political reputation.

Perceptions of one's political activity in the classroom and one's political reputation in the classroom appear to have fundamentally different consequences for

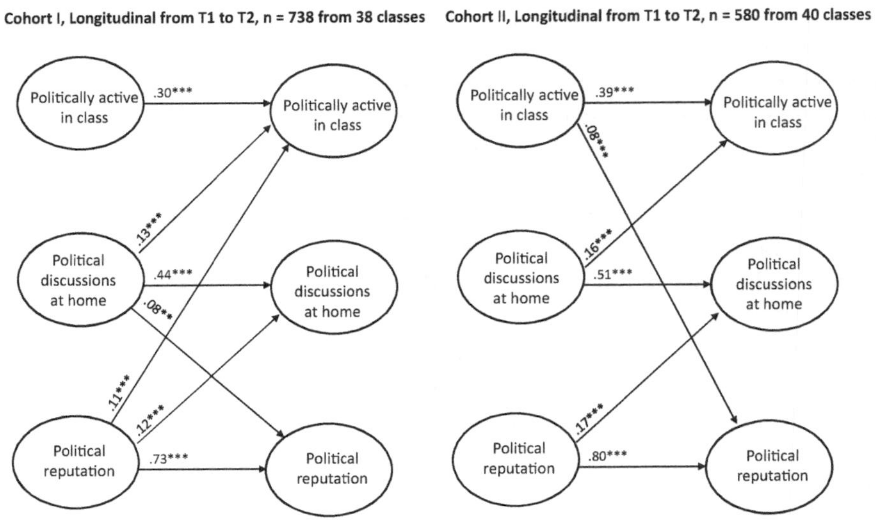

FIGURE 8.5 Analyses of the spillover from political discussions at home to political discussions at school and vice versa.

political discussions at home. First, the more often students discussed political activities with their parents, the more they perceived themselves as politically active in class. But political discussions at home did not affect their political reputation in class. Second, perceptions of being politically active in class were not associated with political discussions at home over time. In contrast, having a political reputation in class was associated with frequent political discussions with parents. These associations over time were found for both age cohorts.

Conclusion

We examined the spillover effects of political discussions at home on political discussions at school and vice versa. Political discussions at home stimulate adolescents' political discussions at school. The reverse was not found. It is probably the case that strong political experiences at school, such as class discussions about an upcoming election, have the consequence that students will bring it up with their parents at home. However, the spillover effects of exposure to strong political information at school, as found in the studies by McDevitt and coauthors (McDevitt & Chaffee, 2000, 2002; Saphir & Chaffee, 2002), are probably not representative of what happens on a daily basis. McDevitt and coauthors' findings represent what *can* happen at home when a current dramatic event is highlighted in school, but in the normal course of events, students are likely to bring their political discussions with parents to political discussions in their classrooms. Further, the students who have a political reputation in their classrooms seem to be the students who do bring input from school to political discussions with parents. Potentially, the classroom context is a special training ground for them. They seem to have the specific personal and social characteristics that make them stand out and deal with potentially negative reactions and lack of support from classmates. The students who have high political reputations in the classroom at one age are largely the same students who will have high political reputations the next year. This political reputation is already crystallized by age 13. Thus, high political interest in early adolescence, as manifested in public recognition of political competence in the classroom (Chapter 4), spills over into political discussions at home. Political reputation in the classroom is an important—but largely unknown to the field of political socialization—social manifestation of a political skill that spills over into the home.

Finally, what is the evidence that young people are active agents in their own political development?

- Adolescents' political interest affects how often they perceive that they talk about politics with their parents. Parents' political interest affects how often they perceive that they talk about politics with their adolescents. Adolescents' perceived emotional relationships with parents are related to how often they perceive that they have everyday conversations with their parents. This is also true for parents. The emotional relationships, perceived by parents, are related to how often parents perceive that they have everyday conversations with their adolescents.
- Adolescents' emotional bonding to school, their perception of teachers' political initiatives in the classroom, or their susceptibility to teachers' political communication in the classroom do not affect how often they consider themselves politically active in the classroom, but their political interest does affect their political activity at school.

PART IV

"We Do Not See Things as They Are, We See Them as We Are"

9

PROJECTION OF LIFE VALUES AND POLITICAL DISCUSSIONS IN FAMILIES

Highlights

When adolescents' values are compared with their parents' values, the associations are typically low. However, when adolescents are asked to report on their parents' values, the associations between their own values and their parents' values are systematically much higher. This chapter tests the idea that adolescents' and parents' perceptions of each other's life values are systematically biased. This bias, or projection, leads adolescents to believe that their parents' values are close to their own. Parents do the same. They believe that their adolescents' values are similar to their own. However, the associations between parents' perceptions of their adolescents' values and their adolescents' reported values are small.

We propose that a similar perceptual bias affects adolescents' and parents' perceptions of their joint political interactions. How often political discussions take place and how politically supportive their parents are is strongly colored by the adolescents' political interest. Similarly, the frequency of political discussions according to parents and the extent to which parents are politically supportive of the adolescent is strongly colored by parents' political interest. In reality, there is little agreement between how adolescents and parents perceive their political interactions.

Projection of Life Values

Adolescents' perceptions of their parents' values are key to their adoption of parental values. Values are considered internalized when children correctly perceive their parents' values and have decided to adopt them as their own (Knafo & Schwartz, 2003, 2009). One problem is that adolescents do not seem to know much about their parents' values. In Chapter 7, we found among 13- and 16-year-olds that there were low correlations between adolescents' and parents' perceptions of their shared political interactions. The same lack of convergence was found for specific socio-political attitudes and values.

In this chapter, we argue that adolescents' views of their parents' values may be systematically biased. Parents' views of their adolescents' values may also be

DOI: 10.4324/9781003371731-13

systematically biased. As a result, the values that adolescents hold and the values that their parents hold will not match. Parents and adolescents will live in different value worlds.

Projection

It is common sense that one's perceptions reflect reality, but the literature suggests that perceptions can be biased. Social psychology has long shown that one's perceptions of the social context contain systematic biases (e.g., Ross et al., 1977; Marks & Miller, 1987; Krueger, 1998; West & Kenny, 2011). One of the most common perceptual biases is projection, the coloring of a person's perception of others' attributes by his or her own attributes (Kenny & Acitelli, 2001; Schul & Vinokur, 2000). As a result of projection, people tend to perceive others as more similar to themselves than they actually are. This bias has been studied using a variety of terms, including assumed similarity (Cronbach, 1955), false consensus (Ross et al., 1977), similarity/attribute projection (Holmes, 1968), pluralistic ignorance (Katz & Allport, 1931), and egocentric attribution (Heider, 1958).

Motivational and cognitive reasons have been proposed to explain why people project (Cameron, 2009; Gniewosz et al., 2008; Marks & Miller, 1987). Motivational reasons for projection focus on the benefits people derive from projecting their own attributes onto others. First, projection can help people maintain and enhance a positive sense of self. It has long been suggested that people seek to validate their own positions by attempting to establish that they are similar to those held by surrounding others (Crano, 1983; Katz, 1960). Because people are likely to feel positive about themselves when their own positions are supported by others (Taylor & Brown, 1988), they construct social support by inflating the perceived similarity between themselves and others (Marks & Miller, 1987). Second, projection may have emotional benefits. When people make inferences about others' attributes, they are likely to experience psychological discomfort due to uncertainty (Hogg & Mullin, 1999) or potential inconsistencies between themselves and others (Cameron, 2009; Festinger, 1957; Harmon-Jones, 2002; Stiff, 1994). Projection then appears to be an easy way for people to alleviate psychological discomfort, as an assumed similarity between oneself and others reduces uncertainty and inconsistency.

The cognitive bases of projection are concerned with cognitive strategies for processing information. From a cognitive-heuristic point of view, projection is a cognitive strategy that provides a shortcut to quick judgments when people make inferences about partially or completely unknown attributes of others (Tversky & Kahneman, 1973). In making such judgments, people rely on a few available cues rather than all available information (Marsh et al., 2004), and these few cues are likely to reflect their own attributes because they are easily accessible (Clement & Krueger, 2000; Marks & Miller, 1987). Egocentric cognitive processes also provide a theoretical explanation for why the similarity between one's own attributes and the perception of others' attributes is inflated. For example, Sherif and Hovland (1961) proposed that people use their own perspective as an anchor when considering the perspective of others. They adjust their perspective according to this anchor, but because the adjustment is usually completed early in the process, it results in greater perceived than actual similarity between themselves and others (Epley et al., 2004). Similarly, Mussweiler (2003) proposed "similarity testing" as a cognitive strategy for social comparison. In similarity testing, people selectively process information in a way that emphasizes similarity. Similarly, some scholars suggest that people tend to expose themselves to information that is consistent with their own positions (Cotton & Hieser, 1980; D'Alessio & Allen, 2002). All of these explanations suggest that there are internal motivational forces and cognitive mechanisms that lead people to see others as similar to themselves.

Projection has a long history in psychology (Holmes, 1968). In developmental research, projection bias has been examined particularly in research on peer deviance. Within the peer deviance literature, a substantial number of studies have reported strong associations between adolescents' own deviance and perceptions of their peers' deviant behavior, concluding that adolescents' deviance is strongly influenced by their friends' deviance and is a socially learned behavior (Akers, 2009). However, only small to moderate associations have been found between adolescents' own deviance and their friends' reports of their deviant behavior (Haynie & Osgood, 2005; Kandel, 1978). Some studies were able to distinguish whether adolescents' perceptions of peer deviance were shared by their friends, whether there was a social influence of friends' values and behaviors over and above shared environmental influences, and whether adolescents projected their own values and behaviors onto their friends (Jussim & Osgood, 1989; Young et al., 2014). These studies found that adolescents projected their own delinquent behaviors onto their friends, that their perceptions of peer deviance were not accurate, and that their perceptions of peer deviance did not influence their own behaviors over time. In short, a central message of these studies is that there is a strong projection effect when adolescents perceive their friends' deviant values.

Accurate Perception and Projection

As we reported in Chapter 7, with the exception of partisan identification, early studies of political socialization found small to moderate correlations between adolescents' values and sociopolitical views and their parents' values and views (Connell, 1972; Jennings & Niemi, 1968, 1974; Tedin, 1974). Similar small to moderate correlations between parents and adolescents have been reported in later studies (Geißler, 1996; Gniewosz & Noack, 2006; Noack, 2001; Oswald & Schmid, 2006; Patterson et al., 2019; ter Bogt et al., 2001; Vollebergh et al., 2001). The implication of these studies is that adolescents' attitudes and values do not strongly reflect their parents' attitudes and values, and that the intergenerational transmission of values from parents to children is limited.

When adolescents report the values and attitudes they perceive their parents to hold, the correlations with the values and attitudes the adolescents themselves hold are often significantly higher (Acock & Bengtson, 1980; Gniewosz & Noack, 2006; Gniewosz et al., 2008; Ojeda & Hatemi, 2015; Whitbeck & Gecas, 1988). Thus, in adolescents' minds, their parents' values are similar to their own. Similarly, in parents' minds, their children's values are similar to their own (Whitbeck & Gecas, 1988). These two very different conclusions require explanation, and a parsimonious explanation seems to be that adolescents tend to project their own values onto their parents, and that parents do the same.

Back in 1980, Acock and Bengtson showed that young people aged 16 to 26 perceived that their mothers' attitudes, a wide range of political attitudes, were close to their own. In reality, the attitudes reported by their mothers showed little correspondence with the young people's attitudes. Commenting on the lack of congruence, the authors speculated that

> if the child's perceptions are accurate, there is less cause for concern on the part of researchers relying on data from only one generation. If, on the other hand, the children do not attribute the correct opinions to their parents, this is of major significance to socialization theory and research practice (p. 507).

Acock and Bengtson suggested that the explanation for the low correspondence was misattribution: "children simply do not know their parents' opinions" (p. 507). Our explanation is different. Youth project their own values and attitudes onto their parents.

To uncover projection, accurate perceptions and projections must be modeled (Tedin, 1974; Westholm, 1999). Projection is typically estimated by the strength of the relationship between one's own attributes and perceptions of others' attributes after accounting for accuracy (e.g., Kenny & Acitelli, 2001; Murray et al., 1996). For example, in a study reported by Gniewosz and Noack (2006), the authors examined adolescents' attitudes toward foreigners and their perceptions of their parents' attitudes. They found a high degree of projection (.78 for mothers and .74 for fathers) and a low degree of accuracy (.15 for mothers and .22 for fathers) in adolescents' perceptions of their parents' attitudes.

If adolescents project their own values onto their parents, this raises the intriguing question of whether parents also tend to project their values onto adolescents. We will model both adolescents' and parents' perceptions of each other's values simultaneously.

Life Values

We focus on broad life values. These values were selected from the values in Shalom Schwartz's theory of fundamental human values (1994, 2016; Schwartz et al., 2012). In this theory, universal values include people's societal concerns, such as protecting the well-being of all people ("universalism-societal concerns") and their desire to protect nature ("universalism-protecting nature"). We examined these values and also included a measure of achievement values. Achievement values include more self-focused values that have the underlying motivation of "personal success through demonstration of competence according to social standards" (Schwartz, 1992, p. 4).

We decided to focus on the 16-year-olds. They should be able to grasp the abstract ideas and value orientations included in our list of universal and achievement values. Following the stem question, "How important is the following to you?" both the 16-year-old adolescents and their parents (n = 518 dyads) were presented with a list of value statements:

Concern for other people's welfare. "Equality, equal opportunities for all people"; "A peaceful world free from war and conflicts"; "Helping other people"; "Social justice, fighting injustice, and caring about the less fortunate in society"; and "Working together with others for a better society."

Concern for nature. "Respecting nature and thinking ecologically"; "Protecting the environment and preserving nature"; and "Preventing pollution of the environment and not wasting resources."

Achievement values. Adolescents reported on the statements "Always doing my best"; "Working hard on school work"; "Studying so that I get good grades"; and "Learning new things." Parents reported on the statements "Always doing our best"; "Working hard to achieve the goals we have set"; "Getting better at what we do"; "Being among the better ones at what we do"; and "Learning new things."

The response scale ranged from 1 (*not at all important*) to 5 (*very important*).

Analyses and Results

Using MPlus (Muthén & Muthén, 1998–2012), four confirmatory factor analyses were conducted in which the three life values (concern for other people's welfare, concern for nature, and achievement values) were constructed as latent variables: adolescents' own values, their perception of parents' values, parents' own values, and parents' perception of adolescents' values. We then tested two models. One was where adolescents' and parents' perceptions of each other's life values could be explained by their accurate perceptions (Figure 9.1, model a), and the second model added projection coefficients to the first model (Figure 9.1, model b). For all three types of values, the differences in the χ^2 tests between the two models were significant at the $p < .001$ level, indicating that adolescents' and parents' perceptions represent both accurate perception and projection bias. The results for model b are shown in Figure 9.2.

As shown in Figure 9.2, adolescents tend to project their life values onto their parents, and they did not accurately report their parents' values. All associations

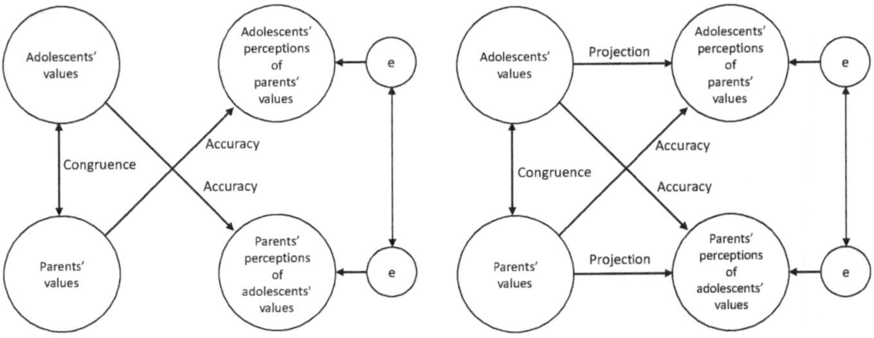

Model a. Perception as a reflection of accurate perception.

Model b. Perception as a combination of accuracy and projection.

FIGURE 9.1 Competing value models.

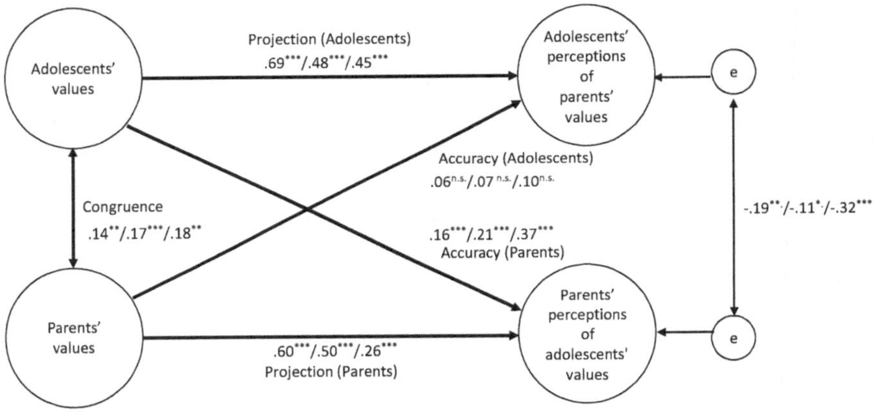

FIGURE 9.2 Final model for interpersonal value perceptions between parents and adolescents. Coefficients are standardized and are shown in order: Concern for other' welfare, Concern for nature, and Achievement values.

n.s., not significant.

$^{*}p < .05$, $^{**}p < .01$, $^{***}p < 001.$

between their perceptions of their parents' values and their own values were not significant. Parents also failed to accurately report their adolescents' values, but the associations in these cases were all significant—but small. For parents, projection was high for the values of concern for others' welfare and concern for nature, with projection estimates of .60, $p < .001$, and .50, $p < .001$, and low accuracy estimates of .16, $p < .001$, and .21, $p < .001$. However, less evidence for projection was found for achievement values. The projection estimate was only .26, $p < .001$, and the accuracy was higher, at .37, $p < .001$.

Discussion

Parents and adolescents do not accurately perceive each other's views on life values. In our study, levels of accuracy were low. For the most part, adolescents projected their own life values onto their parents, and parents did the same, but to a lesser extent. This means that the intergenerational transmission of values from parents to children does not work as expected. The value socialization model also seems problematic in that it assumes that children must accurately perceive their parents' values before they can choose to adopt those values or not (Grusec & Goodnow, 1994). We have reported in previous chapters that adolescents tend to be open to their parents' views, and if they can identify these views, they are likely to internalize them. The problem with the value socialization idea is that adolescents do not seem to know much about their parents' life values. In fact, the agreement in values between adolescents and parents was low, ranging from .02 to .14 for 13-year-olds and from .09 to .40 four years later. These findings of low accuracy and high degree of projection are consistent with an earlier study by Gniewosz and Noack (2006), and also with Westholm's (1999), both of which found that adolescents see a close correspondence between their own and their parents' views, but have views that are not very consistent with their parents' views.

The striking finding is that parents also project their life values onto their adolescents. This was the case for the values of concern for others and concern for nature, but less evidence of projection was found for achievement values. It may be surprising to find that parents project their life values onto their children. Note, however, that projection is most likely to occur in close relationships, such as between spouses. The literature on intimate relationships suggests that the effort to attend to each other's arguments diminishes in long-term relationships, in part because partners assume they know each other fairly well (Gagne' & Lydon, 2004; Kenny & Acitelli, 2001).

Projection is likely to be stronger for broader and more abstract life values than for more concrete and familiar issues. The life values of concern for the welfare of all people and concern for nature are more abstract values than specific achievement values, and it is for achievement values that we see that parents' projection bias is lower than for concern for the welfare of all people and concern for nature. It should be particularly important for parents to be involved in their adolescents' academic performance. Recall that in Chapter 5, parents reported that the most frequent topic of conversation with their adolescents was "school, school work, and homework." However, the level of accurate assessment of their adolescents' achievement values is rather low, given the high level of discussion of these topics at home.

In speculation, projection bias may undermine adolescents' and parents' accurate perceptions of each other's values and undermine adolescents' adoption of their parents' values. That projection may be a barrier to successful attitude transmission was originally proposed by Gniewosz et al. (2008). If adolescents believe that they are quite similar to their parents, they are likely to consolidate their current value orientations and have little incentive to make efforts to explore and adapt to their parents' orientations. Thus, projection runs the risk of leaving adolescents to their own value worlds.

The same is true for parents, of course. They also run the risk of becoming stuck in their biased perceptions of their adolescents' life values. If parents see their adolescents as largely similar to themselves, they may view their efforts to teach values as successful and see no need for intervention. In short, parents may refrain from engaging in values discussions with their adolescents because they perceive their adolescents as having roughly the same values as they do.

The overall conclusion is that adolescents' and parents' perceptions of each other's life values are affected by projection biases that undermine accurate perceptions. Biased perceptions lead adolescents and parents to believe that the world as they see it is also the world as the other person sees it. They fail to see the differences and risk becoming trapped in their own value worlds.

Therefore, researchers need to recognize that adolescents' and their parents' reports of their shared interactions—about everyday life and political issues—might be idiosyncratic psychological experiences that often do not converge and are not unbiased indicators of those interactions. It is a common bias in research to attribute what happens in the family to either children's or parents' reports. The problem of using only one family member's perceptions as a valid indicator of the other is not unique to political science research, but extends to the social sciences in general, for example, a recent study in psychiatry entitled "Parents Still Matter! Parental Warmth Predicts Adolescent Brain Function and Anxiety and Depressive Symptoms 2 Years Later" (Butterfield et al., 2021). In this study, parents did not report on their warmth. It was the adolescents in the study who provided information about their parents' warmth. Perhaps not surprisingly, when their parents do not express much warmth toward them, these adolescents generally become more anxious and depressed over time.

Projections of Political Discussions in Families

Let us go one step further. A key conclusion from research on parent-adolescent political discussions is that adolescents' interest in politics benefits from political discussions with their parents and from the support they receive from their parents for their political development. In their discussions about politics and society with their adolescents, parents transfer their political interests, attitudes, and values to their offspring (Andolina et al., 2003; Lake Snell Perry and Associates, 2002; McIntosh et al., 2007). The more often parents engage in joint political discussions, the more adolescents benefit from parents' political knowledge and experience. Empirical studies show that these discussions about politics and society in the home affect several aspects of adolescents' political attitudes and behaviors. The more often political issues are discussed in the family, the more politically literate adolescents become. Here, we will examine an alternative interpretation to this common belief about the role of political discussion, namely that adolescents tend to project their own political interests onto their political interactions with their parents, both in terms of the frequency of joint political discussions and their perceptions of parental support for their political activities.

First, consider the convergence between adolescents' and parents' reports of the frequency of political discussions at home. As we have seen earlier in this book, these are typically small (Meadowcroft, 1968; Meeusen, 2014; Pacheco, 2008), and there are also small correlations between communication styles related to political discussions in the family between adolscents' and parent reports (Ritchie & Fitzpatrick, 1990; Saphir & Chaffee, 2002; Tims & Masland, 1985). None of the studies reported strong convergences. In short, adolescents' perceptions of the frequency of family discussions of political issues and family communication orientations do not converge significantly with those of their parents.

Next, consider the predictive power of the frequency of political discussions between adolescents and parents on adolescent attitudes and behaviors. The frequency of discussions about political and social issues at home has been significantly associated with adolescents' political interest (Levinsen & Yndigegn, 2015; Warner & Warner Colander, 2016); attention to news (Shehata & Amnå, 2017); political knowledge (McIntosh et al., 2007); volunteering, civic engagement, and political participation (Boyd et al., 2011; Wray-Lake & Sloper, 2016); and later voting (Anderson & Goodyear-Grant, 2008). Overall, there seems to be strong empirical support for the idea that engaging in political discussions with parents makes adolescents more politically sophisticated.

The problem with these studies is that they are all based on adolescent reports. Adolescents report how often they discuss political issues with their parents, and they report their own political interest, attention to news, political knowledge, and political activity. In adolescents' minds, the frequency of political discussions at home is consistent with their political interest.

The key question is: How do we simultaneously explain the low convergence of adolescents' and parents' opinions about the frequency of political discussions while accepting the various findings in the literature that adolescents' perceptions of the frequency of these discussions are indeed strongly related to many different characteristics of adolescents' political sophistication? The low concordance between adolescents' and parents' perceptions has been explained by adolescents' lack of precise definitions of political issues (Fitzgerald, 2013) and by social desirability (Prior, 2019). However, we argue that a good reason for the differences between adolescents' and parents' perceptions is projection, the idea that people tend to believe that other people have similar attitudes, values, beliefs, and perceptions to their own (Krueger, 1998).

Previous research on projection shows that people's own motivations and ideals color their interpersonal perceptions (Lemay et al., 2010; Maner et al., 2005). This has been the explanation in the peer deviance literature: adolescents project their own deviance onto their friends (Jussim & Osgood, 1989; Young et al., 2014). We propose that adolescents' own political interest colors their perceptions of family political discussions and the political support they receive from their parents, and that the same perceptual bias applies to parents. Thus, both parents' and adolescents' political interest will drive their perceptions of the frequency of their political interactions with each other, but adolescents' and parents' perceptions will show low agreement. This perceptual bias may explain the finding in previous studies that adolescents' perceptions of the frequency of family communication about political issues have limited agreement with parents' perceptions, but on the other hand, there is high agreement between adolescents' perceptions of their own political interest and their perceptions of how often they have political discussions with their parents.

We will examine adolescents' and parents' perceptions of the frequency of joint political discussions and their perceptions of parental political support for adolescents' political development (see Figure 9.3), and we make the following three hypotheses:

- Adolescents' perceptions of the frequency of political discussions in the family and of their parents' political support derive mainly from their own political interest.
- The same projection bias applies to their parents.
- There is only limited overlap between adolescents' and parents' perceptions of their joint political discussions and parents' political support.

Information from the two youngest cohorts was used. All students in school records included 960 13-year-olds and 1,052 16-year-olds. The analysis samples were 904 in the younger cohort and 892 in the older cohort. In the younger cohort, 571 parents returned our questionnaires, and in the older cohort, 581 parents returned our questionnaires. Complete parent and youth data were available for 509 individuals in the younger cohort (56% of the analytic sample) and 541 in the older cohort (60%).

The following measures were used.

Political interest. In line with the notion that political interest has both cognitive and affective components (Prior, 2019; Silvia, 2008), we used two questions. First, the participants were asked "How interested are you in politics?" with response options ranging from 1 (*totally uninterested*) to 5 (*very interested*). Second, they were asked, "People differ in how they feel about politics. What are your feelings?" Here, the participants answered on a six-item response scale ranging from (1) *loath* to (6) *great fun*. The "interest" question was rescaled into a six-point scale and the two item scores were aggregated.

Parents were asked the following questions: "How interested are you in politics or societal issues? and "People in a household differ regarding what they feel about politics. What are your feelings?" The response scales were same as those for the

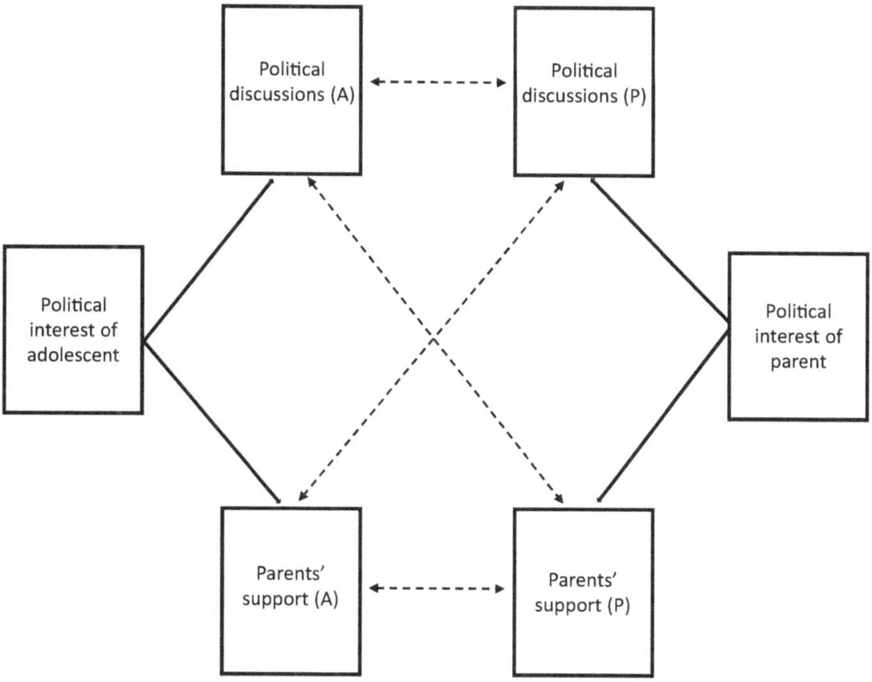

FIGURE 9.3 The conceptual model. Y represents adolescent reports and P represents parent reports. Solid lines represent our expectation of strong associations and dotted lines represent our expectation of weak associations.

adolescents. Questions about mothers' and fathers' interest and feelings about politics were asked separately. If only one parent participated in the study, he or she also provided responses for the non-participating parent.

Political discussions. The adolescents and their parents reported how often they discussed "What they had heard on the news about what is going on in Sweden and around the world" and "Politics or societal issues." The response scale ranged from 1 (*never*) to 4 (*very often*).

Parental support. A five-item scale reported by the adolescents measured the support of the parents for the political interest and involvement of the adolescents. First, it was designed to measure whether parents try to *raise the adolescents' awareness*: "Do your parents try to make you more aware of environmental issues?" and "Do your parents try to make you more aware of what is going on in the world?" Second, it tapped into whether parents were making *concrete suggestions for action*: "Suggest newspapers, books or websites where you can read about politics or societal issues," "Give me information about activities or organizations in which you can get engaged," and "Want me to sit down and watch the news on television with them." The response scale for the raising-awareness questions ranged from 1 (*no, never*) to 5 (*yes, almost always*) and for making concrete proposals for action from 1 (*definitely doesn't apply*) to 5 (*applies very well*). Factor analyses of the standardized items produced one factor with high factor loadings for both age cohorts.

Parents responded to the same five items, slightly reframed to assess their attempts to *raise their adolescents' awareness* and to establish whether they *make concrete proposals* for action (e.g., "We suggest newspapers, books or websites where our child can read about politics or societal issues"), with the same response scales as for the adolescents. Factor analyses of the standardized items produced one factor with high factor loadings in each age cohort.

Covariates. The main analyses controlled for parents' education, ranging from 1 (*less than 9 years*) to 5 (*university*), sex of participants (0 = female, 1 = male), and which parent(s) answered the questionnaires (47% mother, 10% father, 42% both parents together).

Results

A structural equation model was constructed in which adolescents' own political interest predicted their reports of political discussions with parents and parental support, while parents' own political interest predicted their reports of political discussions with their adolescents and their political support (see Figure 9.3). The effect of adolescents' political interest on both parents' views of political discussion and parental support and the effect of parents' political interest on both adolescents' views of political discussion and parental support were fixed at zero. All of these variables were included as latent variables generated by confirmatory factor analyses. Latent variables have the advantage of compressing many variables into a single factor representing the common variance of the variables under consideration and estimating measurement error. Latent variables can be interpreted as latent constructs underlying the set of observed variables under consideration. The model controlled for adolescent gender, age cohort, parental education, and source of parental report (mother, father, with "both" as the reference category). The model fit was good: $\chi^2(248) = 796.649$, $p < .001$, CFI = .923, TLI = .902, RMSEA = .046 [90% CI = .042, .049].

As shown in Figure 9.4, politically interested youth reported a high frequency of political discussions with their parents ($R^2 = .54$) and a high level of parental support for their political development ($R^2 = .31$). Similarly, politically interested parents reported frequent political discussions with their adolescents ($R^2 = .68$) and support for their political development ($R^2 = .46$). Apparently, both politically interested adolescents and parents tend to perceive a high frequency of political discussions and a high level of political support from their parents.

The residual correlations between adolescent-reported and parent-reported political discussions and support represent the degree of congruence between adolescent and parental reports after controlling for adolescent and parental political

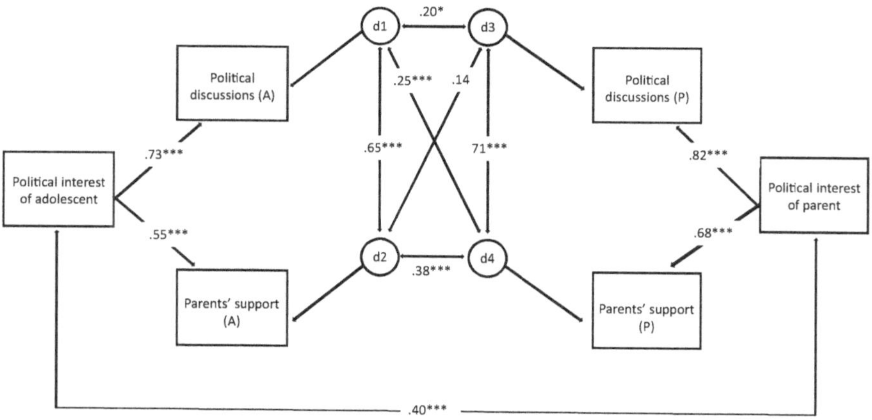

FIGURE 9.4 Multivariate multiple regression model. Standardized coefficients are shown.

* $p < .05$, ** $p < .01$, *** $p < .001$.

interest, adolescent gender, parental education, and the source of the parental report. These residual correlations show rather low congruence between parent- and adolescent-reported discussions and reported parental support for political development. This suggests that adolescents and parents have quite different views about how much they discuss politics with each other. Adolescents and parents show relatively greater agreement on the level of parental support for political development. However, the magnitude of the correlations between adolescents' and parents' reports are small. These findings are what would be expected if there were a projection bias in adolescents' and parents' reports.

Discussion

In Chapter 7, we reported that adolescents do not perceive their political interactions with parents in the same way that parents do. When adolescents were asked to report on their parents' political interest and knowledge, the frequency of political discussions at home, their parents' attempts to influence them politically, their parents' political support, and their own attempts to influence parents politically, there was little convergence between adolescents' and parents' perceptions on these issues. This was also the case for several sociopolitical issues such as attitudes toward immigrants, basic values such as concern for the welfare of others, concern for nature, and achievement values. Our findings do not differ from what has been reported previously in the literature. Empirical studies suggest that there is little agreement between the sociopolitical views of adolescents and their parents. In contrast, other studies have found moderate to high associations between the frequency of political discussions with parents and adolescents' political interest (Koskimaa & Rapeli, 2015; Oswald & Schmid, 1998; Schmid, 2012; Warner & Warner Colander, 2016).

The difference between these two sets of seemingly opposite findings can be explained by who is reporting. When adolescents report on their political discussions with parents and also report on various aspects of their political sophistication, high associations are found. However, when adolescents report on their political interactions with their parents and on various sociopolitical attitudes and values, there is little convergence with parents' reports. In essence, when information comes solely from adolescents' perceptions, various indicators of political sophistication are significantly associated with adolescents' political interest, but do not match their parents' reports.

We proposed that projection, a biased perception, can provide a parsimonious explanation for both sets of findings when it comes to joint political interactions. Here, adolescents' own political interest colors their perceptions of their political interactions with their parents—how often they have political discussions with their parents and their parents' political support. Thus, high associations are expected between adolescents' political interest and their perceptions of political interactions with parents. We suggested that the same projection might hold for parents. Parents' political interest will color their perceptions of how often they have political discussions with their adolescents and their own political support. However, because of the low to modest relationships between parents' and adolescents' political interest, their perceptions of joint political interactions will show low associations. In short, adolescents will not perceive their political interactions with parents in the same way that parents do. These suggestions were empirically confirmed, and no significant differences were found between the first and second cohorts.

The study goes beyond suggesting caution in expecting high levels of agreement between adolescents and parents in perceptions of the frequency of political discussion in the family. It adds to the literature an explanation for the divergences that have repeatedly been found between parents' and adolescents' reports of their joint political interactions. Previously, these low convergences have been explained by different definitions of what "politics" means to adolescents and parents (Fitzgerald, 2013; Tims & Masland, 1985) and by poor reliability of measures (Ritchie & Fitzpatrick, 1990). The projection explanation is a new, testable hypothesis that can be cross-validated in existing databases.

That political interest may color both adolescents' and parents' perceptions has implications for the broader issue of adolescents' internalization of their parents' views. For example, key to value socialization theory is adolescents' accurate perceptions and acceptance of their parents' views (Grusec & Goodnow, 1994). This model may not be fully applicable to political socialization research because, as we have argued here, adolescents' perceptions of and receptivity to their parents' political messages may be biased by their own political interests, and, as reported in Chapter 7, their perceptions of joint political interactions with their parents do not converge with their parents' perceptions.

There are two limitations to the idea of biased perceptions that we have proposed: the assumption of causality and support based on inference. First, the results of the tests of the projection hypothesis that we have presented are based on cross-sectional data. This precludes interpretations about directions of influence. However, according to the notion of projection, a projection bias that is present at one point in time is likely to be present at another point in time. Second, the analyses of projection effects were based on comparing parents' and adolescents' own unique perceptions of their joint interpersonal interactions with the correspondence that existed between their perceptions. Here, projection is based on inference. We infer projection from the expectation that adolescents' perceptions of how often they had political discussions with their parents and that their parents' political support will be strongly related to adolescents' own interest in politics, but will show less similarity to how often their parents report having political discussions with their adolescents and their political support. This is the same analytical approach that has been used previously in research on peer and partner relationships (Jussim & Osgood, 1989; Kenny & Acitelli, 2001; Young et al., 2014). Nevertheless, the conclusions about projections are inferred and not based on direct tests. Despite these limitations, what is undeniable from the analyses is that both parents' and adolescents' perceptions of their shared political interactions are colored by their own interest in politics and that there is little convergence in opinions about these shared interactions. The findings reported in this chapter are consistent with a biased perception hypothesis. The study conveys the message that practitioners, parents, and adolescents need to be aware of projection effects, and that projection applies to both parents and adolescents.

Finally, what evidence was presented in this chapter that young people are active agents in their own political development?

It seems that projection, a perceptual bias, risks locking parents and youth into their own idiosyncratic understandings of each other. Adolescents misperceive their parents' values as close to their own, and apparently their parents do the same. Politically interested adolescents are likely to believe that they have frequent political discussions with their parents and that their parents are politically supportive. A similar projection bias holds for parents. Parents' political interest also influences their perceptions of their shared political interactions. With low to moderate associations between adolescents' and parents' political interest, there is little agreement between adolescents' and parents' perceptions of their shared political interactions.

10

OPENNESS TO OTHERS' INFLUENCE

Highlights

Projection, a biased perception, explains why adolescents' and parents' political interests color their perceptions of their observed common political interactions—the frequency of political discussions and the extent of parents' political support. It also explains the low accuracy that exists in adolescents' and parents' perceptions of their shared political interactions. The lack of shared perceptions of observed behaviors does not preclude adolescents from being open to political socialization attempts by their parents and others.

Here, we tested the idea that adolescents' perceptions of their political interactions with significant others overall are influenced by their own political interests to a greater extent than perceived political interactions influence adolescents' political interests. The 13- and 16-year-olds were followed for 1 year. We found that adolescents' perceptions of important others' (parents, teachers, friends) political views, political interest, political influence and support, and their own susceptibility to others' political communication were all influenced by their own political interest. These findings suggest that adolescents' political interest is an input to their political development, making politically interested adolescents active agents in their political interactions with significant others.

A Broader Interpretation

In the previous chapter, we hypothesized that adolescents' political interest would color their perceptions of their political interactions with their parents—overt behaviors such as political discussions and supportive behaviors by parents. Similarly, we hypothesized that parents' political interest would color their perceptions of their political interactions with their adolescents. Because of the lack of convergence in adolescents' and parents' political interest, we expected that adolescents' and parents' perceptions of political discussion and political support would show little similarity. We attributed these differences to projection: biased perceptions. This interpretation appears to be valid, but there is a broader interpretation that includes not only observable behaviors but also other features of the joint political

DOI: 10.4324/9781003371731-14

interactions. This interpretation, with its direct focus on adolescents' political agency, is tested here.

Consider an agentic perspective. This is the idea that adolescents' political interest opens them up to the political views and influence of other important people in their lives—parents, friends, and teachers. The perception of important others as politically influential stems from the adolescent's own political interest. Such an agentic perspective would suggest that politically interested adolescents are curious to know more about other people's thoughts about what is happening in the world and in their society. It is an agentic idea in that adolescents' awareness of others' political views, perception of others' political interests, identification of others as providing them with political information, recognition of others as trying to influence them politically, and susceptibility to these others' political influences all stem from adolescents' own political interests. Here, adolescents' high political interest makes them sensitive to others' political communication. They try to remain open to the views and political influence of others. In such an interpretation, adolescents must have a certain level of political interest in order to perceive the political views and interests of important others, to identify and recognize the attempts of important others to exert political influence, and to be susceptible to the attempts of others to do so. From the opposite perspective, adolescents who are not politically interested are unlikely to be motivated to engage in political discussions initiated by politically interested others about issues in which they have little insight or interest, or to be susceptible to the political communication of others.

Look at it from a learning perspective. Then we would expect that if some adolescents experience that the most important people in their lives are politically interested, that these people provide them with political information, that they try to influence them, and that they are susceptible to the views of these people, then these adolescents would be more likely to increase their political interest over time than other adolescents. They encounter other people who seem to have a lot of insight into politics, and they are susceptible to the political influence of these people. We argue that it is the other way around. It is adolescents' political interest that makes them sensitive to the political input of others.

This idea that high political interest sensitizes adolescents to others' political communication and makes them aware of others' political interest, influence, and sources of political inspiration is tested here with a longitudinal design. Adolescents in the first two cohorts—samples of 908 13-year-olds and 869 16-year-olds—were followed for one year. T2 data were available one year later for 793 (87%) in cohort 1 and 682 (78%) in cohort 2.

The adolescents reported on their political interactions with their parents, friends, and teachers. Questions were asked about the following:

If participants knew the political views of their parents and friends,
If parents and friends were interested in what was happening in society,

If parents, friends, and teachers provided political information,
If parents and friends tried to influence the adolescents politically, and
If the adolescents were receptive to political communication from parents, friends, and teachers.

In the analyses we controlled for sex and immigrant background.

Table 10.1 summarizes the specific questions and measures. Four measures had lower reliability than .70, but the inter-item correlations, ranging between .49 and .53, were adequate.

TABLE 10.1 Scales measuring adolescents' perceptions of the political influence of parents, friends, and teachers and adolescents' susceptibility to these influences.

Content	*Response scale*		*Scale reliabilities*			
			T1		*T2*	
			Age 13	*Age 14*	*Age 16*	*Age 17*
Awareness of others' political views: How much do you know about your parents' (best friends') views on and ways of looking at societal issues?	1 (*I don't know anything about what they think*) 5 (*I think I know most of what they think*)		–	–	–	–
Perception of others' political interest: My parents (best friends) are interested in what is going on in the world My parents (best friends) keep track of the news	1 (*doesn't apply at all*) 4 (*applies very well*)	Parents:	.68	.74	.75	.77
		Friends:	.72	.69	.73	.74
Perception that others provide concrete information: My parents (teachers) suggest newspapers, books, or websites where you can read about politics or societal issues My best friends (teachers) provide information on pages on the Internet where you can read about politics or societal issues	1 (*definitely doesn't apply*) 5 (*applies very well*)	Parents:	.64	.68	.73	.70
		Friends:	.78	.83	.84	.86
		Teachers:	.84	.86	.85	.87

Content	*Response scale*		*Scale reliabilities*			
			T1		*T2*	
			Age 13	*Age 14*	*Age 16*	*Age 17*
My parents (best friends) give me information about the activities of organizations that you can contact or get engaged in (they talk about what these organizations do and how you get in contact with them)						
Perception that others try to exert influence:						
Do your parents (best friends) try to get you to become more aware of what is going on in the world?	1 (*no, never*) 5 (*yes, almost always*)	Parents: Friends:	.79 .87	.70 .81	.74 .83	.65 .77
Do your parents (best friends) try to get you to become more aware of environmental issues?						
Susceptible to others' influence:						
My parents (best friends, teachers) talk about politics and societal issues in a way that makes them fun and interesting	1 (*definitely doesn't apply*) 5 (*applies very well*)	Parents: Friends: Teachers:	.80 .85 .87	.84 .87 .89	.83 .97 .88	.86 .90 .89
My parents (best friends, teachers) talk about things that happen in the world and in society in such a way that I become curious and want to know more						
My parents (friends, teachers) tell me about the news they have heard on TV or read about in a way that evokes strong feelings in me						

Note: For the three-items measures we report Cronbach's alpha reliabilities, and for the two-item measures Spearman-Brown reliability coefficients.

Analyses

We used latent change models to test the idea that adolescents' political interest affects their perceptions of their parents, peers, and teachers, rather than vice versa. In these models, the intercept reflects the mean level of the variable at the first assessment, while the slope reflects the amount of linear change that occurs between the two points in time. We estimated the initial level (intercept) and the rate of change (slope) for each family of variables considered, that is, knowledge of others' views, others' political interest, others' provision of political information, others' attempts to influence, and susceptibility to others' political communication. We then used equality conditions to test whether baseline levels and rates of change differed between the two age cohorts. The same type of model was discussed in Chapter 3.

Results

Figure 10.1 shows the structure of the model that was tested, using perceptions of parents' political interest as an example. In the first set of analyses, we compared models in which all cross-lagged effects were freely estimated (model 1) with models in which the effects of others' perceptions on political interest at T2 were fixed at 0 (model 2). These model comparisons showed that model 2 was preferred for four of the five measures, indicating that adolescents' political interest affected their perceptions of significant others, but not vice versa. Model 1 was preferred for perceiving others' political views.

Table 10.2 shows the estimates of the latent change models with multiple group comparisons. We present the effects in the models that should be preferred on the basis of the model comparisons. The first three rows of the table show the effects of initial interest on changes in adolescents' perceptions of others. In particular, adolescents' political interest positively and significantly predicted changes over time in

- perceptions of significant others' political views,
- perceptions of others' political interest,
- perceptions of others providing political information,
- perceptions of others as trying to influence, and
- susceptibility to political communication from others.

We also found a significant effect of adolescents' political interest on parents' attempts to influence their adolescents politically, although the effect was limited ($p = .03$). In terms of the other direction of effects, reported in the table under the label "From others to interest", there were significant effects of adolescents' perceptions of political interactions with their parents on changes in adolescents' political interest. These effects were not as strong as those in the opposite direction. We also found very little evidence to support the idea that young people's interest stems from interactions with their peers. (Only two significant cases were found:

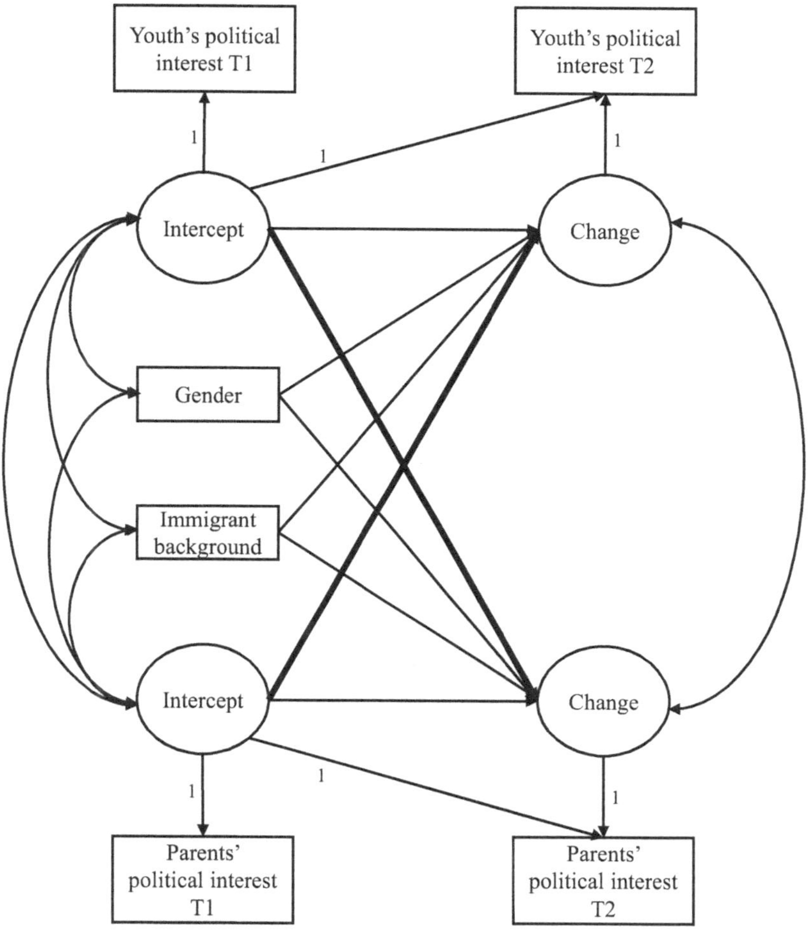

FIGURE 10.1 The structure of the tested models.

Friends' political interest and perception of friends providing political information. Also, awareness of friends' political views tended to increase adolecents' political interest over time, but only in the older cohort.) Nor was there any evidence that political interactions with teachers increased young people's political interest. In short, in 11 of the 12 longitudinal analyses, young people's political interest strongly influenced perceptions of their political interactions with others (with $p < .001$), but none of the 12 effects of perceptions of political interactions with others on changes in young people's political interest reached the same level of significance. Where bidirectional effects were found, the results showed that it was more likely that young people's political interest influenced their perceptions of important others' political influence than that others' political influence influenced young people's political interest over time. Additional support for our conclusion comes from the proportion of variance explained in our dependent variables (R^2). When

TABLE 10.2 Unstandardized coefficients for the multi-group latent change models.

	Others' political views		*Others' political interest*		*Others provide information*		*Others try to influence*		*Being susceptible*	
	Coeff. (95% CIs)	*p*	*Coeff. (95% CIs)*	*p*	*Coeff. (95% CIs)*	*p*	*Coeff. (95% CIs)*	*p*	*Coeff. (95% CIs)*	*p*
From interest to others										
I—Interest → S—Parents	.18(.15/.22)	< .001	.04(.02/.06)	.001	.12(.08/.15)	< .001	.04(.01/.06)	.03	.15(.11/.18)	< .001
I—Interest → S—Peers	.18(.15/.22)	< .001	.07(.05/.09)	< .001	.13(.09/.16)	< .001	.12(.09/.15)	< .001	.16(.12/.20)	< .001
I—Interest → S—Teachers	–	–	–	–	.14(.10/.18)	< .001	–	–	.14(.10/.17)	< .001
From others to interest										
I—Parents → S—Interest	.07(.02/.11)	.02	.14(.06/.22)	.003	.08(.03/.13)	.005	.08(.02/.14)	.02	.08(.02/.13)	.02
I—Peers → S—Interest	.00(−.06/.06)^{y}	1.00	.10(.03/.18)	.02	−.08(−.13/−.02)	.03	−.00(−.06/.05)	.94	−.03(−.09/.03)	.38
	.11(.05/.17)^{o}	.003								
I—Teachers → S—Interest	–	–	–	–	.02(−.02/.07)	.43	–	–	.04(−.00/.09)	.12
From initial levels to slopes										
I—Interest → S—Interest	−.43(−.49/−.37)^{y}	<.001	−.44(−.49/−.38)^{y}	<.001	−.42(−.48/−.36)^{y}	<.001	−.43(−.49/−.37)^{y}	<.001	−.43(−.49/−.37)^{y}	<.001
	−.31(−.36/−.26)^{o}	<.001	−.29(−.34/−.25)^{o}	<.001	−.27(−.31/−.22)^{o}	<.001	−.27(−.32/−.23)^{o}	<.001	−.29(−.34/−.24)^{o}	<.001
I—Parents → S—Parents	−.76(−.82/−.71)^{y}	<.001	−.64(−.72/−.57)^{y}	<.001	−.60(−.64/−.56)	<.001	−.58(−.63/−.52)^{y}	<.001	−.54(−.58/−.50)	<.001
	−.63(−.69/−.57)^{o}	<.001	−.48(−.54/−.41)^{o}	<.001			−.43(−.48/−.38)^{o}	<.001		
I—Peers → S—Peers	−.70(−.74/−.66)	<.001	−.63(−.68/−.59)	<.001	−.71(−.76/−.66)	<.001	−.62(−.66/−.57)	<.001	−.65(−.70/−.61)	<.001
I—Teachers → S—Teachers	–	–	–	–	−.76(−.80/−.71)	<.001	–	–	−.66(−.70/−.62)	<.001
Covariates										
Sex → S—Interest	.04(−.04/.12)	.42	.05(−.04/.13)	.35	.04(−.04/.13)	.38	.04(−.04/.13)	.40	.06(−.03/.14)	.26
Immigrant → S—Interest	.08(−.10/.26)^{y}	.49	.08(−.10/.26)^{y}	.47	.07(−.11/.25)^{y}	.53	−.08(−.21/.04)	.27	−.10(−.23/.02)	.16
	−.21(−.37/−.04)^{o}	.04	−.24(−.41/−.07)^{o}	.02	−.24(−.41/−.07)^{o}	.02				
Sex → S—Parents	.04(−.05/.12)	.47	−.05(−.10/−.00)	.08	.17(.09/.24)	<.001	−.02(−.08/.04)	.65	−.06(−.13/.01)	.15
Immigrant → S—Parents	.09(−.03/.20)	.22	.17(.08/.27)^{y}	.002	.34(.22/.46)	<.001	.27(.18/.36)	<.001	.13(.03/.23)	.03
			.03(−.07/.13)^{o}	.64						
Sex → S—Peers	−.07(−.15/.02)	.19	.02(−.03/.07)	.58	.19(.11/.26)	<.001	.10(.01/.20)^{y}	.07	−.05(−.12/.03)	.29
							−.06(−.16/.03)^{o}	.26		
Immigrant → S—Peers	−.03(−.15/.10)	.70	−.04(−.10/.03)	.39	.20(.08/.31)	.005	.20(.10/.30)	.001	.00(—.11/.11)	.99
Sex → S—Teachers	–	–	–	–	.05(−.04/.13)	.34	–	–	.06(−.02/.13)	.23
Immigrant → S—Teachers	–	–	–	–	.11(−.01/.23)	.14	–	–	.01(−.10/.12)	.88

Model fit					
χ^2 (df), p	42.17(16), p <.001	45.77(19), p < .001	105.62(35), p <.001	33.63(20), p = .03	72.77(36), p <.001
CFI–TLI	.989–.962	.985–.956	.974–.936	.994–.983	.990–.975
RMSEA (95% CIs)	.040(.026,.055)	.037(.024,.051)	.045(.035,.055)	.026(.008,.041)	.032(.021,.042)
***R*²** (young and old cohorts respectively)					
S–Interest	.17–.16	.17–.15	.17–.14	.18–.13	.17–.14
S–Parents	.39–.34	.32–.25	.30–.31	.31–.26	.27–.27
S–Peers	.37–.38	.31–.33	.37–.34	.32–.33	.31–.30
S–Teachers	–	–	.38–.41	–	.33–.37

When multiple group comparisons indicate significant differences between age cohorts, we report the coefficient for each group: The superscript ^{y} indicates coefficients for the younger cohort (age 13), ^{o} indicates coefficients for the older cohort (age 16). *N* is 2020.

Note: Sex is coded 1 = male, 0 = female; Immigrant background is coded 1 = immigrant, 0 = not immigrant (native). I, Intercept; S, Slope.

predicting latent changes in adolescents' perceptions of their political interactions with others based on their initial level of political interest, we were able to explain on average 30% of the variance but only about 15% of the variance in the change in political interest. This is a clear indication that our models were better at explaining changes in young people's perceptions of political interactions with others than changes in young people's own political interest. Overall, the results suggest that high political interest makes young people more aware of others' political views, interests, and influence and more susceptible to being influenced by others.

Discussion

Politically interested adolescents are seemingly not stuck in their perceptual worlds because of distorted perceptions of parents' values and everyday political interactions. They appear to be open and receptive to the political views of parents and other important people—friends and teachers.

Two tendencies seem to characterize politically interested adolescents' perceptions of their parents. On the one hand, as reported in Chapter 9, adolescents' political interest affects their perceptions of the frequency of political discussions at home and of their parents' political support. Parents' political interest also affects parents' perceptions of how often they discuss politics with their adolescents and their political support. Parents and adolescents do not have very similar perceptions of the frequency of these discussions and of parental support. These findings, based on a comparison of adolescents' and parents' views, suggest that politically interested adolescents and parents do not see a shared political world at home. They see their own.

But the findings reported in this chapter suggest that politically interested adolescents are willing to go a long way to understand how their parents think about political issues. They perceive themselves as knowledgeable about their parents' political views, think they know a lot about their parents' political interests, recognize that their parents try to provide them with concrete political information, and recognize that their parents provide political support and try to influence them to a greater extent than do politically uninterested adolescents. Perhaps most importantly, they see themselves as receptive to their parents' political communication. This openness to parents appears to be matched by a similar openness to their friends and teachers. In sum, adolescents' political interests make them open to other people's political views, interests, and the political support of significant others.

We found mostly monodirectional relationships in which adolescents' political interest influenced their perceptions of the political influence and support of important others, but not vice versa. We had expected at least some influence of adolescents' perceptions of their political interactions with others. But perceptions of parents', friends', and teachers' political knowledge and interest, attempts to influence them, provision of political information, political support, and attempts to influence them politically had little effect on their political interest. The classic literature emphasizes the unilateral influence of significant others on adolescents' political development (Jennings et al., 2009). However, adolescents' perceptions of others' views and influence did not significantly affect their political interest over time. We conclude that adolescents' political interest sensitizes them to the political views of others. It appears to be an input to their political development, making politically interested adolescents active agents in their political interactions with their significant others.

In value socialization theory, adolescents must be open to the values and attitudes of others if political socialization is to function as expected (Grusec & Goodnow, 1994; Grusec & Kuczynski, 1997). In the family context, they need to accurately perceive and accept their parents' views in order to internalize their parents' views. In order to accurately perceive parents' views, adolescents must be open to these values and attitudes. Indeed, as shown earlier, politically interested adolescents are open to and seem to be influenced by political information from significant others in their everyday environment. However, as we also saw earlier, this does not fit well with the lack of convergence in the attitudes and views of adolescents and parents. We attributed this to a projection bias. The findings of a perception bias do not refute the argument that politically interested adolescents are open to the political influence of significant others.

More broadly, developmental theories in psychology converge on the idea that the way people appraise situations and interactions with others they encounter in everyday life determines their reactions and actions. The psychological meanings of these situations and interactions are determinants of their behaviors (Magnusson & Stattin, 2006). It is oftentimes the person's perception, more than friends' or parents' perceptions of the person, that links to behavior and wellbeing (Janssen et al., 2021). This insight is valuable for the studies discussed in previous chapters that have attempted to examine how adolescents and young adults perceive political interactions with others. In Chapter 9, we showed that when 16-year-old adolescents were asked to report on their parents' core values—concern for the welfare of others and concern for nature—and achievement values, they reported their parents' values as close to their own. The adolescents' reports of these values did not match their parents' reports. In the same chapter, we found that adolescents' political interest was strongly related to their perceptions of the frequency of family political discussions and their parents' political support. Again, there was little agreement between parents' and adolescents' reports of these discussions and parental support. There appears to be a general tendency for adolescents to view their parents' values and political interactions as similar to their own, and also a general tendency for parents to view their adolescents' values and political interactions as similar to their own. As Anaïs Nin (1903–1977) famously said, "We don't see things as they are, we see them as we are."

But the findings discussed in this chapter suggest that adolescents are not stuck in their perceptual worlds. Their political interest seems to make them open to the political input of others.

Finally, what evidence has been presented in this chapter that young people are active agents in their own political development?

Politically interested youth are more likely than less interested youth to recognize the political knowledge and interest of others, their political support and influence, and to be inspired by their political communication with others. The often taken-for-granted assumption in the literature that the development of adolescents' political interest is largely under the influence of parents, peers, and teachers through social learning is not self-evident. Adolescents' political interest seems to act as a filter for their perceptions of political communication with others, making them far from passive recipients of others' political influence. The most obvious conclusion to be drawn from this chapter is that politically interested adolescents appear to be open to the political influences of others, regardless of the environmental context, whether it be in the peer group, at school, or at home. This openness does not translate into having similar perceptions as others.

PART V

Why a Person-Oriented Approach Is Needed

11

WHY SOME ADOLESCENTS, BUT NOT OTHERS, ARE OPEN TO THEIR PARENTS' POLITICAL COMMUNICATION

Highlights

Based on a reformulation of the perceptual accuracy argument (Tedin, 1974), that is, that children's accuracy in perceiving their parents' political values and attitudes can explain why parents' political socialization attempts succeed or fail, we found that the group of adolescents who accurately perceived their parents' high political sophistication was particularly aware of their parents' political socialization attempts, were receptive to their parents' political communication, considered their parents' political views important, talked about political matters frequently, and were more politically interested than other adolescents.

A Broader Interpretation

According to Abraham Maslow's Law of Tools, "If the only tool you have is a hammer, you tend to see every problem as a nail." Let's apply this law to the lack of convergence that exists between adolescents' and parents' sociopolitical values and shared political interactions. Sample statistics show that there is little correspondence between adolescents' and their parents' sociopolitical values and their judgments about how often joint political interactions occur. These analyses are concerned with relationships between variables across individuals, where the relationships between the variables and how they operate are the same for all individuals and reflect what is characteristic of the average person (Bergman et al., 2003). But some of the low associations between parents' and adolescents' views on sociopolitical issues and joint political interactions that we have reported earlier may mask the fact that some adolescents in a given sample may indeed correctly perceive their parents' political sophistication. To examine this, we need to move away from linear analyses for the full sample. In this chapter, we discuss a specific group of adolescents who accurately perceive their parents' high political sophistication.

DOI: 10.4324/9781003371731-16

Interpersonal communication is a central concept in most past and current models of political socialization (Lee et al., 2012; Shah et al., 2009). Classical family political socialization emphasizes the social learning process by which adolescents acquire their political interests, values, ideologies, and opinions through their parents (Jennings et al., 2009; Jennings & Niemi, 1968). Studies of political socialization have traditionally assumed a unidirectional transmission of political interests and attitudes from parents to children. This assumption implies that children conform to and adopt their parents' views, and that the roots of adolescents' political and social interests lie largely in the views, values, and attitudes transmitted by their parents (Barrett & Brunton-Smith, 2014). Research in this tradition has not paid much attention to whether adolescents are open to parental political influence (nor whether learning is the correct explanation). The failure of parents to express their values consistently over time has been one explanation for why adolescents do not accurately perceive their political messages (Jennings et al., 2009). The problem with this argument is that parents' messages and influences must pass through adolescents' perceptions.

The need for adolescents to pay attention to their parents' socialization attempts is the hallmark of value socialization theory (Grusec & Goodnow, 1994)—a theory that we have referred to several times. This theory is concerned with how adolescents internalize their parents' views, and the theory outlines this as a two-step process. For adolescents to successfully internalize their parents' values and attitudes, they must first accurately perceive their parents' messages. If they accurately perceive their parents' values and attitudes, then they can choose to adopt those values and attitudes as their own. Applied to the political sphere, in order for adolescents to adopt their parents' interest in politics, society, and the world, they must first recognize that their parents are politically interested and have political messages to communicate.

This raises the question of how accurately adolescents perceive their parents' political interests, values, and attitudes. As we have seen repeatedly in previous chapters, analyses of the full sample of an age group show that adolescents do not seem to accurately perceive their parents' way of thinking about shared political interactions, and they have quite different views about specific sociopolitical attitudes and values. If adolescents do not accurately perceive their parents' views, how can they be internalized? The usefulness of value socialization theory seems limited. But even if adolescents' openness to their parents' attempts at political socialization is not true for all, it may be true for some. What are the characteristics of families in which adolescents might be expected to be more open to their parents' political socialization than in other families?

Early in political science, Kent Tedin (1974) suggested that children's perceptual accuracy in recognizing their parents' political values and attitudes might explain why parents' attempts at political socialization succeed or fail. In developmental psychology, as we have seen, the same perceptual accuracy argument was raised in value socialization theory (Grusec & Goodnow, 1994; Knafo & Schwartz, 2003, 2009) and later in political science in research on adolescent-parent correspondence (Ojeda & Hatemi, 2015). In these models, decisions to accept parents' political interests, values, and attitudes depend on adolescents' accurate perceptions of them. Applying the perceptual accuracy argument to parental political socialization, we propose that adolescents' attention to their parents' political communication is facilitated when they correctly perceive their parents' high political interest and knowledge—a high political sophistication. This is the case when parents are highly politically interested and knowledgeable and adolescents report that their parents are highly politically interested and knowledgeable. These adolescents should be particularly likely to perceive their parents' political support and influence and to be more receptive to their political communication than other adolescents. In addition, adolescents who correctly identify their parents' high political sophistication should be more likely than other adolescents to perceive that they have had political discussions with their parents. Adolescents who fail to recognize their parents' political sophistication are less likely to recall such discussions.

The ability to perceive one's parents as politically interested and knowledgeable requires some level of political interest on the part of the adolescent. We do not expect adolescents who are not interested in politics or who dislike politics to recognize their parents' political interest and knowledge. Thus, the ability to recognize their parents' high political sophistication, political interest, and knowledge should be related to the adolescents' own political interest.

In sum, whereas the learning position (Jennings et al., 2009) proposes that it is parents' ability to consistently communicate their political values, beliefs, and opinions that influences their adolescents' political development, our reformulated perceptual accuracy hypothesis suggests that it is precisely those adolescents who correctly perceive their parents' high political sophistication who will recognize their parents' socialization messages and be open to their views. This ability to recognize their parents' high political sophistication should be related to adolescents' own political interests.

Participants and Analyses

We needed independent information from the adolescents and their parents and used the second cohort: the 16-year-olds. The target sample consisted of 1,052 students according to class lists. Of these, 866 students (82%) completed the questionnaires at school. Parents completed the questionnaires at home ($N = 580$). Complete responses from parents and adolescents were available for 516 participants (67% of the analytic sample). We will also use data from the next year, T2. Of the 516 participants at T1, 420 (81%) of the adolescents and parents were available 1 year later at T2.

As seen in Table 11.1, we measured the following:

- *Parents' political sophistication:* Adolescent- and parent-reported
- *Political interest:* Adolescent-reported
- *Perceptions of parental political support*: Adolescent- and parent-reported
- *Perceptions of parental attempts to influence adolescents politically:* Adolescent- and parent-reported
- *Perceptions that parents' views are important:* Adolescent-reported
- *Susceptibility to political communication from parents:* Adolescent-reported
- *Political discussions:* Adolescent- and parent-reported
- *Covariates:* Parental education level, immigrant status, and participants' sex

TABLE 11.1 Scales and items used in the chapter.

Concept	*Items*	*Response scale*
Parents' political sophistication: Parent-reported		
Political interest and knowledge:		
"How interested are you in politics or societal issues (mother/father)?"	2	1 (*totally uninterested*) 5 (*very interested*)
Follow the news:		
"To what extent does this apply to you?" "Can be described as a person who tries to keep informed about what is going on in the world," "Follows the news daily to know what other people are talking about."	2	1 (*doesn't apply at all*) 5 (*applies very well*)
Parents' political sophistication. Adolescent-reported		
Interest:		
"My parents are interested in what is going on in the world" "My parents keep themselves in touch with the news," My parents don't care so much about what is going on in the world (reversed coded)." "My parents are not particularly interested in politics or societal issues (reversed coded)."	4	1 (*doesn't apply at all*) 5 (applies very well)
Knowledge:		
"Are your parents knowledgeable about what is going on in Sweden and in the rest of the world?"	1	1 (*they have no knowledge of what is going on*) 5 (*they have very good knowledge of what is going on*)
Political interest: Adolescent-reported:[a]		
"How interested are you in politics?"	2	1 (*totally uninterested*) 5 (*very interested*)
"People differ in how they feel about politics. What are your feelings?" The interest question was re-scaled to range between 1 and 6, and the two items were then aggregated.		1 (*loathe*) 6 (*great fun*)

Concept	Items	Response scale
Parents' provision of political support: Adolescent- and parent-reported:[b]		
My parents: "Suggest newspapers, books, or websites where I can read about politics or societal issues;" "Give me information about activities or organizations in which I can get engaged;" "Want me to sit down and watch the news on television with them."	3	1 (*definitely doesn't apply*) 5 (*applies very well*)
Parents responded to the same three items, slightly reframed (e.g., "We suggest newspapers, books, or websites where our child can read about politics or societal issues.")	3	1 (*definitely doesn't apply*) 5 (*applies very well*)
Parents' attempts to politically influence their adolescents: Adolescent- and parent-reported:[c]		
"Do your parents try to get you to become more aware of environmental issues?" "Do your parents try to get you to become more aware of what is going on in the world?"	2	1 (*no, never*) 5 (*yes, almost always*)
The same two questions were also posed to the parents.	2	1 (*no, never*) 5 (*yes, almost always*)
Parents' views are important: Adolescent-reported		
"Are your parents' views on and ways of looking at societal issues important to you?" The adolescents responded on a scale ranging from *no, not at all* (1) to *yes, very* (4).	1	1 (*no, not at all*) 4 (*yes, very*)
Susceptibility to parents' political communication: Adolescent-reported		
My parents ". . . talk about politics and societal issues in a way that makes them fun and interesting," ". . . talk about things that happen in the world and in society in such a way that I become curious and want to know more," ". . . tell me about the news they have heard on TV or read about in a way that evokes strong feelings in me."	3	1 (*doesn't apply at all*) 5 (*applies very well*)
Political discussions: Adolescent- and parent-reported:[d]		
The participants were asked how often they and their parents discussed: "What you have heard on the news about what is going on in Sweden and around the world?" "Politics or societal issues?"	2	1 (*never*) 4 (*very often*)

(*Continued*)

TABLE 11.1 (Continued)

Concept	*Items*	*Response scale*
Covariates:		
The educational level of the parents, immigrant status, and sex were controlled for at T1. The questions about mothers' and fathers' scores on educational level were averaged. Immigrant status was a dichotomous measure Sex was coded 0 = female, 1 = male. Educational level was reported by parents and immigrant status and sex were adolescent reported.	4	1 (less than 9 years of education) 5 (college/university education) 1 (students both of whose parents were born outside the Nordic countries) 0 (other students)

[a] The interest question was re-scaled to range between 1 and 6, and the two items were then aggregated. The correlation between the two items at T1 was .59, $p < .001$.
[b] Alpha reliability was .70 for the adolescents and .67 for the parents.
[c] The correlation between the two adolescent-reported questions was .54 at T1. The correlation for parent reports at T1 was .46.
[d] The correlation between the two question responses for the adolescents was .53 at T1 and was .46 for the parents at T1.

First, the responses to the questions about parents' political interest and political knowledge, which were asked of both parents and adolescents, were factor analyzed. As shown in Table 11.2, two factors emerged, labeled "*Parents' political sophistication* "and "*Adolescents' perceptions of parents' political sophistication.*" These factors are the main measures in the study.

Next, to avoid the problems of conducting multiple comparisons, which increases type 1 errors, adolescents' reported measures of perceptions of their political interactions with parents (parents' provision of political support, parents' attempts to politically influence their adolescents, parents' views are important, susceptibility to parents' political communication, and political discussions) were factor analyzed. One factor emerged with factor loadings between .76 and .82. At T2, the same measures again yielded a factor with factor loadings ranging from .71 to .82. We refer to this factor as "*adolescents' perceptions of open political interactions with parents*." The three parent-reported measures of their political interactions with adolescents (providing political information, trying to influence their adolescents politically, and having political discussions) also yielded one factor with factor loadings ranging from .72 to .83. The factor is labeled "*parents' political socialization attempts*." These two factor scores were used in the Results section.

Cluster analysis was used to distinguish groups of adolescents based on both parents' own reports of their political sophistication and adolescents' reports of

TABLE 11.2 Principal component analysis of measures of parents' political interest and knowledge and adolescents' perceptions of parents' political interest and knowledge.

	Parents' sophistication	*Adolescents' perceptions of parents' sophistication*
Parent reports: Politically interested	.65	.04
Parent reports: Follow the news	.60	−.02
Adolescent reports: Parents are interested	.03	.73
Adolescent reports: Parents are knowledgeable	−.04	.67

their parents' political sophistication. We expected that one of the clusters would contain adolescents whose parents reported high political sophistication and adolescents who also reported that their parents had high political sophistication. The resulting factor scores for the factors "*Parents' political sophistication*" and "*Adolescents' perceptions of parents' political sophistication*" in Table 11.2 were standardized and then cluster analyzed. First, a hierarchical cluster analysis using Ward's method was used to determine the number of clusters for these two measures. The lower explanatory limit was set at 67% of the total error sum of squares for the number of clusters selected (Bergman et al., 2003). Second, as recommended by Kinder and colleagues (1991), with the number of clusters known, a non-hierarchical cluster analysis, *K*-means clustering, was used to arrive at the final cluster solution. Ordinary ANOVAs were then used to examine differences between the cluster groups on the two measures of parent-adolescent political interactions (reported by adolescents and parents, respectively) and adolescents' own political interest, controlling for participants' sex, immigrant status, and parents' level of education.

Results

Cluster Results

According to the hierarchical cluster analysis, five clusters explained 77% of the total error sums of squares at T1. A subsequent non-hierarchical cluster analysis yielded the clusters shown in Table 11.3. Consistent with our expectations, the final cluster, hereafter referred to as the HH adolescents, contained adolescents whose parents expressed High political sophistication and whose adolescents also reported that their parents had High political sophistication. This group comprised 26% of all adolescents in the sample. We conclude that HH adolescents emerge as a naturally occurring cluster group in this sample of 16-year-olds. There was also a

TABLE 11.3 Cluster analysis of measures of parents' political sophistication and adolescents' perceptions of their parents' political sophistication.

Parents (T1): *Adolescents (T1):* *Label:*	*Low* *Low* *LL*	*Low* *Medium* *LM*	*Medium* *Medium* *MM*	*High* *Low* *HL*	*High* *High* *HH*
Parents' political sophistication	−0.74	−1.86	−0.42	0.80	0.79
Adolescents' perceptions of parents' sophistication	−1.66	−0.30	0.12	−0.59	1.13
N (%)	55 (11)	45 (10)	163 (32)	109 (22)	133 (26)
% girls[a]	51	49	54	44	55
% immigrants[b]	13	7	13	10	15
Parents' education (*z*-scores)[c d]	−0.33[a]	−0.42[a]	−0.13[a]	0.21[b]	0.35[b]

Low values (L): lowest value through −.70; Medium values (M): −.69 through .69; High values (H): .70 through highest value.

[a] χ^2 (4 df) = 3.57, $p = .468$; [b] χ^2 (4 df) = 2.38, $p = .667$; [c] F (4, 499) = 10.22, $p < .001$.

[d] For parents' education, across rows, the superscripts represent significant differences ($p < 0.05$) between clusters in SNK post-hoc tests.

group in which parents reported High political sophistication, but their adolescents reported that their parents had Low political sophistication. We refer to this group as HL adolescents. This cluster contained almost as many individuals, 22%, as the HH adolescents. For the rest, three clusters emerged in which both parents and adolescents reported low or medium parental political sophistication (the LL, LM, and MM adolescents). Note that the correlation between parents' political sophistication and adolescents' perceptions of their parents' political sophistication was .29, $p < .001$, for the full sample. Excluding the HH adolescents, the correlation was −.04, $p = .437$. Thus, it is only by chance that adolescents in clusters other than HH correctly perceive their parents' political sophistication as high or low. As reported in Table 11.3, we tested whether there were differences in gender and immigrant status for the five cluster groups, as well as differences based on parents' education level. There were no significant differences for gender and immigrant status, but parental education was higher among HH, HL, and MM adolescents than among the other two cluster groups.

A similar cluster analysis at T2 yielded five clusters that explained 73% of the total variance. Because two of these included adolescents who correctly identified their parents' low political sophistication, and one of these was more extreme than the other, it was decided to report a four-cluster solution (65% of the total variance). Again, a cluster of HH adolescents (13% of the sample) and a cluster of HL adolescents (28% of the sample) were found (see Table 11.4). There were no differences by gender or immigrant status, but there was a significant effect of parents' educational status. The LL adolescents (parents have low political sophistication

TABLE 11.4 A cluster analysis of measures of parents' political sophistication and adolescents' perceptions of their parents' political sophistication at T2.

Parents (T2): *Adolescents (T2):* *Label:*	*Low* *Low* *LL*	*Low* *High* *LH*	*High* *Low (medium)* *HL*	*High* *High* *HH*
Parents' political sophistication	−0.98	−0.50	0.78	0.95
Adolescents' perceptions of parents' sophistication	−0.76	0.76	−0.60	1.17
N (%)	112 (31)	77 (21)	101 (28)	72 (13)
% girls[a]	44	56	52	54
% immigrants[b]	11	9	9	13
Parents' education (*z*-scores)[c d]	−0.32[a]	0.11[b]	0.01[b]	0.25[b]

Low values (L): lowest value through −.70; Medium values (M): −.69 through .69; High values (H): .70 through highest value.

[a] χ^2 (3 df) = 2.85, $p = .415$; [b] χ^2 (3 df) = 0.80, $p = .849$; [c] F (3, 357) = 5.82, $p < .001$.

[d] For parents' education, across rows, the superscripts represent significant differences ($p < .05$) between clusters in SNK post-hoc tests.

and adolescents also report low political sophistication of their parents) had lower levels of education than the other three cluster groups of youths. Overall, there is confirmation of the existence of groups of adolescents who correctly identify their parents' high political sophistication and who fail to identify their parents' high political sophistication.

Stability and Change in the Cluster Solutions

An overall χ^2 is often used to provide a general test of independence between two variables when they are cross-tabulated. However, sometimes it is necessary to analyze whether a particular cell frequency is larger or smaller than would be expected according to an independence model. EXACON serves this purpose (Bergman & El-Khouri, 1987). The program computes exact one-sided probabilities of observed cell frequencies according to the Fixed Margins model, using the hypergeometric distribution. The EXACON program, with a Bonferroni adjusted *p* value of .05, was used to determine which specific cells occurred more often (a type) and less often (an antitype) than expected by chance when the results of the clustering solution at T1 were cross-tabulated with the clustering solution at T2. The results are shown in Table 11.5.

This analysis showed a high stability of the T1 clusters. The contingency coefficient was 0.59, $p < .001$. Aside from the "types" where the T1 clusters appeared more often than expected by chance at T2 (indicating high stability over time for

TABLE 11.5 Cross-tabulation of clusters between T1 and T2.

		T2			
		LL	*LH*	*HL*	*HH*
T1	LL	15[t]	0	9	0
	LM	16[t]	3	3	0
	MM	33	25	19	12
	HL	13	10	36[t]	5[a]
	HH	2[a]	18	8[a]	41[t]

Note: The first figure is parents' political sophistication and the second is adolescents' perceptions of parents' political sophistication. L = low, M = medium, H = high.

[a] antitype: the cell frequency is smaller than expected by change.
[t] type: the cell frequency is larger than expected by chance.

this particular cell), the most notable observations are that the HL adolescents at T1 were less likely than expected by chance to appear in the HH cluster at T2, and the HH adolescents at T1 were less likely than expected by chance to appear in the HL cluster at T2. In essence, the participants in these two clusters appear to show opposite developmental trends over time.

Parents' Socialization Attempts

We had hypothesized that the HH adolescents at T1 would perceive more open political interactions with their parents (i.e., frequent political discussions with their parents, awareness of their parents' political socialization attempts, openness to their parents' political communication, susceptibility to parents' political communication, and awareness of joint political discussions) than the other adolescents. As can be seen in Table 11.6, which reports the results of ordinary ANOVAs, this also seemed to be the case. There were highly significant differences between the cluster groups, with HH adolescents scoring highest on the aggregated factor of open political interactions with parents. The η^2 is a measure of effect size, and the value of 0.18 indicates a large effect size for the differences that exist between the five cluster groups. The reports of the HL adolescents were below the average for the entire sample. It should be noted that the HH adolescents had significantly higher mean scores than the adolescents in the other clusters also when all four original indicators were examined individually. Regarding the effects of the control variables, parental education and immigrant status were significant ($p < .001$) for adolescents' reports of political interactions with their parents. High levels of political interactions were more common among highly educated parents and less common among adolescents with immigrant parents.

The measure of Parents' reports of political interactions with their adolescents was a factor score covering parents' attempts to politically socialize their

TABLE 11.6 Differences between the five cluster groups on adolescent- and parent-reported measures of their political interactions (factor scores) and adolescent political interest. Z-scores.

Cluster group	*1*	*2*	*3*	*4*	*5*	*F*	*p*	η^2
Parents	Low	Low	Medium	High	High			
Adolescents	Low	Medium	Medium	Low	High			
Label	LL	LM	MM	HL	HH			
Open political interactions (A)	-0.83^{a}	-0.29^{b}	0.05^{c}	-0.22^{bc}	0.69^{d}	22.66	<.001	0.18
Political socialization attempts (P)	-0.50^{ab}	-0.71^{a}	-0.21^{b}	0.35^{c}	0.51^{d}	17.52	<.001	0.15
Political interest (A)	-0.40^{a}	-0.23^{ab}	0.08^{b}	-0.05^{ab}	0.52^{c}	9.00	<.001	0.07

Note: All measures in the table are standardized. Across rows, superscripts represent significant differences ($p < .05$) between clusters in SNK post-hoc tests.

A, adolescent reports; P, parent reports.

adolescents (providing political information, attempting to politically influence, and frequently discussing political issues with their adolescents—one factor in a principal component analysis). The effect size for the differences between the cluster groups was about large ($\eta^2 = 0.15$). The most active parents were the parents of HH adolescents. In line with the high political sophistication of the parents, the parents of HL adolescents also reported relatively strong attempts to politically socialize their adolescents. Significantly higher means were found for the three original indicators for both HL and HH adolescents than for adolescents in the other clusters. This suggests that politically sophisticated parents do indeed try to politically socialize their children more than other parents. However, among the adolescents in these families, it is mainly the HH adolescents who are able to recognize and be open to their parents' political communication. None of the covariates were significant at the .001 level.

Adolescents' Political Interest

We had expected that a certain level of political interest would be necessary for adolescents to be able to perceive their parents' high political sophistication. As can be seen in Table 11.6, HH adolescents also stand out in this respect, while HL adolescents have average scores. The effect size for the differences between the cluster groups was medium ($\eta^2 = 0.07$). None of the control variables were significant at the .001 level.

Four Years Later

Of the 505 participants in the cluster analysis at age 16, 242 (48%) participated again in a data collection four years later, when they were 20 years old. All scales/

items that made up the factor Adolescents' perceptions of open political interactions with parents (parents' provision of political support, parents' attempts to influence their adolescents politically, parents' views are important, susceptibility to parents' political communication, and frequency of political discussions) at age 16 were factor analyzed again at age 20. One factor emerged with factor loadings ranging from 0.50 to 0.72 (explaining 50% of the variance). This factor and the political interest of the participants at age 20 were compared between the original cluster groups at age 16. Covariates were sex and immigrant status. The results from this ANOVA are reported in Table 11.7.

Now, at age 20, when most of the participants were no longer living at home with their parents, there were still significant differences between the age 16 clusters. Again at this age, the youth in the HH cluster reported significantly higher perceptions of open political interactions with their parents than did youth in the other four clusters. The effect size was medium. The differences among the five clusters for political interest were significant, but none of the clusters differed from each other. The effect size was small. However, the youth in the HH cluster had the highest mean score. Neither of the two covariates were significant. We conclude that the differences in perceptions of open political interactions with parents and political interest that existed among the five clusters at age 16 were reproduced to a large extent four years later.

Discussion

Tedin (1974) argued that if parents are to be successful in transmitting their values and attitudes to their children, children must have accurate perceptions of their parents' values and attitudes. We reformulated this argument to suggest that adolescents' attention to their parents' political communication and influence would be facilitated if they correctly perceived their parents' high political sophistication—high interest and knowledge. To identify the constellation of adolescents whose parents had high political sophistication and where adolescents perceived their

TABLE 11.7 Differences between the five cluster groups on adolescent-reported measures of their political interactions (factor scores) and their political interest at age 20. Z-scores.

Cluster group	*1*	*2*	*3*	*4*	*5*	*F*	*p*	η^2
Parents	Low	Low	Medium	High	High			
Adolescents	Low	Medium	Medium	Low	High			
Label	LL	LM	MM	HL	HH			
N	28	20	76	58	60			
Open political interactions	-0.51^{a}	-0.26^{ab}	-0.08^{ab}	0.04^{b}	0.50^{c}	7.18	<.001	0.12
Political interest	-0.16^{ab}	-0.48^{a}	0.11^{ab}	0.04^{ab}	0.40^{ab}	3.84	.005	0.06

Note: All measures in the table are standardized. Across rows, superscripts represent significant differences ($p < .05$) between clusters in SNK post-hoc tests.

parents to have high sophistication, we cluster analyzed parents' reports of their political sophistication simultaneously with 16-year-old adolescents' reports of their parents' political sophistication. Five clusters were extracted, one of which contained adolescents whose parents had high political sophistication and whose adolescents also perceived the parents to have high political sophistication (labeled HH adolescents). This group of adolescents represented 26% of the sample at age 16. An almost equally large group (22%) was a cluster in which parents reported high political sophistication but their adolescents reported that their parents had low political sophistication (referred to as the HL adolescents). Three other clusters emerged in which both parents and adolescents reported low or medium parental political sophistication. Not surprisingly, what characterized the HH and HL clusters relative to the other three groups was that their parents had significantly higher levels of education.

Despite this similarity between HH and HL adolescents, these two groups of adolescents had quite different experiences of political interaction with their parents. The HH adolescents reported greater awareness of and openness to their parents' political socialization attempts than adolescents in the other cluster groups. (They recognized that their parents tried to provide them with political support, that their parents tried to influence them politically, that their parents' political views were important to them, that they had frequent political discussions at home, and that they were receptive to their parents' political communication.) Overall, these findings support the first study hypothesis that adolescents who accurately identify their parents' high political sophistication also recognize their parents' efforts to politically socialize them and are receptive to these political socialization efforts. It is noteworthy that the differences in perceptions of open political interaction with parents and personal political interest that existed among the five clusters at age 16 were largely reproduced four years later—at a time when the majority were no longer living at home with their parents.

In addition to the high level of education of the parents of the HH and HL adolescents, when parents reported on their political interactions with their adolescents, both the parents of the HH and HL adolescents reported higher levels of political socialization attempts than the parents of the other three cluster groups (more than other parents they provided political support, tried to influence their adolescents politically, and had frequent political discussions with their adolescents). This is what we should expect from highly educated parents with high political skills (Patterson & Pahlke, 2021). They should be particularly concerned with the political socialization of their adolescents. But apparently the parents of the HL adolescents were less successful.

Why? Either the parents of the HL adolescents were less able to transmit their political enthusiasm and knowledge to their children. They lacked the necessary communication skills that the parents of the HH youth had. This is one explanation. Jennings et al. (2009) proposed and found support for the idea that parents need to express their attitudes consistently over time for the transmission of their attitudes and values to take place. Another explanation for the different perceptions of HH and HL adolescents is that this difference is more a function of adolescent characteristics. In this study, we argued that adolescents need to have a certain level of political interest in order to perceive their parents' high political sophistication. This hypothesis was supported. The HH adolescents had significantly higher political interest than the other cluster groups of adolescents. In contrast, the political interest of the HL adolescents was at the average level of the entire sample.

Perhaps one would expect that HL adolescents would become more similar to HH adolescents over time as a result of their parents' socialization efforts. However, there is little empirical support for this idea. When we cross-tabulated the cluster solution that the 16-year-olds had one year later, the HL adolescents were less likely than expected by chance to appear in the HH cluster, and the HH adolescents were less likely than expected by chance to appear in the HL cluster one year later. Thus, their political development over time appears to be in opposite rather than similar directions. Future studies are needed to identify the conditions, both on the part of parents and adolescents, that significantly increase the likelihood over time that adolescents will adopt their parents' political interests and views.

The main strength of this study is that it applies and largely confirms a model of how adolescents' perceptions of their parents' high levels of political interest and knowledge are related to their perceptions of their parents' political support and influence, and to their acceptance of their parents' political messages. Another strength of the study is its multi-informant design, which includes both parental and adolescent reports. The main limitation of the study is that it cannot draw causal conclusions. The study's hypothesis is that an accurate perception of one's parents' high political sophistication benefits adolescents in recognizing their parents' political support and influence and makes them susceptible to their parents' political communication. This is not to say that the causal sequences cannot be reversed.

Nevertheless, a general conclusion is that adolescents' correct perception of their parents' high political sophistication seems to pave the way for the recognition of parents' political socialization attempts and an openness to parents' political communication. This openness suggests that these adolescents are more likely than other adolescents to accept their parents as political role models.

Parental education seems to affect parents' own attempts to politically socialize their adolescents, but this does not mean that the educational effect translates into more political interactions and higher political interest among adolescents. Both HH and HL adolescents had parents with higher levels of education than the other cluster groups. Both HH and HL parents also reported more attempts to politically socialize their adolescents compared to parents of adolescents in the other cluster groups. Adolescents reported on their political interactions with their parents. This was a factor score covering their perceptions of parents' provision of political information, parents' attempts to politically influence their adolescents, whether parents' views were important, susceptibility to parents' political communication, and having political discussions with parents. Despite higher levels of parental education in the HH and HL clusters, adolescents in the HH cluster reported significantly higher levels of openness to political interaction with parents than adolescents in the other clusters, and also higher levels of political interest than adolescents in the other clusters. This suggests that higher levels of parental education do not necessarily mean that young people benefit from their family background. This seems to be related to young people's perceptions of their parents' political sophistication.

Subgroup studies are needed for more precise theory building. If this study had been based on a correlational design, it would have started with the finding that the correlation between parents' political sophistication and adolescents' perceptions of their parents' political sophistication was .29, $p < .001$ when the adolescents were 16 years old and .25, $p < .001$ one year later. From these low correlations, one would not expect to distinguish a group of adolescents who were highly receptive to their political socialization attempts from a group of adolescents who were much less receptive. Interactions could have been tested in a regression design, but it is difficult to confirm hypotheses that predict interaction effects. The person-centered approach used here was preferred to correlational analyses for testing the specific hypothesis about the reformulation of the perceptual accuracy argument.

Finally, what evidence has been presented in this chapter that young people are active agents in their own political development?

When we clustered parents' reports of their political sophistication and adolescents' reports of their parents' political sophistication, we found five clusters, including two clusters in which parents reported high political sophistication. In one of these clusters, adolescents accurately reported that their parents had high political sophistication. In the other cluster, adolescents reported that their parents had low political sophistication. In both clusters, parents' reported attempts to politically socialize their adolescents were significantly higher than parents' reports in the other cluster groups.

If parents' attempts at political socialization were successful, then adolescents in these two clusters should report high levels of openness to political interaction with their parents. This was not the case. High levels of openness to political interaction with parents were particularly concentrated in the cluster where parents report high political sophistication and their adolescents accurately report that their parents have high political sophistication. This is strong evidence that adolescents need to accurately perceive their parents' high political sophistication in order to be open to political communication from their parents. To be able to perceive their parents' high political sophistication, adolescents need to have some level of political interest. We found that adolescents in this cluster group had higher levels of political interest than adolescents in the other cluster groups. In conclusion, if parents' attempts at political socialization are to be successful, adolescents need to be able to understand that their parents are politically interested and knowledgeable about political issues. How adolescents perceive their parents' political sophistication seems to matter a great deal for their political interactions with their parents.

12

POLITICALLY INTERESTED ADOLESCENTS ARE NOT A HOMOGENEOUS GROUP

Highlights

What role do basic human values play in the political values, attitudes, and behaviors of politically interested adolescents?

We used cluster analysis of 16-year-old adolescents' political interest and concern for the welfare of others, expecting to find a group of adolescents with high political interest and high concern for the welfare of others (HH adolescents) and a group of highly politically interested adolescents with low concern (HL adolescents). Five cluster groups were obtained, two of which matched the expected characteristics. Hypotheses about differences between the HH and the HL adolescents were developed. HH adolescents reported higher environmental values, more inclusive attitudes toward immigrants, higher evaluations of democratic principles, and a greater willingness to intervene if something endangered the welfare of others than adolescents in the other clusters. The HL adolescents were uniformly below average on all of these comparison measures, and they had particularly low environmental values. The HH adolescents had higher political efficacy and were more involved in civic organizations and offline political activities than the other adolescents. Both HH and HL were more engaged in online political activities than other cluster groups of adolescents. It seems that the main channel for political activities for HL adolescents is the Internet. We conclude that the basic human value of concern for the welfare of others translates the high political interest of adolescents into various attitudes and behaviors.

Using the same clustering technique, about the same types of clusters were found when we examined parents' political interests and their concern for the welfare of others. The results of comparing measures of concern for others and nature between the parent cluster groups were similar to the differences between the adolescent cluster groups. Among both parents and adolescents, the HH cluster group was significantly more involved in civic organizations, had more inclusive attitudes toward immigrants, were more willing to engage in political action if they felt it was necessary, and had higher environmental values.

Although the outcome measures are similarly related to the adolescent and parent cluster groups, it is almost by chance that individual families contain parents and adolescents who have the same cluster combination. The exception is the combination of high political interest and high concern for the welfare of others.

DOI: 10.4324/9781003371731-17

A Concern for Other People's Welfare

Throughout this book, we have considered a high level of political interest to be a desirable characteristic in young people. For developmental psychologists, a young person's political interest indicates positive youth development (Sherrod, 2007). In political science, a high level of political interest is considered vital to society: "Political interest is key to the founding of a country because it promotes good citizenship" (Prior, 2019, p. 352). This is not necessarily the case. Politically interested adolescents and young adults may be politically distrustful, have conspiracy theories, and hold undemocratic views and racist attitudes (Wray-Lake, 2019). They may become politically radicalized and have ideas that show little concern for others. In short, they do not necessarily have characteristics associated with good citizenship. In this chapter, we will compare politically interested adolescents with high concern for the welfare of others to politically interested adolescents with low concern. We will use cluster analysis, and we expect these two groups to emerge as naturally occurring clusters. Further, we expect these two groups of adolescents to differ profoundly on basic values, attitudes, and behaviors that reflect their high or low concern for others and nature.

Thinking and caring about others can be seen as fundamental assets in society (Bardi & Schwartz, 2003). In both individualistic and collectivistic cultures, parents try to teach their children to treat others with respect and dignity. Parents' socialization efforts must be seen in the light of their children's ability to understand their parents' values. It seems that values related to concern for the welfare of others tend to stabilize already in childhood (Döring et al., 2015; Vecchione et al., 2020). van Deth et al. (2011) found that four out of five children were able to endorse helping others as a desirable quality of citizenship as early as the first year of primary school. Thus, from the perspective of political socialization, young people seem to be able to reflect on values related to caring for others at a fairly early age.

This characterization of values is elaborated in Shalom Schwartz's theory of basic human values (1994, 2016; Schwartz et al., 2012), which was introduced in Chapter 9. Schwartz argues that values express people's desirable goals, are organizing principles for their behavior, and guide their attitudes and activities in everyday life. His theory includes 10 motivational values that are thought to differentiate people around the world. One of these universal values is that of societal concern, which refers to a "commitment to equality, justice, and protection for all people" (Schwartz et al., 2012, p. 669). This value, referred to here as *concern for the welfare of others*, will be analyzed in this study simultaneously with the political interest of adolescents. In the context of politically interested adolescents, this will essentially involve comparisons between those with high concern for others' welfare and those with low concern. Since these two groups are expected to differ in their values of concern for others' welfare, they can be expected to differ in other values, attitudes, and behaviors as well.

Minority groups. Concern for the welfare of others among politically interested adolescents is expected to be associated with inclusive attitudes toward minority groups. Substantial associations between universalist values and inclusive attitudes toward minority groups have been reported previously (Kuntz et al., 2015; Sagiv & Schwartz, 1995; Vecchione et al., 2012). In the present study, we examine the attitudes of politically engaged adolescents toward immigrants and expect that those who are more concerned about the welfare of others will have more inclusive attitudes than those who are less concerned.

Democratic principles. Social justice and equality are key features of the value of caring for others. They are also basic democratic principles (Miller, 1978). In this chapter, we expect that positive attitudes toward democratic principles will be stronger among politically engaged youth with high concern for others than among those with low concern.

Standby citizens. Democracies need people who are knowledgeable and can monitor the consequences of political actions and then act on their moral convictions (Schudson, 1998). The term "standby citizens" was coined by Amnå and Ekman (2014) to emphasize the willingness to intervene in politics when people are treated unfairly. Standby citizens should be a societal asset because their values make them vigilant and easily trigger their macro concern that other people may be treated unfairly (Boehnke & Schwartz, 1997; Schwartz et al., 2000). Our hypothesis is that politically interested adolescents with high concern for the welfare of others are the adolescents who should be more likely to intervene and manifest their values when they perceive the welfare of others to be at risk than politically interested adolescents with low concern.

Nature. In Schwartz's model (Schwartz et al., 2012), concern for the welfare of others is closely related to concern for nature, and these two values form a broader set of universalist values. Thus, people who hold values about equality, justice, and helping other people also tend to respect and protect nature. This is also likely to be the case for politically interested adolescents. If politically interested adolescents endorse concern for the welfare of others, they are likely to endorse concern for nature. Furthermore, if adolescents' environmental values are organizing principles for their behavior, then these values should guide their environmental activities and thinking in everyday life (Bardi & Schwartz, 2003; Schwartz & Butenko, 2014). For example, adolescents with high political interest who report high concern for the welfare of others should be more likely than politically interested adolescents with low political concern to engage in pro-environmental behaviors in their daily lives and to feel a strong sense of collective environmental effectiveness—that is, a sense that they can address the threat of climate change together with others (Jugert et al., 2016).

Political Engagement

Specifically, our hypotheses concern differences in the content of politically interested adolescents' opinions, attitudes, and behaviors related to caring for people.

These are expected to differ between politically interested adolescents with high and low concern for the welfare of others. But how do politically interested adolescents with high or low concern for others translate their interest in politics into political action? There is reason to believe that there are links between adolescents' concern for people and their involvement in civic organizations and political activities that share the same motivational values.

It might be expected that politically interested adolescents who place a high value on the welfare of others would be more involved in civic associations than politically interested adolescents who place a lower value on the welfare of others, and would also be more involved in civic activities offline: associations and activities that are often based on concern for people and nature. Whether the two groups of adolescents differ in their online political activities is an open question. Moreover, from the 1980s (Finkel, 1985) to the present (Oser, 2021), internal political efficacy has emerged as one of the stronger predictors of political behavior and participation. Potentially, differences in political behavior between politically interested adolescents who are high or low in concern for the welfare of others can be seen in differences in their sense of political efficacy.

Universal values tend to be held more strongly by women than by men (Schwartz & Rubel-Lifschitz, 2009). Therefore, gender was controlled for in the main analyses. We also controlled for immigrant status because values, attitudes, and behaviors may differ between youth whose parents were born in the country and those whose parents were not. In a final set of analyses, gender differences were examined for all measures in the study.

Finally, confirmation of the hypotheses raises the question of whether civic knowledge and political visibility differ between the politically engaged adolescents with high and low concern for the welfare of others. Therefore, a test of participants' civic knowledge and a measure of political reputation in the classroom were used to examine potential differences between the two groups of adolescents.

Sample and Analyses

The 16-year-old cohort was used. The target sample consisted of 1052 students in 57 classes, and the analytic sample consisted of 857 people (81%). The scales we used are listed in Table 12.1.

Political interest and concern for the welfare of others were the two basic measures that were clustered. Both measures were standardized. Standardized values above 2.5 were set to 2.5 and values below −2.5 were set to −2.5. First, a hierarchical analysis (Ward's method) was used to determine the number of clusters. The criterion was that the number of clusters should account for at least 67% of the total error sums of squares (Bergman et al., 2003). Five factors were found, explaining 71% of the total error sums of squares. Second, a non-hierarchical cluster analysis, *K*-means clustering, was used to arrive at the final cluster solution (see Kinder et al., 1991).

TABLE 12.1 Scales and items used in the chapter.

Concept	*Items*	*Response scale*
Political interest [a]:		
"How interested are you in politics?"	1	1 (*totally uninterested*) 5 (*very interested*)
"People differ in how they feel about politics. What are your feelings?"	1	1 (*loathe*) 6 (*great fun*)
Concern for other people's welfare:		
"Equality, equal opportunities for all," "A peaceful world free of war and conflict," "Helping other people," "Social justice, removing injustice, and caring for the less fortunate in society," and "Working together with others for a better society"	5	1 (*not at all important*) 5 (*very important*)
Trust in societal movements:		
How much trust do you have in "Societal movements (e.g., organizations for human rights, environmental organizations, the Animal Rights Movement)?"	1	1 (*no trust at all*) 4 (*a lot of trust*)
Member of a civic association:		
The participants were asked if they were a member of any of two types of associations: environmental association, or an association for peace or human rights (e.g., the peace movement, Amnesty International).	3	1 (*no*) 2 (*yes*)
Standby citizenship [b]:		
Stem question: "How active should people be on political issues? What do you think? For me it is important to . . .:" "Protest when people are treated unfairly," "React when something important is at stake," "Give up my time when others ask me to step in," and "Keep an eye on what is going on, so that I can do something if needed."	4	1 (*not important at all*) 4 (*very important*)
Inclusive attitudes toward immigrants:		
"Our culture is enriched when people from other countries move here," "In the future, Sweden will be a country offering exciting encounters between people from different parts of the world," "Immigrants should have same rights as people born in Sweden."	3	1 (*doesn't apply at all*) 5 (*applies very well*)
Positive attitudes toward democratic principles:		
"There are different views on how society should function. What is your view?" followed by statements about democratic rights, "All citizens are free to choose their leaders," "Women should have the same rights as men," and "Everyone should have the right to publicly criticize the government," and about democratic obligations, "You must follow the laws determined by the majority," "Violence must never be used in political protests," and "You have to pay taxes that are democratically determined."	6	1 (*disagree completely*) 4 (*agree completely*)
Environmental values:		
Concern for nature ("Respecting nature and thinking ecologically," "Protecting the environment and preserving nature," and "Preventing pollution of the environment and not wasting resources")	3	1 (*not at all important*) 5 (*very important*)
Pro-environmental behaviors [c]:		
"Help my parents to sort at source," "Use public transport, cycle, or walk rather than being taken by car," "Turn off the light when I leave an empty room"	6	1 (*almost never*) 5 (*always*)

Collective environmental efficacy:		
The stem question: "How well do the following apply to what you think?" followed by two statements: "If we all pitch in, we can solve many environmental problems" and "If we work together, we can do something about climate change."	2	1 (*doesn't apply at all*) 5 (*applies very well*)
Internal political efficacy:		
Covers nine items which refer to a domain-specific efficacy belief in the capacity of one's own actions to effect change in society (Bandura, 2006). After the stem, "If I really tried, I could manage to . . ., " the participants responded to nine statements, such as "Take on responsibility in a political youth organization" and "Discuss politics with people with more experience than I have."	9	1 (*I could definitely not manage that*) 4 (*I could definitely manage that*).
Political activities offline:		
"Worked voluntarily for a good cause," "Attended a meeting concerned with political or societal issues," "Collected signatures," "Distributed leaflets with a political content," "Took part in a legal demonstration or strike," "Donated money to a good cause," "Boycotted or bought certain products for political, ethical or environmental reasons," "Donated money to support the work of a political group or organization," "Wore a badge or a t-shirt with a political message."	8	1 (*no*) 3 (*yes, several times*)
Member of a civic association:		
The participants were asked if they were a member of any of two types of associations: environmental association, or an association for peace or human rights (e.g., the peace movement, Amnesty International).	3	1 (*no*) 2 (*yes*)
Political activities online:		
"Discussed societal or political questions with friends on the Internet," "Linked news to my friends," "Chatted with friends on the Net about something I've seen on the news," "Sent friends music that I think has a good political and societal message," "Sought information about politics or societal issues on the Internet," "Read about politics in a blog," "Viewed videos or film clips about societal issues or politics."	7	1 (*no*) 3 (*yes, several times*)
Political reputation in class:		
"Here, different types of people are described. Which of your classmates fit the two descriptions? The participants could report up to three classmates for each of the two descriptions. "Keeps track of what is going on in Sweden and in the world" "Often starts discussions about societal issues in class."	2	
Test of civic knowledge:		
"Of which American state was the actor Arnold Schwarzenegger the governor?" "Which of the following countries are not members of the EU?" "What does 'development assistance' mean?" "All but one of these people have been Sweden's prime minister. Which one?"	8	
Covariates:		
Immigrant status was a dichotomous measure differentiating between students whose parents were born outside the Nordic countries (coded 1) and other students (coded 0). Sex was coded 0 = female, 1 = male.	2	

[a] The interest question was re-scaled to range between 1 and 6, and the two items were then aggregated. The correlation between the two items was .59, $p < .001$.

[b] (Amnå & Ekman, 2014).

[c] Ojala (2010).

TABLE 12.2 A cluster analysis of adolescent political interest and concern for the welfare of others.

Clusters	*LL*	*LA*	*AA*	*HL*	*HH*
Political interest	−1.18	−1.05	0.07	0.73	0.95
Concern for others	−1.30	0.51	−0.03	−1.37	0.79
N	123	166	234	78	256
%	14.4	19.4	27.3	9.1	29.9
% boys [a]	66.7	39.2	41.5	74.4	44.9
% immigrants [b]	10.6	16.4	11.5	5.2	19.5

Note: Low values (lowest to −.70); average values (>−.69 to 0.69); high values (>.70).

[a] F (df = 4) = 48.88, $p < .001$.
[b] F (df =4) = 14.46, $p = .006$.

Results

Cluster Analysis

The cluster solution is shown in Table 12.2. The five clusters were as follows: LL (low interest and low concern), LA (low interest, average concern), AA (average interest, average concern), HL (high interest, low concern), and HH (high interest, high concern). We confirm the existence of two groups of politically interested adolescents. One has low concern for the welfare of others (HL) and the other has high concern for the welfare of others (HH). Of these two groups of politically interested adolescents, most showed high concern for the welfare of others ($n = 256$) and fewer expressed low concern ($n = 78$). It is noticeable that the cluster with high political interest and low concern for others (the HL cluster) was predominantly composed of males (74%). The HH cluster was more evenly divided between boys and girls.

Differences Between the Main Two Cluster Groups

Hypothesized differences. Table 12.3 reports differences between the five cluster groups for measures that were hypothesized to differentiate between the two groups of adolescents with high political interest. Without exceptions, these one-way ANOVAs showed that the highly politically adolescents with high concern for others scored significantly higher on all comparison measures than the other four cluster groups. They had more positive attitudes toward immigrants, had more trust in social movements, were more involved in civic organizations, had more positive attitudes toward democratic principles, and scored higher on the measure of standby citizen, that is, a higher willingness to act politically if something bad were to happen to other people. They expressed greater concern for the environment, had

TABLE 12.3 Differences between the five cluster groups on measures of concern for others and for nature. Z-scores.

Clusters	*LL*	*LA*	*AA*	*HL*	*HH*	*F*	*p*	η^2
Care for others:								
Trust in societal movements	-0.60^{a}	-0.25^{b}	0.10^{c}	-0.39^{ab}	0.48^{d}	35.85	<.001	0.15
Member of civic association	-0.13^{a}	-0.18^{a}	-0.16^{a}	-0.01^{a}	0.34^{b}	10.42	<.001	0.05
Standby citizen	-0.76^{a}	-0.33^{b}	0.07^{c}	-0.16^{b}	0.57^{d}	29.87	<.001	0.11
Attitude immigrants	-0.70^{a}	-0.14^{bc}	0.03^{c}	-0.34^{a}	0.49^{d}	31.90	<.001	0.12
Attitude democratic principles	-0.49^{a}	-0.15^{b}	0.02^{b}	-0.17^{b}	0.35^{c}	15.77	<.001	0.07
Care for nature:								
Environmental values	-0.91^{a}	0.15^{b}	0.08^{b}	-0.79^{a}	0.52^{c}	68.32	<.001	0.24
Pro-environmental behaviors	-0.57^{a}	-0.25^{b}	0.09^{c}	-0.20^{b}	0.40^{d}	23.51	<.001	0.10
Environmental efficacy	-0.59^{a}	-0.22^{b}	0.16^{c}	-0.27^{b}	0.43^{d}	30.55	<.001	0.12

Note: All measures are standardized. Across rows, superscripts represent significant differences ($p < .05$) between clusters in SNK post-hoc tests.

higher pro-environmental behaviors, and higher environmental efficacy. Compared to these adolescents, the cluster group of highly politically interested adolescents with low concern for the welfare of others scored low on these measures. The effect size was high for environmental values and medium for the other measures.

Political efficacy and political activities. Table 12.4 shows the differences between the cluster groups for political efficacy and political activity. The effect size across cluster groups for political efficacy was high. The adolescents with high political interest and high concern for others had the highest political efficacy score. This cluster group also reported more frequent offline political activity. Here, the differences between the cluster groups were small. In contrast, engaging in online political activities was equally common among both groups of highly politically interested adolescents with high and low concern for others. The effect size was large. Thus, the differences between the two study groups are related to whether the political activities take place offline or online. For offline activities, the group of politically interested adolescents with high concern for others scored highest. For online political activities, they, and the HL adolescents were both more active than the other three cluster groups.

Robustness of results. To examine the robustness of the differences among the cluster groups, the comparison measures at age 16 (Tables 12.3 and 12.4) were exchanged for the same comparison measures two years later, at age 18. As can be seen in Table 12.5, political interest was significantly higher among HH and HL adolescents than the other two cluster groups, and the highest levels of concern for the welfare of others were found among HH adolescents, while the HL cluster group still scored very low. Furthermore, although the average η^2 decreased from 0.12 to 0.08 over the two years for the 10 comparison measures in Table 12.5, the

TABLE 12.4 Differences between the five cluster groups on internal political efficacy and offline and online political activity. Z-scores.

Clusters	*LL*	*LA*	*AA*	*HL*	*HH*	*F*	*p*	η^2
Political efficacy	−0.53^{a}	−0.46^{a}	−0.08^{b}	0.27^{c}	0.55^{d}	44.02	<.001	0.18
Offline political activities	−0.24^{a}	−0.18^{a}	−0.09^{a}	−0.06^{a}	0.33^{b}	11.07	<.001	0.05
Online political activities	−0.47^{a}	−0.47	−0.09^{b}	0.38^{c}	0.48^{c}	39.33	<.001	0.16

Note: All measures are standardized; Across rows, superscripts represent significant differences ($p < .05$) between clusters in SNK post-hoc tests.

TABLE 12.5 Differences between the five cluster groups on measures of concern for others and nature, and on political efficacy and political activity two years later, at age 18. Z-scores.

Clusters	*LL*	*LA*	*AA*	*HL*	*HH*	*F*	*p*	η^2
Political interest	−0.69^{a}	−0.55^{a}	−0.04^{b}	0.58^{c}	0.61^{c}	54.61	<.001	0.26
Concern for others' welfare	−0.79^{a}	0.16^{b}	−0.00^{b}	−0.70^{a}	0.50^{c}	40.28	<.001	0.21
Care for others:								
Trust in societal movements	−0.39^{a}	−0.02^{bc}	−0.04^{b}	−0.33^{a}	0.29^{c}	8.96	<.001	0.06
Member of a civic association	−0.12^{a}	−0.10^{a}	−0.05^{a}	0.06^{a}	0.15^{a}	1.66	.158	0.00
Standby citizen	−0.61^{a}	−0.11^{b}	−0.08^{b}	0.08^{b}	0.43^{c}	17.93	<.001	0.11
Attitude immigrants	−0.51^{a}	−0.08^{bc}	0.03^{c}	−0.30^{ab}	0.42^{d}	16.00	<.001	0.10
Care for nature:								
Environmental values	−0.49^{a}	−0.00^{b}	0.04^{b}	−0.56^{a}	0.36^{c}	17.57	<.001	0.11
Pro-environmental behaviors	−0.42^{a}	−0.02^{bc}	0.07^{bc}	−0.19^{ab}	0.23^{c}	7.24	<.001	0.05
Environmental efficacy	−0.18^{a}	.0.14^{a}	−0.03^{a}	−0.19^{a}	0.29^{b}	5.83	<.001	0.04
Political efficacy and activities:								
Political efficacy	−0.56a	−0.33a	−0.01b	0.25bc	0.46c	23.24	.001	0.13
Offline activities	−0.41^{a}	−0.33^{a}	−0.01^{b}	0.11^{b}	0.43^{c}	15.94	<.001	0.09
Online activities	−0.33^{a}	−0.34^{a}	−0.11^{a}	0.31^{b}	0.35^{b}	15.56	<.001	0.09

Note: All measures are standardized. Across rows, superscripts represent significant differences ($p < .05$) between clusters in SNK post-hoc tests.

Some items in the scale Attitude toward democratic principles was not measured at age 18, so the scale was dropped.

HH adolescents consistently had the highest scores, and in 6 cases out of 12 these scores were significantly higher than those of the other cluster groups. We conclude that the differences between the HH and HL adolescents persist over a considerable period of adolescence. Again, as in Table 12.4, both the HH and the HL adolscents scored high on online political activities.

TABLE 12.6 Differences between the five cluster groups on political reputation in the classroom and a test of adolescents' political/societal knowledge. Z-scores.

	LL	*LA*	*AA*	*HL*	*HH*	F^{1}	*p*	η^2
Political reputation	−0.22[ab]	−0.32[a]	−0.04[b]	0.39[c]	0.26[c]	13.38	<.001	0.06
Civic knowledge	−0.18[ab]	−0.41[a]	−0.04[b]	0.48[d]	0.23[c]	14.49	<.001	0.07

Note: All measures are standardized; Across rows, superscripts represent significant differences ($p < .05$) between clusters in SNK post-hoc tests.

Reputation and Knowledge

Do HH and HL adolescents differ in the way their political interest and knowledge are visible to others and in their knowledge of politics and society as revealed by an "objective" knowledge test? As reported in Table 12.6, both the highly politically interested with high and low concern for others had higher political reputations in their classes than the other three cluster groups. This was also the case for the civic knowledge test. Here, the cluster group with high political interest and low concern for others actually had significantly higher reputation and knowledge scores than the politically interested youth with high concern for others.

Civil Society Organizations, Trust in Institutions, Radical Groups, and Use of Violence for Political Purposes

We made a more in-depth analysis of which of the most common civil society organizations in Sweden were approved by the young people in the five cluster groups. The value orientation of these organizations parallels the high value of concern for the welfare of others among members of the HH cluster. Therefore, we expected that especially the HH youth would approve of these CSOs. We also made a comparison in another direction. We examined the approval of more radical forms of groups, but did not have explicit hypotheses about this approval. Finally, we examined which of the cluster groups of adolescents would consider using violence for political purposes.

Adolescents were asked "There are many groups and organizations in society. Which ones do you like?" and were presented with six different types of nonprofit organizations or groups.

- *Environment-protection associations*, such as Climax, Greenpeace, Friends of the Earth
- *Animal-rights groups*, such as the Animal Rights Alliance, Animal Rights Sweden, the Animal Liberation Front
- *Equality issues and feminism*, such as the Women's Front in Sweden, Young Women's Empowerment Centers, the Women's Political Forum
- *Aid organizations*, such as the Red Cross, Save the Children, and Doctors Without Frontiers

- *Peace activism and peace work*, such as the Ofog Network (against different forms of militarism in Sweden), Sweden's Peace and Arbitration Association, the Plowshares Movement
- *Solidarity with refugees and other exposed groups*, such as the No One Is Illegal Network, the Network against Racism, the International Solidarity Movement, Palestine Group

Trust in institutions was measured asking the participants "How much trust do you have in the parliament, the government, the courts, the political parties, with response scales ranging from (1) *no trust at all* to (4) *a lot of trust*. Alpha reliability for the four items was 0.92.

Some adolescents in the five cluster groups might approve of radical groups or be positive about the use of violence for political purposes. Therefore, we examined differences between the cluster groups for approval of radical left and radical right groups and approval of violence for political purposes:

- *Left-wing radical groups*, such as Counterforce (Motkraft.net), the Young Socialists, Anti Fascist Action (AFA)
- *Right-wing radical groups*, such as Info 14, the Swedish Resistance Movement, the Party of the Swedes (formerly the National Socialist Front)

The response options for nonprofit organizations and radical groups were 1 (*don't like*), 2 (*like a lot*), and 3 (*don't know or am uncertain*). We differentiated between the adolescents who liked each of the organizations/groups at lot versus was those who were uncertain or didn't like these organizations.

- *Approval of violence for political purposes* was measured with two items. The first had the stem question "There are different conceptions of what society should be like. What do you think yourself?" and the specific question was: "Violence should never be used at political protests." The response scale ranged from 1 (*disagree absolutely*) to 4 (*agree absolutely*). The second item had the stem question "What do you think about breaking rules in order to change something in society?" The response continued with the statement "If I think that something is wrong:" and the response options were 1 (*I will stay within the law. Swedish law says what is right and proper. If we have decided on laws together, we must stick to them. If something is to be changed, it must be done within the law*), 2 (*I can imagine breaking the law. If the decisions made by politicians are wrong, it is right to go against the laws. So I can imagine going against the law if necessary*), and 3 (*I can imagine breaking the law even if other people are harmed. If a law is wrong, you sometimes have resort to drastic measures*). The two items were standardized and aggregated.

Table 12.7 reports the differences between the cluster groups for the civic organizations that the young people liked a lot and their approval of radical groups and

TABLE 12.7 Differences among the five cluster groups for approval of civic organizations, radical groups, and willingness to use political violence (z-score).

	LL	*LA*	*AA*	*HL*	*HH*	F^1	*p*	*eta*^{2}
Non-profit organizations								
Environment-protection	-0.40^{a}	-0.26^{a}	0.09^{b}	-0.13^{ab}	0.33^{c}	16.08	<.001	0.07
Animal-rights	-0.35^{a}	-0.08^{bc}	0.10^{cd}	-0.25^{ab}	0.21^{d}	8.77	<.001	0.04
Equality and feminism	-0.46^{a}	-0.04^{b}	0.17^{b}	-0.40^{a}	0.23^{b}	15.36	<.001	0.07
Aid	-0.59^{a}	-0.21^{b}	0.17^{c}	-0.14^{b}	0.32^{c}	22.96	<.001	0.10
Peace work	-0.45^{a}	-0.13^{b}	-0.02^{b}	-0.13^{b}	0.37^{c}	16.80	<.001	0.07
Solidarity	-0.29^{a}	-0.13^{a}	-0.12^{a}	-0.02^{a}	0.34^{b}	11.81	<.001	0.05
Trust in institutions, approval of radical groups and readiness to use violence and break the law:								
Trust in institutions	-0.37^{a}	0.03^{b}	0.07^{b}	0.07^{b}	0.32^{b}	4.92	<.001	0.04
Radical-left	-0.13^{b}	-0.13^{b}	0.03^{bc}	-0.21^{a}	0.20^{b}	4.76	<.001	0.02
Radical-right	-0.06^{a}	-0.02^{a}	0.03^{a}	0.16^{a}	-0.03^{a}	0.71	0.587	0.00
Use of violence	0.34^{a}	0.04^{bc}	-0.07^{c}	0.26^{ab}	-0.19^{c}	7.56	<.001	0.04
Break the law	0.36^{c}	0.12^{ab}	-0.12^{bc}	0.16^{ab}	-0.18^{c}	7.85	<.001	.004

Note: All measures in the table are standardized. Across rows, superscripts represent significant differences (p < .05) between clusters in SNK post-hoc tests.

approval of violence for political purposes. For ease of comparison with previous results, the response scales were transformed into *z*-scores.

There were significant differences at the .001 level between the cluster groups for all CSOs. The η^2 values indicate that the effect sizes were small to moderate. The general pattern of results is that HH adolescents reported the highest approval of all these types of organizations, and they had significantly higher approval scores than all other cluster groups for environmental protection, animal rights, peace, and solidarity organizations. The negative *z*-scores for HL cluster members indicated that they were not particularly interested in these CSOs. Finally, trust in institutions was highest among the HH participants, but they differed significantly only from one of the other cluster. There were small effect sizes when comparing the five cluster groups on approval of radical groups, willingness to use violence for political purposes, and willingness to break the law. The HL youth showed less approval of left-wing radical groups than the other cluster groups, and the use of violence for political purposes and the willingness to break the law were highest among the HL and LL cluster groups.

Sex Differences

What remains to be understood are the differences between boys and girls for the measures we have examined in this chapter. As shown in Table 12.8, which shows ordinary *t*-tests for these measures between boys and girls, there were no differences for political interest. Girls scored significantly higher than boys on concern

TABLE 12.8 Gender differences in the measures examined in the chapter (means).

	Total	*Boys*	*Girls*	*t*	*p*	*Cohen's d*
Political interest	3.04	3.04	3.03	0.11	.913	0.01
Concern for the welfare of others	4.19	4.02	4.35	−7.39	<.001	0.50
Trust in societal movements	2.46	2.23	2.68	−7.67	<.001	0.53
Member of a civic organization	2.03	2.03	2.04	−0.05	.964	0.01
Standby citizenship	2.76	2.61	2.89	−5.44	<.001	0.37
Attitudes toward immigrants	2.93	2.74	3.11	−7.45	<.001	0.51
Attitudes toward democratic principles	3.06	3.06	3.06	0.28	.781	0.01
Environmental values	3.74	3.60	3.87	−4.29	<.001	0.29
Pro-environmental behaviors	3.04	2.82	3.25	−6.78	<.001	0.46
Environmental efficacy	4.13	3.92	4.33	−5.76	<.001	0.39
Political efficacy	2.57	2.61	2.53	1.55	.123	0.11
Offline political activities	1.27	1.26	1.27	−0.44	.663	0.03
Online political activities	1.47	1.53	1.41	4.31	<.001	0.29
Political reputation	1.69	1.71	1.66	3.87	<.001	0.27
Knowledge test	6.46	8.27	4.71	4.18	<.001	0.28

for the welfare of others. Girls also scored higher on all environmental measures—environmental values, pro-environmental behavior, and environmental efficacy. In addition, girls scored higher on trust in social movements, inclusive attitudes toward immigrants, and willingness to act politically when something bad happens to other people. The effect sizes ranged from 0.29 to 0.53. Similar sex differences in caring for others were reported by Oswald and Schmid (1998). There were no sex differences in attitudes toward democratic principles and membership in a political/civic association.

There were no sex differences in political efficacy and offline political activity. Boys were more involved in online political activities, had higher political reputations in their classes, and scored higher on the civic knowledge test. The effect sizes were 0.29, 0.27, and 0.28, respectively.

Overall, girls reported being more concerned about the two universal values of caring for others and caring for nature. They also had more positive attitudes toward immigrants and democratic principles, and would intervene if people were in danger or being treated unfairly. On the other hand, boys were more likely to discuss politics with their friends on the Internet. Boys also had a higher level of civic knowledge and were seen by their classmates as someone who knew a lot about political issues and often brought this up in class.

Sex Differences: Civil Society Organizations, Radical Groups, and Use of Violence for Political Purposes

Sex differences were calculated for the measures in Table 12.7 (see Table 12.9). Given the significant sex differences we found in the value placed on concern for

TABLE 12.9 Differences between boys and girls for benevolent groups, trust in institutions, and more radical groups that the youth liked a lot[a] and for using violence[b] and breaking the law[c].

	Total	*Girls*	*Boys*	*t*	*Sign.*	*Cohen's d*
Environment protection	1.35	1.43	1.27	4.99	<.001	0.34
Animal rights	1.49	1.62	1.35	8.20	<.001	0.56
Equality issues and feminism	1.40	1.58	1.22	11.47	<.001	0.79
Aid	1.71	1.84	1.57	8.74	<.001	0.61
Peace work	1.32	1.34	1.30	1.18	.238	0.09
Solidarity	1.24	1.28	1.21	2.26	.024	0.16
Trust in institutions	2.44	2.53	2.34	3.73	<.001	0.26
Radical left	1.09	1.06	1.12	−2.89	.004	0.28
Radical right	1.05	1.03	1.09	−2.93	.004	0.23
Use of violence	1.86	1.68	2.04	−5.80	<.001	0.90
Break the law	1.61	1.49	1.74	−6.04	<.001	0.60

[a] 1 = *don't like*, or *don't know or am uncertain*, 2 = *like a lot*.
[b] 1 = *disagree absolutely to* 4 = *agree absolutely*.
[c] Three-point scale, see text.

the welfare of others, we expected that girls would be more likely than boys to approve of the various civil society organizations. As shown in Table 12.9, this was the case for all six organizations (except peace work), with medium effect sizes for environmental, animal rights, gender equality and feminism, and aid organizations. Less trust in societal institutions with small effect size was reported by boys. For the two more radical groups, the radical right and the radical left, significantly more boys than girls approved of these radical groups. The effect sizes were small. Boys also scored highest for using violence for political purposes and breaking the law. The two effect sizes here were large and medium.

Discussion

Politically interested adolescents are more knowledgeable, more interested in political and civic engagement, and more willing to mobilize than other adolescents (Prior, 2019). However, politically interested adolescents are not a homogeneous group. We used Schwartz's theory of core human values (Schwartz et al., 2012), specifically the value of caring for the welfare of others, to identify the diverse values, attitudes, and behaviors of politically interested adolescents. A cluster analysis was conducted for the 16-year-old cohort based on these adolescents' political interest and concern for the welfare of others. Two of the five clusters extracted included adolescents who were highly politically interested. In the largest cluster (n = 256), these politically interested adolescents expressed high levels of concern for the welfare of others (the HH adolescents), and in the other cluster they expressed low levels of concern (n = 78) (the HL adolescents). In the first group, there were as many girls as boys. In the HL group, three out of four were boys.

As hypothesized, the two cluster groups differed in several ways. First, the politically interested adolescents with high concern for others reported greater willingness to protect the environment and showed higher pro-environmental behaviors and environmental efficacy. They showed more trust in social movements for human rights, environmental organizations, and animal rights than adolescents in the other cluster groups. Consistent with previous studies linking universal values to concern for minority groups (Kuntz et al., 2015; Sagiv & Schwartz, 1995; Vecchione et al., 2012), the politically interested adolescents with high concern for others had more positive attitudes toward immigrants. Universal values include social justice and equality, which are fundamental democratic principles (Miller, 1978). We hypothesized and confirmed that the politically engaged adolescents with high concern for others scored higher on democratic principles than the politically interested adolescents with low concern for others. Finally, we also found that the politically interested adolescents with high concern for others were more likely to intervene in a future situation if something threatened the welfare of others. In all of these respects, the high concern for others group scored significantly higher than adolescents in any of the other four cluster groups. The politically interested adolescents with low concern for the welfare of others reported consistently low scores on these measures. In short, we confirm these study hypotheses. Highly politically interested adolescents do not appear to be a homogeneous group. Our finding that a global value such as concern for others' welfare has strong specific implications for politically interested adolescents' attitudes, behaviors, and willingness to act in certain circumstances in the future is striking. HH adolescents report greater concerns for other people and nature than do HL adolescents.

Because of their concern for the welfare of others, we hypothesized that HH adolescents would have more opportunities to participate in political activities and civic associations than other adolescents because these activities and associations are often aimed at caring for others. Indeed, HH adolescents were more likely than adolescents in the other four cluster groups to be members of various types of civic associations, to be more engaged in offline political activities, and to report the highest levels of political efficacy, a key predictor of political engagement, than adolescents in the other cluster groups. However, both HH and HL adolescents were more politically active online than adolescents in the other cluster groups. The results regarding the frequency of various political activities suggest that the two groups of highly politically interested adolescents channel their political interest in different ways, with the exception of their high political activities on the Internet.

One of the most striking findings in this chapter is that males dominate the cluster of adolescents who are politically interested and report low concern for the welfare of others. Adolescents in this cluster are less likely than the HH cluster to be concerned about the environment, to have positive attitudes toward immigrants, to be concerned about demographic principles, to be willing to act politically if something bad were to happen to other people, to engage in offline political activities, to express high political efficacy, and to be less likely to engage in offline political activities. However, they are just as politically active on the Internet as HH youth. According to civic knowledge tests, they are significantly more politically knowledgeable than HH adolescents, and according to their peers, they are somewhat more politically competent as HH adolescents. Nevertheless, in most of the areas examined in this chapter, the politically interested adolescents with low concern for the welfare of others—mostly males—do not seem to translate their political interest into civic associations or political activities offline. Their political activities are limited to the Internet. It should also be added that there is little evidence in our findings that the HL adolescents are attracted to political violence. They do not seem to be interested in radical groups, left or right, nor are they more likely than other young people to break the law to get their ideas accepted.

Finally, the findings reported in this chapter regarding differences between HH and HL youths appear to be robust over time. When the comparison measures at age 16 were replaced with the same comparison measures collected two years later, roughly the same results were obtained.

Sex Differences

The main findings in this chapter say almost as much about gender differences as they do about what characterizes cluster groups of adolescents who differ in their political interest and concern for the welfare of others. The strongest sex differences appear in universal values. On all measures of concern for others and for nature, girls show more positive attitudes and more behavioral commitments than boys. This is consistent with what has been reported previously in the literature. Stronger universal values in the Schwartz tradition have previously been found to characterize females more than males (Ardenghi et al., 2021; Döring et al., 2015; Schwartz & Rubel-Lifschitz, 2009). Other studies conclude that females tend to express more concern and report stronger environmental attitudes and behaviors than boys (Gifford & Nilsson, 2014; Zelezny et al., 2000). Girls' stronger other-orientation and social responsibility than boys (Zelezny et al., 2000; Strohmeier et al., 2017) may explain their stronger adherence to democratic principles, more positive attitudes toward immigrants, and willingness to act when others' welfare are at risk. It was hypothesized that these domains would particularly characterize politically interested adolescents with high concern for the welfare of others. They did. But these domains also characterize girls more than boys. Apparently, care for the vulnerable, social justice, and solidarity seem to be closer to the concerns of females than of males.

There are some other gender differences in political activity that stand out. Boys are more politically active on the Internet, but in other respects—membership in a civic association and offline political activity—there are no differences between boys and girls. However, in terms of political reputation in class and scores on a test of civic knowledge, boys are more politically reputable and knowledgeable.

Implications

Broad, general values such as valuing human dignity and human rights have been said to underpin citizens' political participation (Barrett, 2016), but research linking values to political participation has focused primarily on narrower values (see Heath et al., 2022). The finding that a global value such as concern for the welfare of others has strong implications for politically interested adolescents' attitudes, behaviors, offline political action, and willingness to act in certain circumstances in the future raises practical questions. Apparently, the broad universal value of concern for others seems to have high explanatory power to differentially shape adolescents' political activity and willingness for future political action. Perhaps one strategy for mobilizing youth for political action, such as volunteering, is to provide clear value-based motivations that link young people's high political interest to their genuine concern for the needs of others.

There are potentially three lessons to be learned from the application of the findings. First, high levels of political interest among 16-year-olds are not necessarily good for welfare and democratic principles. Second, for those involved in recruiting volunteers for civic and political organizations and campaigns, the study underscores the importance of emphasizing motivations related to basic human values such as helping others, equality, justice, and giving back to society (Gage III & Thapa, 2012; Chambré, 2020). Third, for educators in general and civic educators in particular, a human values perspective on adolescent citizenship is needed to support orientation to the social conditions of others, as recently discussed by Veugelers (2021).

Parents' Cluster Combinations

In principle, there is little reason to believe that the findings reported in this chapter for 16-year-olds are unique to this age group. In fact, the general pattern of results may also apply to other age groups, perhaps even to the parents of the adolescents. Parents who are characterized by high levels of political interest and concern for others may also be more likely to protect the environment, to have more inclusive attitudes toward immigrants, to be members of civic organizations, and to express a greater willingness to become politically active if they see a need to do so. In short, caring for people and nature and being willing to get involved in politics when necessary may also apply to parents who have high levels of political interest and concern for the welfare of others. If this is the case, we need to know whether similar types of HH and HL clusters are found among parents as among adolescents when a cluster analysis simultaneously includes parents' political interest and concern for the welfare of others.

Two cluster measures for parents were selected:

- *Parents' political interest.* This was a four-item measure that combined mothers' and fathers' separate reports of political interest on a 5-point scale and their feelings about politics on a 6-point response scale. The items made up one factor. Alpha reliability was .76.
- *The values of concern for others' welfare.* Totally five items made up one factor in parent reports. Parents reported on the same statements as described for the adolescents. Alpha reliability was .82.

The two measures, parents' political interest and their concern for others, were standardized. Standardized scores above 2.5 were set to 2.5 and scores below −2.5 were set to −2.5. First, a hierarchical cluster analysis was conducted. Five clusters were extracted. The five-cluster solution explained 68.4% of the total error sums of squares. Next, a non-hierarchical cluster analysis, *K*-means clustering, produced the final cluster solution, which is shown in Table 12.10.

As can be seen in Table 12.10, the cluster solution for the parents was surprisingly similar to the cluster solution for the adolescents (compare with Table 12.2). First, the different clusters for adolescents were reproduced in the cluster analysis for parents: LL (low interest and low concern), LA (low interest, average concern), AA (average interest, average concern), HL (high interest, low concern), and HH (high interest, high concern). Second, the percentages of parents for each of the five clusters were also similar to the percentages for the adolescents.

TABLE 12.10 A cluster analysis of parents' political interest and concern for the welfare of others.

Clusters	*LL*	*LA*	*AA*	*HL*	*HH*
Political interest	−0.85	−1.36	−0.12	0.78	0.87
Concern for others	−1.41	0.60	0.20	−0.92	0.80
N	80	80	172	92	148
%	14	14	30.1	16.1	25.9

Note: Low values (lowest to −.70); average values (>−.69 to 0.69); high values (>.70).

We do not have the same comprehensive information to compare the clusters for parents as we do for adolescents. We used the following parent-reported measures:

- *Member of a civic association.* Parents were asked if they were a member of an environmental association or an association for peace or human rights (the peace movement, Amnesty International, and the like).
- *Standby citizen* was a four-item measure. After the stem question "How active should people be on political issues? What do you think as parents? For me it is important to:" Parents responded on the statements "Give up time when asked by others to step in," "React when something important is at stake," and "Get

involved if I see a possibility to exert influence." Note that the adult version of the standby citizen measure does not explicitly mention the risk for other people's harm. The response scale ranged from 1 (*not important at all*) to 4 (*very important*). The alpha reliability was low, .58. As well, the inter-item correlation was low, .32.

- *Inclusive attitudes toward immigrants* was the same measure that the adolescents responded to. Alpha reliability was .74.
- *The value of concern for the nature* was built on three items. They were the same as previously reported for the adolescents. Alpha reliability was .90.
- *Pro-environmental behaviors* was a three-item measure with the stem questions "How often do you do the following things for environmental reasons? "Buy environmentally friendly products," "Take public transport, cycle, or walk rather than traveling by car," and "Turn off the TV and the computer completely when they are not being used (by using the power switch not just the stand-by button)." The response scale ranged from 1 (*almost never*) to 5 (*almost often*) The alpha reliability was .46 and the inter-item correlation was .23. The reliability is evidently not adequate.
- *Political activities offline*. After the stem question "Have you done any of the following things during the last 12 months?" parents responded to five political activities "Signed a petition," "Attended a meeting concerned with political or societal issues," "Worked voluntarily for a good cause," "Contacted a politician or public official" and "Donated money to support the work of a political group or organization." The response scale ranged between 1 (*no*) and 3 (*yes, several times*). Alpha reliability was .73.
- *Political activities online*. With the same stem question and response scale the parents responded to the single statement "Discussed societal or political issues on the Internet."

As can be seen in Table 12.11, there were significant differences between the five parent clusters for all of the measures covering care for others and care for nature we used for comparison. The effect size was large for the environmental concerns and mostly medium or near medium for the other comparison measures. Parents in the HH cluster scored highest on all of these comparison measures in Table 12.11. They had significantly higher scores than all other cluster groups on civic organization membership, inclusive attitudes toward immigrants, the standby citizen measure, and concern for the nature. Both the HH and HL clusters had significantly higher scores than the other three cluster groups on offline and online political activity.

We conclude that there are similarities in the study results between the HH and HL youth clusters (Table 12.2) and the HH and HL parent clusters (Table 12.11). The HH adolescents and HH parents have stronger environmental values, are more likely to be members of civic organizations, have more inclusive attitudes toward immigrants, and express more willingness to take action if necessary in the future than the HL adolescents and HL parents. In the case of the adolescent clusters, the differences between the HH and HL clusters were stronger on all comparison measures than

TABLE 12.11 Differences between the five cluster groups for the comparison measures used for parents. Z-scores.

Clusters	*LL*	*LA*	*AA*	*HL*	*HH*	*F*	*p*	η^2
Care for others:								
Member of civic organization	-0.23^a	-0.24^a	-0.15^a	-0.01^a	0.41^b	9.85	<.001	0.07
Standby citizen	-0.70^a	-0.02^b	-0.08^b	0.04^b	0.47^c	20.83	<.001	0.13
Attitude immigrants	-0.71^a	-0.31^b	0.18^{cd}	0.02^c	0.34^d	19.96	<.001	0.12
Care for nature:								
Concern for the environment	-0.94^a	0.47^d	0.11^c	-0.62^b	0.52^d	58.00	<.001	0.29
Pro-environmental behaviors	-0.47^a	-0.05^b	-0.05^b	0.09^b	0.28^b	7.93	<.001	0.05
Political activities:								
Political activities offline	-0.41^a	-0.42^a	-0.11^b	0.23^c	0.42^c	17.16	<.001	0.11
Political activities online	-0.25^a	-0.21^a	-0.25^a	0.20^b	0.43^b	13.50	<.001	0.09

Note: All measures in the table are standardized. Across rows, superscripts represent significant differences ($p < .05$) between clusters in SNK post-hoc tests.

between the HH and HL parent clusters. To some extent, this is due to the better psychometric properties of some of the measures reported by the adolescents. Finally, while HH adolescents were more engaged in offline political activities than HL adolescents, HH and HL adolescents were equally engaged in online political activities. Cluster comparisons for parents showed that both HH and HL parents reported more offline and online political activities than other cluster groups of parents.

Comparison Between the Clusters of Adolescents and Those of Parents

If parents are politically interested, they should be more likely to want to discuss political issues and support their adolescents' political interests than parents who are not politically interested. The HH and HL clusters are the clusters where we should expect political discussions to take place and where parents should be more likely to offer their political support than in other cluster groups (at least from the parents' perspective). We decided to test the validity of this hypothesis. In these analyses, we decided to examine both adolescents' and parents' reports of political discussion and parental support for both parents' and adolescents' cluster combinations. Two key measures were reported by both parents and adolescents.

- *Frequency of political discussions* was related to two questions about how frequently parents and adolescents discussed about "What you have heard on the news about what is going on in Sweden and around the world" and "Politics or societal issues." The response scale ranged from 1 (*never*) to 4 (*very often*). The correlation between the two discussion items was .46, $p < .001$ for adolescents' reports and .53 for parents' reports.
- *Providing political support* was a three-item measure asking the adolescent and the parents if the parents Suggest newspapers, books, or websites where our

child can read about politics or societal issues; Give information about activities or organizations that one can contact or get engaged in; Suggest that the children sit down with us and that we watch the news together. The response scale ranged from 1 (*definitely doesn't apply*) to 5 (*applies very well*). Alpha reliability for adolescents' reports was .70 and the reliability for parents' reports was 67. The respective inter-item correlations were .43 and .40.

As can be seen in the top two rows of Table 12.12 (S1), there were significant differences between the parent cluster groups, with near-high effect sizes, when parents themselves reported political discussion and support. Both HH and HL parents reported more frequent political discussions than parents in the other clusters, and particularly high levels of parental support were reported by HH parents. The two rows below (S2) show differences in adolescents' perceptions of political discussion and parental political support across the five cluster groups of parents. There were medium effects for joint political discussions and small differences in adolescents' perceptions of parental political support. In particular, a high frequency of joint political discussions was reported by adolescents of HH parents.

Moving to the combinations of adolescent clusters, as shown in the next two rows (S3), there were strong differences between the five adolescent cluster groups when adolescents themselves reported joint political discussions and parental support. In particular, HH adolescents reported a high frequency of political discussions and parental support compared to youth in the other cluster groups. As shown in the last two rows (S4), when their parents reported joint political discussions and parental support, there were few differences among the five cluster groups of adolescents, and highest means for parents' HH cluster. Overall, the table shows a mismatch between parents' and adolescents' reports of how often politics is discussed

TABLE 12.12 Differences across cluster groups of both adolescents and parents when adolescents and their parents report the frequency of political discussions and the political support of parents. Z-scores.

Parents' clusters:	*LL*	*LA*	*AA*	*HL*	*HH*	*F*	*p*	*eta²*
(S1) Political discussions (P)	-0.49^{a}	-0.48^{a}	-0.10^{b}	0.30^{c}	0.46^{c}	22.53	<.001	0.14
(S1) Political support (P)	-0.58^{a}	-0.30^{b}	-0.08^{bc}	0.14^{c}	0.45^{d}	18.65	<.001	0.13
(S2) Political discussions (A)	-0.24^{ab}	-0.38^{a}	-0.06^{ab}	0.01^{b}	0.48^{c}	14.56	<.001	0.10
(S2) Political support (A)	-0.14^{a}	-0.08^{a}	-0.10^{a}	0.03^{a}	0.24^{a}	3.20	.013	0.02
Adolescents' cluster:	*LL*	*LA*	*AA*	*HL*	*HH*	*F*	*p*	*eta²*
(S3) Political discussions (A)	-0.81^{a}	-0.53^{b}	0.03^{c}	0.29^{d}	0.60^{e}	76.06	<.001	0.27
(S3) Political support (A)	-0.46^{a}	-0.40^{a}	-0.03^{b}	0.02^{b}	0.48^{c}	32.41	<.001	0.13
(S4) Political discussions (P)	-0.09^{ab}	-0.25^{a}	-0.01^{ab}	0.18^{b}	0.26^{b}	4.18	.002	0.03
(S4) Political support (P)	-0.10^{a}	−0.14a	-0.10^{a}	-0.07^{a}	0.23^{a}	2.59	.036	0.02

Note: All measures are standardized. Across rows, superscripts represent significant differences ($p < .05$) between clusters in SNK post-hoc tests.

A= Adolescent reports P = Parent reports

in the family and parents' political support when comparing the different cluster combinations of political interest and concern for others. When parents' clusters are compared, both parents in the HH and the HL clusters report that political discussions take place more often than parents in the other clusters. When the adolescents report, the adolescents in the HH cluster report more frequent discussions than the adolescents in the other parent clusters. When adolescents' clusters are compared, the adolescents in the HH cluster report more frequent political discussions than adolescents in the other clusters. But when parents report, there are no difference in political discussions between the HH and the HL clusters.

A general lack of concordance in the adolescent and parent cluster groups is shown in Table 12.13. Here we cross-tabulated the adolescent and parent cluster groups and found a significant effect but weak effect size: χ^2 (16 df) = 38.44, p = .001, contingency coefficient = 0.27. A subsequent analysis using the EXACON program (Bergman & El-Khouri, 1987) aimed to find cluster cells with a higher or lower frequency than would be obtained by chance alone. This analysis showed that adolescents in the HH cluster were more likely to be found in their parents' HH cluster group than expected by chance, and less likely to be found in their parents' LL cluster group (low political interest and low concern for others). These were the only types and antitypes. The concentration of similarities with the HH clusters probably reflects the finding in Table 12.12 that adolescents in their parents' HH cluster report a high frequency of political discussions. In summary, there are similar combinations of political interest and concern for the welfare of others for parents and adolescents. With the exception of the combination of high levels of political interest and concern for others, we rarely find that adolescents and parents have similar types of combinations of political interest and concern for others in individual families. We find a lack of correspondence.

TABLE 12.13 A cross-tabulation of cluster solutions of adolescents and parents.

Clusters		*Parents*				
		LL	*LH*	*AA*	*HL*	*HH*
	LL	12	8	25	14	9
	LA	14	21	28	10	16
Adolescents:	AA	27	20	34	23	39
	HL	8	2	17	11	10
	HH	10[at]	19	46	29	55[t]

Note: [a], antitype, [t], type.

Conclusion

What role do basic human values play in the political values, attitudes, and behaviors of politically interested adolescents? When we clustered adolescents' political interest and their concern for other people's welfare, five clusters were extracted, and two of them were politically interested adolescents with high concern for other people (the HH adolescents) and politically interested adolescents with low concern for other people (the HL adolescents). The HH and HL adolescents differed profoundly on values, attitudes, and behaviors measuring concern for other people and nature. The HH adolescents had highest means for all three measures of concern for nature, as well as trust in social movements, membership in civic organizations, inclusive attitudes toward immigrants, positive attitudes toward democratic principles, and a higher willingness to get involved in politics when other people are harmed.

A similar cluster analysis for their parents extracted five cluster groups similar in content to the adolescent clusters. Again, the HH and HL cluster groups were found. We did not have the full range of measures or as high psychometric properties as for the adolescents, but the HH parents had the highest means on all comparison measures, and they differed from the HL parents by expressing higher levels of environmental values, more involvement in civic associations, more inclusive attitudes toward immigrants, and greater willingness to influence politics if it seemed necessary.

With these similarities in the content of the adolescent and parent cluster groups and in the comparison measures, we turned our attention to the political interactions between parents and adolescents. This is where the similarities end. When comparing the cluster groups, it is primarily the HH cluster of the adolescents that stands out. Adolescents in this cluster report a significantly higher frequency of political discussions with their parents and a higher level of political support from their parents than adolescents in all other clusters. However, when we examine whether there are differences in parents' reports of shared political interest and political support, we find small differences among the five adolescent clusters. Furthermore, when we compare the five parent clusters, parents perceive the highest frequency of political discussions in the HH and HL clusters, and it is primarily the HH parents who report strong attempts to politically support their adolescents. However, when we examine whether there are differences in adolescents' reports of shared political interest and political support, only for the HH cluster of parents do adolescents report higher levels of political discussion, and there are no differences between the five cluster groups of parents for adolescents' reports of parental political support. Within individual families, there appears to be a discrepancy between both cluster group membership and reports of political discussion and parental support. It should be added that we examined whether the results differed depending on whether the mother, father, or both parents completed the questionnaire. No differences were found.

Finally, what evidence has been presented in this chapter that young people are active agents in their own political development?

- Politically interested adolescents are not a homogeneous group. If some of them express concern for the welfare of others, it follows that their attitudes and behaviors are consistent with this broad concern for others. If they do not, their attitudes and behaviors are consistent with lower levels of this value of concern for others. As active agents in their own development, the two groups of politically interested adolescents have come to different conclusions about the value of concern for others in their interactions with others, and, as a result, their attitudes and behaviors follow different paths.

PART VI

What Have We Learned?

13

TIE THE THREADS TOGETHER

It is time to summarize the main idea of this book, namely, that young people's political interest shapes their political development. We have developed two main hypotheses.

The First Proposition

Young People's Political Interest Is Both Push and Pull in Their Political Development

The evidence for this hypothesis is the following.

Setting Long-Term Goals

Our initial research was grounded in the theory of planned behavior (Ajzen, 1985, 1991; Fishbein & Ajzen, 1975). In Chapter 2, we reported that as early as mid-adolescence, by age 16, adolescents set goals for their future political and civic engagement, and that these goals moderated the association between their political interest and their political activities of various kinds four years later—offline and online political activities, membership in political/civic organizations, and public support for a party before and after a national election. Particularly high levels of political activity and voting in a national election four years later were found among 16-year-olds who had high levels of political interest and high goals for their future political and civic engagement. These goals appear to be early rational plans for future political and civic activism.

DOI: 10.4324/9781003371731-19

Attention to Political Information

Political interest has been defined as an intrinsic motivation to attend to political information (Lane, 1959; Lupia & Philpot, 2005; van Deth, 2000). We hypothesized that there is a dynamic interplay between political interest and political information, in which adolescents' own political interest makes them more attentive to political information over time, and attention to political information increases their political interest. We believe that these dynamic processes are central to understanding the growth of adolescents' political interest over time.

In Chapter 3, we reported that about one in five 13- and 16-year-old adolescents reported experiencing events in the past year that had increased their political interest. These adolescents already had elevated political interest and positive feelings about politics 2 years earlier, and this interest and feelings seemed to facilitate the identification of these interest-raising events. Based on self-determination theory (Deci & Ryan, 1991, 2000; Ryan & Deci, 2000, 2006), we found that the adolescents who had experienced interest-triggering events years earlier had engaged in behaviors that reflected their needs for autonomy (following the news, setting personal goals), relatedness (having political discussions with parents, initiating political discussions at home, and talking to others about political issues on the Internet), and competence (internal political efficacy) more than other students. Finally, exposure to interest-triggering events increased adolescents' political interest one year later. This is an example of the dynamic interplay between political interest and attention to political information.

We also asked participants in all five cohorts whether they thought it was important to be informed about what was going on in the world. Cross-lagged analyses showed that political interest significantly predicted changes over two years in perceptions of the importance of staying informed for all age groups covered (14 to 16, 16 to 18, 18 to 20, 20 to 22, 22 to 24, 24 to 26, and 26 to 28). The belief that it is important to stay politically informed significantly predicted changes in political interest over two years in seven of nine analyses. Our analyses indicate, again, that political interest predicts changes in future beliefs about staying informed, and, to a lesser extent, believing it is important to keep up with what is happening in the world predicts changes in political interest.

Political Reputation in the Classroom

As a result of their political interest, some adolescents gain a reputation among others as politically competent, and this reputation may further enhance their political interest, knowledge, and behavior. We used Nick Emler's (1990, 2013, 2019) theory of reputation enhancement to develop our hypotheses. Students who combined a recognition as having good political knowledge together with bringing up political issues in class were defined as students with a high political reputation in their class.

In chapter 4 we examined the relationship between political reputation and students' political interest, self-efficacy, and perceptions of their own political activity in the classroom. According to Emler's reputation enhancement theory, one would expect that students who have an identity as someone who is politically active in the classroom would be likely to have a political reputation among their classmates. Political interest was the strongest positive cross-sectional predictor of classroom political reputation among 13-year-olds. Political interest, political efficacy, and self-perceived political activity in class predicted political reputation among 16-year-olds. In the latter age group, political reputation was particularly high among politically interested students with high internal political efficacy. Among 16-year-olds, perceiving oneself to be politically active in class and having political interest were longitudinal predictors of political reputation.

What are the consequences of political reputation in the classroom? In the short term, over one year, political reputation predicted an increase in political interest among students in both the first and second cohorts, as well as an almost equal increase in students' political efficacy in both age groups. In sum, political interest in particular was a strong predictor and also a significant longitudinal predictor of political reputation in the classroom among 16-year-olds. Conversely, students' political reputation predicted increases in both political interest and political efficacy over a one-year period.

In terms of longer-term effects, we focused on the 16-year-olds and found that students with a political reputation in the classroom were more likely than other students to engage in collective political activity 4 years later, that is, political activity with or in front of others—such as attending a meeting about political or social issues, volunteering for a good cause, contacting a politician or public official, or participating in a legal demonstration or strike. We also found that these students were more likely than others to be members of political, environmental, peace, or human rights organizations. Finally, we also found that, when the students now were 20 years old, those with a political reputation in the classroom were more involved in collective forms of political activity related to the ongoing national election (Working on a nonprofit basis for a party in the general election, for example, by handing out flyers for the party, and supporting a party by wearing its badge or t shirt) rather than solitary forms of political activity (Using the Internet to support the parties they like, and Following and "liking" parties on social networks) such as Twitter and Facebook).

Second, we argued that other characteristics observed by their classmates might facilitate or hinder the future political activities of individuals who had a political reputation in class. We found that being popular among classmates facilitate these students' engagement in future political activities that involve contact with other people, while being a student with a political reputation and simultaneously being seen as a person who gets angry easily and causes trouble discourage themselves or others from engaging them in collective political activities.

Consistent with our first hypotheses, political reputation in the classroom at age 16 significantly predicted all three forms of collective political activity and did not predict individual election-related activity four years later. Political interest, as a unique predictor, significantly predicted all four outcome measures. Consistent with moderator hypotheses, two of the collective activities were higher for individuals with high political reputation and high class popularity than for individuals with high political reputation and low class popularity. As well, two of the collective activities were lower for politically reputed persons who were perceived to be quick to anger than for politically reputed persons who were not perceived to be quick to anger.

The take-home message is that what once began as a strong interest in politics and high political efficacy developed, for some, into a political reputation through group processes in the classroom. We believe that this study provides good evidence that early interest in politics creates specific channels for becoming politically active several years later.

Time to Bring in Parents

Interactions With Parents in Adolescence

The first indication of the role of parents in adolescents' political development comes from adolescents' own reports of their political interactions with their parents (see Chapter 5).

Most adolescents viewed their parents as politically competent. Most adolescents thought their parents' views were important to them and that they and their parents had similar views. Many adolescents talked to their parents about societal and political issues. Most adolescents were aware of parents' influence attempts. Most adolescents perceived themselves as susceptible to their parents' political communication. Some adolescents had tried to politically influence their parents and they were generally met with positive reactions. We believe that adolescents' responses to these questions show that they recognize, respect, and are receptive to their parents' political competence. However, the openness to parents' political views revealed in these cross-sectional analyses does not imply that adolescents' political development is shaped by their parents.

Interactions in Early Adulthood

The second indication comes from young adults' perceptions of their political interactions with their parents, reported in Chapter 6. Even if they had left home, young adults talked to their parents about political issues more often than adolescents did; they viewed their parents as politically competent at least as often as adolescents did; they recognized the importance of their parents' political views; and they perceived themselves as having similar views to their parents as much as adolescents did. In the comparisons between adolescents and young adults, there is little to suggest that parents are less important to the political development of young people than they are to adolescents.

We asked members of all five cohorts and all ages to respond to the following two statements: "My parents are interested in what is going on in the world" and "My parents keep up with the news." The response scale was 1 (*not at all true*), 2 (*not so much true*), 3 (*somewhat true*), and 4 (*very true*). The percentage of respondents who answered "somewhat true" or "very true" that their parents are interested in what is going on in the world is shown in Figure 13.1. Here, between about 90% of adolescents and young adults in all age groups agreed with the statement that their parents are interested in what is going on in the world. As shown in Figure 13.2, again about 90% agreed that their parents keep up with the news. Clearly, if adolescents and young adults want to share their thoughts about political and social issues with others, they should feel comfortable discussing them with their parents, who they perceive as knowledgeable.

In Chapter 6, we discussed whether common transition events in early adulthood—such as leaving home, getting married, and having children—reduce political discussions with parents. We found little evidence that they do. But do people who are closer in age to young adults—such as friends, college peers, coworkers, and the romantic partner—emerge as new sources of political discussion? First, our analyses showed that young adults discussed political issues with their parents at least as often as they discussed politics with their friends, college peers, and work colleagues. But at this stage in their lives, young adults discussed politics most often with their romantic partners. This was an unexpected finding.

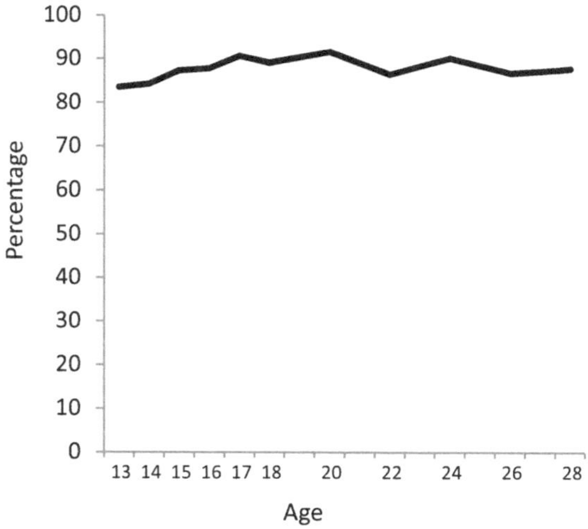

FIGURE 13.1 Young people's reports on the statement "My parents are interested in what is going on in the world." Percentage of respondents in different ages who answered "applies quite well" or "applies quite well," rather than "doesn't apply at all" or "doesn't apply so well."

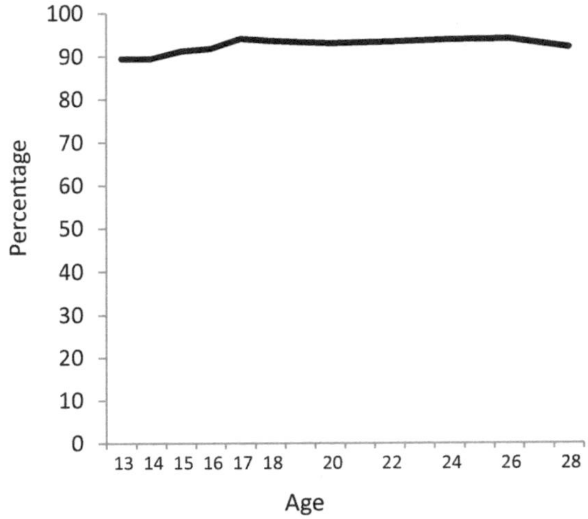

FIGURE 13.2 Young people's reports on the statement "My parents keep themselves in touch with the news." Percentage of respondents in different ages who answered "applies quite well" or "applies quite well," rather than "doesn't apply at all" or "doesn't apply so well."

Longitudinal analyses that linked political discussions with parents to political discussions over time with peers, college peers, coworkers, and romantic partners generally showed that the more often young adults discussed politics with their parents, the more often they discussed politics with their college peers and coworkers. In contrast, the frequency of political discussions with college peers and work colleagues generally did not affect the frequency of political discussions with parents. These findings do not support the idea that other people take over parents' role as political discussion partners in early adulthood. One exception was romantic partners. The more often young adults had political discussions with their romantic partners, the more often they had discussions with their parents. It appears as political discussions with romantic partners stimulate political discussions with parents. But conversely, we do not find that political discussions with parents had any effect over time on political discussions with romantic partners. We suggest that the romantic partner may be the last person in many people's lives who can more systematically thwart or enhance people's political interest (Stattin & Korol, 2020). Meeting a romantic partner in early adulthood opens a window for changes in young adults' political interests, as they must adapt to their partner's political interests.

We conducted the same types of analyses for adolescents' and young adults' best friends. Adolescents had more frequent political discussions with parents than with friends. This was especially true in early adolescence. Later, in early adulthood, young adults talked as much with their parents as with their friends. Do discussions with parents spill over into discussions with peers over time, or is it the other way around? We found that there are bidirectional relationships, with political discussions with parents spilling over into political discussions with friends, and political discussions with friends spilling over into political discussions with parents.

Interactions With Parents Versus Friends

With these earlier analyses, we have already begun to uncover the role that friends play in young people's political development. In addition to being less likely to discuss political issues with friends than with parents during adolescence, we found that 13- and 16-year-olds were less receptive to political communication from friends than from parents. Compared to parents, adolescents perceived their friends as less politically knowledgeable, perceived their friends as less likely to keep up with the news, were less aware of their friends' views and perspectives on social issues, and reported that their friends were less likely to try to influence them politically. This more limited role of friends relative to parents in political interactions has also been found in previous research (Dostie-Goulet, 2009). We have conducted several other analyses not reported earlier comparing the political socialization roles of parents and peers, and they converge in showing that parents are more important than peers in young people's political development. Despite the challenge of integrating information from different settings and individuals outlined here, we have focused primarily on parents in this book.

It Seems as If . . .

Adolescents and young adults recognize their parents' political knowledge, perceive that their parents' political views are important to them, and, most important, report that they are receptive to their parents' political communication. However, the fact that parents are the preferred discussion partners of adolescents and young adults does not imply a unidirectional political influence of parents or that the political views, attitudes, and behaviors of adolescents and young adults converge with those of their parents.

The Second Proposition

Young People's Political Interest Affects Their Perceptions of the Political Interactions They Have With Other People

Evidence for this hypothesis includes the following:

A Bidirectional Relationship Between Political Discussions With Parents and One's Own Political Interest

The classic literature on political socialization (Beck & Jennings, 1982, 1991; Jennings et al., 2009; Jennings & Niemi, 1968) views parents as the primary socialization agents, and the idea that parents are the special gateway to the political world of youth is still widely held (Bacovsky & Fitzgerald, 2023; Fitzgerald & Caughlin, 2002). Through discussion, modeling, and reinforcement, parents shape their children's political views, values, and attitudes.

In Chapter 7, we looked into evidence that the political discussions adolescents and young adults have with their parents influence their political interest. We used information from all the cohorts. We found bidirectional associations, with effect sizes of similar magnitude in both directions. These results are a disappointment for unidirectional socialization models. It is true that having political discussions with one's parents affects adolescents' and young adults' interest in politics—and particularly in early adolescence. But this is not the whole story. Political interest stimulates adolescents' and young adults' political discussion with their parents, and political discussion with parents stimulates adolescents' political interest. There are bidirectional relationships.

Attitudes and Values of Young People Do Not Necessarily Correspond to Those of Their Parents

Are parents' attitudes reflected in adolescents' attitudes? Proponents of the intergenerational transfer of worldviews, attitudes, and values from parents to children would assume that there should be a high degree of convergence between parents' and adolescents' sociopolitical views. Proponents of the learning position would assume the same. They would assume that parents' political views, attitudes, and behaviors become adolescents' views, attitudes, and behaviors through direct parental messages, modeling, and reinforcement. This does not appear to be the case.

Early studies found overwhelmingly low correlations between parents and adolescents on a wide range of sociopolitical issues (see Connell, 1972), but these findings seem to have been forgotten later on. Convergence between the frequency with which parents and adolescents reported discussing political issues or parents' communication patterns was low to modest (Pacheco, 2008). We found in chapter 7 a correlation of .15 ($p < .001$) between 13-year-old adolescents' and their parents' reports of the frequency of shared political discussions. The same correlation was .38 ($p < .001$) four years later for this sample.

There was also a lack of agreement between adolescents' and parents' views on specific sociopolitical issues (environmental protection, concern for the welfare of others, concern for nature, achievement values, active citizenship, social trust, positive attitudes toward immigrants, negative attitudes toward immigrants). Overall, these low associations between adolescents' and parents' reports of shared political interactions and sociopolitical attitudes do not support a case for a strong transfer of parents' political attitudes to the next generation or a hypothesis that parents' direct communication, modeling, and reinforcement of their political views, attitudes, and behaviors become adolescents' views, attitudes, and behaviors. The lack of convergence between adolescents and parents on shared political interactions and sociopolitical issues may mask the fact that at least some families have children whose views on their shared political interactions and attitudes are closer to those of their parents. Some would say that good emotional relationships in some families might contribute to higher convergences. But as we saw in Chapter 8, the emotional relationships between parents and adolescents did not affect their discussions about political issues, nor did they moderate adolescents' interest in politics and their discussions with parents about politics. Instead, emotional relationships influenced parents' and adolescents' conversations about everyday, non-political topics. The lack of convergence between adolescents and parents on various sociopolitical issues and their joint political interactions is evident throughout this book and poses a serious problem for theoretical models that rely on unilateral parental influence on adolescents' political views, attitudes, and behaviors. Parents and adolescents seem to have little insight into each other's perceptual worlds when it comes to politics. In a sense, they seem to live in different perceptual worlds when it comes to political issues and values. This calls for special attention to the particular complexity of political communication.

Different perceptual worlds have also been reported for younger samples. After interviewing parents and their 5- to 8-year-old children about the 2016 U.S. presidential election, Patterson and colleagues (2019) concluded that most parents and children were interested in the upcoming 2016 United States presidential election. However, "Unexpectedly, children's interest was not related to their parents' reports of interest in the election or frequency of communication about the election, suggesting that political interest is the result of factors more complex than parental modeling" (p. 140).

Overall, our own findings and those of others point to a lack of congruence between adolescents' and parents' sociopolitical values and attitudes, as well as a lack of shared perceptions of joint political interactions. We have concluded that a central issue is to understand the mechanisms that govern adolescents' perceptions of their political interactions with parents and the mechanisms that govern parents' perceptions of the same interactions with their adolescents.

High Perceptual Accuracy and Low Actual Accuracy

Moderate to high associations have been reported between adolescents' reports of their own values and views and their perceptions of their parents' values and views (Acock & Bengtson, 1980; Gniewosz & Noack, 2006; Gniewosz et al., 2008; Ojeda & Hatemi, 2015; Whitbeck & Gecas, 1988). There are moderate to high associations between adolescents' perceptions of the frequency of political discussions with parents and their political interest (Dostie-Goulet, 2009). In addition, the more frequent adolescents perceive political discussion at home, the higher their political interest, the more they pay attention to the news, and the higher their engagement in civic and political participation, volunteering, civic engagement, political participation, and later voting (Anderson & Goodyear-Grant, 2008; Andolina et al., 2003; Boyd et al., 2011; Dostie-Goulet, 2009; Levinsen & Yndigegn, 2015; McIntosh et al., 2007; Shehata & Amnå, 2017; Wray-Lake & Sloper, 2016).

What the above studies have in common is that all of the information was based on adolescent perceptions. Adolescents' perceptions were both the independent and the dependent variables. For example, the frequency of political discussions with parents, as reported by adolescents, was associated with adolescents' political interest, attention to news, civic and political participation, volunteering, civic engagement, and political participation, also reported by adolescents. Thus, from adolescents' perceptions, a high frequency of political discussions with parents is quite strongly associated with many different characteristics of their political behavior.

It has been argued in both political science (Tedin, 1974; Westholm, 1999; Ojeda & Hatemi, 2015) and developmental psychology (Grusec & Goodnow, 1994; Grusec & Kuczynski, 1997; Knafo & Schwartz, 2003, 2009) that adolescents need insight into their parents' views and opinions in order to adopt or internalize them. Once they know their parents' messages, they can choose to accept them. In short, parents' messages are filtered through adolescents' perceptions of those messages.

This brings us to a central question. How can we simultaneously explain (i) the low convergence in adolescents' and parents' perceptions of their shared political interactions and (ii) the finding that adolescents' perceptions of political discussion with parents are quite highly associated with many other features of their reports of political attitudes, values, and behaviors? The search for cumulative knowledge requires new theoretical ideas.

A Projection Interpretation

This has been a key question for us. We hypothesized that biased perceptions, a projection effect, could explain the simultaneous occurrence of high associations between adolescents' political attitudes and behaviors and their perceptions of how often political discussions occur with parents, while low actual accuracy exists. Projection is a biased perception because people typically assume that others perceive the world as they do (Krueger, 1998; Schul & Vinokur, 2000). They assume that other people's attitudes and values are close to their own attitudes and values. If projection is an explanation for the low correspondence between adolescents' attitudes and their parents' attitudes, on the one hand, and the much higher correspondence between adolescents' attitudes and their perceptions of their parents' attitudes, on the other hand, we would expect adolescents to perceive that the attitudes they hold are the attitudes their parents hold. However, their perceptions would not match their parents' reports of their values.

To our knowledge, Westholm (1999) was the first to suggest that the associations between adolescents' opinions of their parents' values and their own values might be due to projection. Projection was suggested as a theoretical possibility but was rejected in favor of parental persuasion as the plausible explanation for the association between parents' views and adolescents' perceptions of parents' views.

We first tested this projection idea on broad values such as universal and achievement values in the theoretical framework of Shalom Schwartz (1992). On a list of various values, 12 items related to three types of values: concern for the welfare of others, concern for nature, and achievement values. Adolescents were asked to report how important these values were to them and, separately, how important these values were to their parents. We also examined whether there was a similar projection in parents' perceptions of their adolescents' values. Parents reported how important the three types of values were to them and how important they were to their adolescents. We modeled both accuracy and projection in Chapter 9. Results showed that both parents and adolescents perceived each other's values to be more similar to their own than they actually were. Lower levels of projection existed for parents' perceptions of their adolescents' achievement values, but for the two universal values, concern for others welfare and nature, we found comparable biases in parents' and adolescents' perceptions of each other's values. Despite the belief that parents' values were similar to adolescents' own values and that adolescents' values were similar to parents' own values, there was little agreement between adolescents' and parents' values. Our biased perceptions hypothesis seems to explain (i) why there is high agreement between one's own values and perceptions of the other's values, and (ii) why adolescents and parents tend to misperceive others' values.

Next, we considered adolescents' perceptions of their political interactions with their parents. We hypothesized that adolescents' political interest would color their perceptions of their shared political interactions with their parents—how often they have political discussions with their parents and of their parents' political support. Likewise, parents' political interest would color their perceptions of how often they have political discussions with their adolescents, and of their own political support. We found empirical support for these hypotheses. In addition, we found little agreement between adolescents' and parents' perceptions of the frequency of joint political discussions and the extent of parents' political support.

This is a different framework for active agency than the one we have discussed earlier. Here, it is adolescents' own political interests that influence their perceptions of political interactions with parents. Agency also applies to parents. Parents' political interest also guides their perceptions of how often they discuss politics with their adolescents and how much political support they provide.

That adolescents' perceptions of their parents' and their own behaviors show low to moderate congruence with their parents' perceptions is well known and is not new to the findings in this book (De Los Reyes, 2013; De Los Reyes et al.,

2015; Hou et al., 2020; Korelitz & Garber, 2016). What is new is that we have attempted to explain why parents' and adolescents' perceptions of core values and shared political interactions show low congruence, at the same time as high convergence exist with their own core values and political interests.

Openness to Important Others' Political Communication

At first glance, projection, a biased perception, seems to limit the possibilities for adolescents and parents to properly understand each other's views on shared political interactions. We have taken a broader agentic perspective and advanced the idea that adolescents' political interest indeed opens them up to the political views and influence of other important people—parents, friends, and teachers. The perception of these important others as politically influential stems from the adolescents' own political interest. Adolescents' different levels of political interest make them sensitive or insensitive to others' political communication. In contrast to the projection interpretation, this broader agentic proposal is open to predictions about the future. We have proposed that adolescents' political interest makes them aware of others' political views, leads them to perceive others' political interest, and helps them recognize that others are providing them with political information, that others are trying to influence them politically, and that they are susceptible to the political influence of important others. In short, this openness to the views of others stems from young people's own political interests.

The opposite perspective would be expected from the traditional political socialization literature, including learning theory. This is the idea that adolescents' political interests are likely to increase when they are aware of the political views of important others; perceive that their important others are highly politically interested, provide them with political information, and attempt to influence their political beliefs; and perceive that they are emotionally receptive to political communication from these important others.

We tested in chapter 10 these two opposing perspectives over the course of a year for the two youngest cohorts: 13- and 16-year-olds. We found that adolescents' perceptions of important others' (parents, teachers, friends) political views, political interest, political influence and support, and their own susceptibility to others' political communication were all influenced by their own political interest—and we found little support for the opposite hypothesis. These findings suggest that adolescents' political interest energizes their political development and makes politically interested adolescents active agents in their political interactions with their significant others.

In conclusion, the lack of shared perceptions about political interactions with their parents does not preclude adolescents from being open to parental and others' attempts to politically socialize them. In fact, our findings suggest that adolescents' political interest is an input to their political development, making politically interested adolescents active agents in their political interactions with significant others.

A Political Agency

A central premise of our research has been the following: *Young people need to have at least a nascent political interest and positive feelings about politics in order to recognize and respond to political stimuli in their everyday environments*. If they lack interest, they will not recognize when others raise political issues—or even know that political issues are being raised. Nor will they have the experience of being receptive to the political communication of others or to news in the media. They will not have strong experiences of events that potentially can arouse their political interest, nor will they believe that it is important to keep up with what is happening in the world and in their society. They will not be motivated to seek out political information and will not feel a loss for doing so. If they express their feelings about politics as boring, really boring, or even disgusting, they will turn their ears in another direction when parents, teachers, and friends bring up political issues, will attend to other things in the media, and will not be motivated to engage in anything resembling politics.

If parents' attempts to politically socialize their adolescents are to be effective, adolescents must recognize that their parents are politically sophisticated. If they do not, they have little reason to accept their parents' political views and attitudes. The low accuracy of adolescents' views of their shared political interactions does not preclude the possibility that *some* adolescents have quite accurate perceptions. This insight was the starting point for the ideas we developed in Chapter 11. We proposed that adolescents who can accurately identify their parents' high political sophistication—high political knowledge and interest—will be particularly likely to attend to their parents' political communication and would have particularly high political interest.

A cluster analysis of parents' reports of their political sophistication (high political interest and knowledge) and adolescents' reports of their parents' political sophistication extracted five cluster groups, two of which included parents who reported high political sophistication. In one of these two groups, adolescents correctly reported that their parents had high political sophistication. In the other, they reported that their parents had low political sophistication. The group of adolescents who made correct judgments had high political interest, whereas the adolescents who failed to recognize their parents' high political sophistication had about average levels of political interest. Because they were politically interested, parents in these two groups attempted to politically socialize their adolescents more than parents in other cluster groups. While adolescents who made correct judgments reported being open to their parents' political communication, this was not true for adolescents who did not recognize their parents' high political sophistication. Thus, although parents in these two clusters attempted to influence their adolescents politically, only those adolescents who correctly identified their parents' high sophistication were open to their parents' attempts. A certain level of political interest seems to be necessary to recognize and respond to parents' political information. Another observation: Parents who are politically interested tend to be more educated than other parents (Janmaat & Hoskins, 2022). In fact, parents in the two clusters where parents expressed high political interest had higher levels of education than other parents. However, this higher level of education did not translate into high openness to their parents' political communication among adolescents who did not recognize their parents' high political sophistication.

In the study of cluster groups in Chapter 11, we examined the robustness of the differences that existed at age 16. Four years later, the now 20-year-olds reported on the same measures of open political interactions with their parents and their political interest. The results at age 20 were broadly the same as those four years earlier—at a time when most of the 20-year-olds did not live at home with their parents.

The distinction between high and low political interest youth is also presented in Chapter 12. Here we sought to highlight differences in the values, attitudes, and behaviors of high politically interested adolescents as a function of their concern for the welfare of others. Again, we used cluster analysis and extracted five clusters, two of which were 16-year-old adolescents with high political interest and high concern for the welfare of others and same-age adolescents with high political interest and low concern for the welfare of others. The first group reported higher environmental values, more inclusive attitudes toward immigrants, higher evaluations of democratic principles, and high willingness to intervene when people are treated unfairly compared to other adolescents. They also had higher political efficacy and were more involved in civic organizations and offline political activities. The latter group was mostly below average on these measures, and high online activity was the only political activity in which they stood out. The two groups of highly politically interested youth differ in their attitudes, values, and behaviors.

Now look at these findings from the opposite perspective. One of the five cluster groups included adolescents who were characterized by low political interest and low concern for the welfare of others. One in seven adolescents belonged to this cluster, and two in three of them were boys. There is no evidence that they expressed any form of political engagement. In almost all comparisons, they were the group of adolescents who reported the least concern for others—low trust in social movements, low motivation to stand up when other people's welfare was endangered, negative attitudes toward immigrants, and low attitudes toward democratic principles—the least concern for the environment, and the least political efficacy and offline and online political activity. Four years later, they were still passive.

From a societal perspective, engaging these adolescents in politics is a challenge, perhaps especially for schools. First, nearly half of these students (48%) described their feelings about politics as boring, very boring, or even disgusting, compared to 14% of other students, a difference with a Cohen's d of 0.71.

Second, these students were less likely than other students to recognize when their teachers tried to bring up political and social issues in class. We asked participants about their awareness of their teachers bringing up political issues in class: "There are teachers at my school who often take up the issue of climate change,"

"There are teachers at my school who try to encourage students to become more aware of environmental issues," "There are teachers at my school who try to involve students in discussions about political issues," "There are teachers at my school who try to encourage students to become more aware of what is going on in the world." The students characterized by low political interest and low concern for the welfare of others were significantly different from the students in the other clusters ($t = -3.37$, $p < .001$, Cohen's $d = -0.34$). They did not perceive that they had teachers who brought up political issues in class.

Third, participants were asked about their receptiveness to teachers' attempts at political engagement. They responded to the following statements: "I have teachers who: 'Talk about politics and societal issues in a way that makes them fun and interesting,' 'Talk about things that happen in the world and in society in such a way that I become curious and want to know more,' 'Talk about the news they have heard on TV or read about in a way that evokes strong feelings in me.'" Students in the cluster characterized by low political interest and low concern for the welfare of others were less emotionally receptive than other students to their teachers' attempts at political engagement ($t = -4.05$, $p < .001$, Cohen's $d = -0.41$).

The fourth and final question was about the students' relationship with their teachers: "Most teachers don't like me," "There are scarcely any teachers who I can talk with if I have problems with something at school," "There are scarcely any teachers who praise me when I do a good job." These students had more negative relationships with their teachers than other students ($t = 2.74$, $p = .003$, Cohen's $d = 0.28$).

Overall, it is a long way for teachers to influence the political interest of these young people, who have low political interest, little faith in humanistic and democratic values, negative feelings about politics, and perceive negative attitudes from teachers.

A New Narrative of Shared Political Interactions Is Needed

A new generation of studies based on new narratives is needed to understand political communication between young people—adolescents and young adults—and their parents.

Either the political development of adolescents and young adults is largely in the hands of people who know much more about what is going on in contemporary society than they do or adolescents have their own political views in their interactions with people they consider important—parents, teachers, and friends. It is easy to accept that adolescents are subject to the political influence of their significant others. They do not have the long experience and political knowledge of their parents and teachers. But throughout this book, it is not this message of accepting the influence of their significant others, especially their parents, that stands out. Rather, it is the intrinsic political interest of adolescents and young adults that seems to drive much of their political interaction with others. Political interactions at home with their parents, who undeniably have more social and political experience than they do, are a central training ground for young people's political communication competence. Politically interested young people are not imitators of their parents. A new narrative is needed to describe the political interactions of young people and parents. This is a narrative of parents stimulating their children's curiosity about what is happening in the world in tandem with adolescents' growing political interest. Perhaps the joint political discussions at home are best described as a means of fostering adolescents' political reasoning skills. Political conversations at home provide a relatively safe environment where they develop the ability to formulate political positions and receive feedback. Parents have an important role to play in putting their children's thoughts into questions and arguments.

A new narrative must recognize the role that the respective political interests of young people and their parents play in their political interactions. The perceived frequency of political discussions at home and the perceived support of parents are strongly related to young people's political interest. Similarly, the frequency of political discussions and parents' support for their adolescents' political development are strongly related to parents' political interest. But the relationship between parents' and adolescents' political interest is modest at best, with the consequence that politically interested parents and adolescents perceive their common political interactions rather differently.

The distinction between families practicing socio-oriented versus concept-oriented communication styles (Chaffee et al., 1973; McLeod & Chaffee, 1972; Stone & Chaffee, 1970) and between conversation and conformity orientations (Koerner & Fitzpatrick, 2002; Ritchie, 1991; Ritchie & Fitzpatrick, 1990) were early attempts to characterize families in terms of how political messages were communicated. Parents could be closed to views that challenged their own, or they could be open and encourage their children to develop their own views. These patterns of communication were seen as managed by parents. How adolescents viewed these communication patterns was found to be quite different from how their parents viewed them (Meadowcroft, 1986; Ritchie & Fitzpatrick, 1990; Rauscher et al., 2020; Saphir & Chaffee, 2002; Tims & Masland, 1985). We found little support for these two characterizations of families. A new narrative must recognize that young people may have their own political agendas and that they are an active part of the political dynamics at home. Adolescents' and parents' political interests influence their respective perceptions of political interactions in the family, but adolescents' political interests may not coincide with their parents' political interests. Adolescents develop their own political views, sometimes independently and sometimes through interactions with parents and others.

A new narrative must include the awareness that adolescents are receptive to their parents' political communication. Most adolescent report that they view their parents as politically competent, perceive their parents' views as important to them, are aware of their parents' attempts to influence them, and are receptive to their parents' political communication. They are also open to political communication from their teachers and friends. At the same time, we found that 13- and 16-year-old adolescents' perceptions of important others' (parents, teachers, friends) political views, political interest, political influence and support, and susceptibility to others' political communication were more strongly influenced by their own political interest than perceptions of their political communication with important others influenced their political interest. In short, political interest is a strong contributor to adolescents' perceptions of their political interactions with significant others.

A new narrative must specify when parental political support is most needed. As we concluded in Chapter 5, early adolescence is potentially the most formative time for young people according to their parents. Parents seem to try to influence their 13-year-olds more than their 16-year-olds. Moreover, as shown in Chapter 7, the only age interval in which the relationship between political discussion at home and later adolescent political interest was higher than the opposite relationship, was the 13-to-15 age interval.

We do not have information about earlier ages, but we do know that pronounced changes in political interest occur in early adolescence. The age interval between 13 and 15 is a time when political interest not yet has started to crystalize. Over the years from age 13 to young adulthood, young people change dramatically in their interest in and feelings about politics. In the three oldest cohorts, only 22% reported low political interest (not at all interested or completely uninterested) and 25% expressed negative feelings about politics (bored, very bored, or disgusted). By age 13, however, the majority reported low political interest (54%) and negative feelings (63%). It may be that the parents of the early adolescents in our sample saw an opportunity to educate their children about political issues during this age interval.

A new narrative needs to take into account the very different forms that young people's political interest can take, different from that of their parents and others. Only a limited group translates their high political interest into participation. As a result, the new narrative needs a longitudinal perspective to capture the combination of sustained political interest and more transient action, which may depend, inter alia, on the availability of opportunity structures in different local and national contexts. A new narrative should also be more sensitive to the modes of participation that many in the younger generation seem to prefer. A high level of political interest among young people does not necessarily mean that these young people herald a social pathos and concern for people or nature. Many of them do, but a significant proportion of highly interested young people do not express a high level of concern for the welfare of others and for nature, and do not approve of common organizations working toward this motivating goal. In the narrative, the interactions between political interest, core values, civic norms and action deserve more in-depth analysis.

Finally, a new narrative must recognize the central role that political discussions with parents play in political discussions with others and in other contexts. McDevitt and colleagues, in a series of seminal studies, challenged the conventional parent-adolescent interpretation of family political discussions and proposed that adolescents' political experiences at school can alter family political discussions (McDevitt & Chaffee, 2000, 2002). In these studies, the authors focused on current political events, such as elections, and examined the consequences for parent-adolescent communication of adolescents' exposure to information about these events in school. These studies were limited in their arguments for causal directions because of cross-sectional designs, reliance on individual differences rather than classroom effects, lack of a randomized control design, and failure to control for relevant pretest measures when a longitudinal design was used. Nevertheless, the results generally indicate that child-initiated discussions, generated by political experiences at school, influence changes in parent-adolescent communication patterns and parents' attempts to gain more knowledge through news. In short, when adolescents have strong political experiences outside the home, they can influence parents' communication with their adolescent children and trigger parents' interest in the subject.

Here, students bring their newly awakened political experiences from school to home. Because students' political experiences at school can be manipulated experimentally, the design of the studies provides great opportunities to test the transfer of experiences from school to home conditions. We have questioned the external validity of these studies. *Under normal conditions* political experiences at school are unlikely to influence political discussions with parents. These quasi-experimental studies do not tell us what typically happens when political discussions are transferred between everyday contexts. Nor do they say much about whether these political experiences in school transform from a situational political interest to an intrinsic political interest.

It is more likely that the political discussions adolescents have with their parents are what they bring to political discussions in the classroom. Most adolescents are unlikely to face hostility, insults, or demeaning comments from parents when they discuss their political views. Regardless of their social anxieties, they should feel welcome to express their political ideas. There is a more competitive social climate in the classroom. Because of their social anxiety, some students may be reluctant to express their ideas in front of others. Other students may hesitate because of the risk of strong opposing views, conflict, criticism, and public embarrassment.

In Chapter 8, we examined the transfer of political discussion between home and school over the course of a year. The results showed that there was little evidence that 13- and 16-year-old students' reports of how often they were politically active in class influenced their political discussions with parents. Rather, as hypothesized, political discussions at home with parents stimulated students' political discussions in class for both cohorts. In these analyses, the political reputation that some students had seemed to be an exception. These students can be considered "successful" in communicating their political insights to their classmates. Being seen as politically competent by their peers affected their political discussions with parents in both cohorts over time. These students are perceived as particularly politically competent by their peers, and it is only among these students that we find a spillover from school to home. These are students who do not have a newly awakened interest in political affairs, but who seem to have a persistent intrinsic interest in politics. This is a very different conclusion from the school-to-home direction suggested by earlier political science and civic educational studies.

Five Themes

Five themes stand out in this book.

Active agency

We have said this many times before. The main theme running through this book is that young people are active producers of their political development and that it is their own political interest that shapes their political lives.

- In the past year, some young people have experienced events that they feel have increased their interest. Years earlier, these young people's political interest was significantly higher than that of other young people. The early political interest made it easier to identify these interest-raising events.
- Whether adolescents pay attention to political information in their daily lives depends much on their political interest.
- Some adolescents gain a political reputation in their classes. Political interest is a key factor in explaining why some, but not others, gain this political reputation.
- How young people perceive political interactions with their parents is strongly influenced by their own political interest.
- The frequency of everyday conversations between parents and adolescents depends on parents' and adolescents' perceptions of their emotional relationship, but political conversations are only strongly influenced by the political interests of both parties.
- Some adolescents, but not others, are open to their parents' political communication. High political interest is characteristic of the group of adolescents who have a particular open attitude to their parents.

All this shows that young people's political interests shape their political interactions with parents, friends, teachers and the Internet.

Bidirectional Relationships

A second theme running through this book is that there are bidirectional relationships between adolescents' political interest and their attention to political information. This is supported by longitudinal analyses. More than other adolescents, politically interested adolescents encounter events in their daily lives that trigger their political interest, and having encountered such events positively affects their overall political interest over time. Political interest also shapes the belief that it is important to keep up with information about what is happening in society and the world, and the belief that it is important to keep up with societal, environmental, and political information positively affects political interest over time.

Political interest is also a push and pull in relation to their political discussions with parents. Political interest stimulates adolescents' and young adults' political discussion with their parents, and political discussion with parents stimulates adolescents' political interest. There are bidirectional relationships between political interest and young people's perceptions of political discussion with parents.

A General Openness to Others' Political Communication

Another theme that runs through the book is that adolescents are, on the whole, open to political communication from others. With regard to their parents, most young people think that their parents are politically competent and that their views are important to them, most think that they and their parents have similar views, most talk to their parents about current news and about what is going on in Sweden and in the world, most are aware of their parents' attempts to influence them, and most young people see themselves as receptive to political communication from their parents.

Politically interested adolescents are generally open to political communication from significant others. Thirteen- and 16-year-old adolescents' perceptions of significant others' (parents, teachers, friends) political views, political interest, political influence and support, and their own susceptibility to others' political communication are all influenced by their own political interest. There are no significant opposing directions of effects.

Little Correspondence in Political Views

Openness to the views of parents does not mean that young people have similar political attitudes and values as their parents. A third theme running through the book is that young people's and their parents' perceptions of different sociopolitical attitudes and values, and of their political interactions together, do not match up well. We have tried to explain why this is the case.

It appears that adolescents' own worldviews influence how they perceive their parents' worldviews. First, we found that adolescents perceive their parents to have about the same kind of values—universal and achievement values—as they do. However, adolescents' perceptions of their parents' values do not match the values their parents say they hold. For universal values, but less so for achievement values, parents also, mistakenly, perceive that their adolescents have about the same values as they do. We have explained this as a projection effect. Both adolescents and parents have biased perceptions.

Second, the political interests of both adolescents and parents bias their perceptions of joint political interactions. Adolescents' political interest drives their perceptions of how often they engage in political discussions with their parents and of their parents' political support. However, this perception is not very consistent with that of parents, as parents' political interest also influences their perceptions of how often they engage in political discussions with and politically support their adolescents.

Sex Differences

Contrary to many, but not all, studies in the literature, we do not find substantial differences in males' and females' reports of political interest, interest in what is happening in the world and in their society, and feelings about politics. Developmental trends are about the same. Attention to news is higher among boys than among girls in early and middle adolescence, and analyses of political knowledge among 16-year-olds based on a knowledge test show that boys' political knowledge was higher than girls', with a small effect size. Political reputation was also higher among boys, again with a small effect size. Despite this difference in publicly perceived political competence, boys and girls did not differ in their internal political efficacy.

Sixteen-year-old girls systematically reported higher levels of concern for the welfare of others and for nature. For some of these indicators of concern for people and nature (concern for the welfare of others, trust in social movements, standby citizenship, inclusive attitudes toward immigrants, environmental values, pro-environmental behavior, internal environmental efficacy), these differences showed medium effect sizes (concern for the welfare of others, trust in social movements, inclusive attitudes toward immigrants). Girls also expressed higher levels of trust in institutions dedicated to environmental protection, animal rights, gender equality and feminism, and aid organizations. Indeed, the high political interest, low concern for others cluster group in Chapter 12 was predominantly male.

While reports of offline political and civic engagement do not differ between 16-year-old males and females, boys were more engaged in online political activities, with a small effect size.

Apart from these gender differences, 16-year-old boys reported less trust in institutions (the parliament, the government, the courts, the political parties), a higher approval of radical left and radical right groups, and a greater willingness to use violence and break the law. However, the effect sizes were small.

When comparing the political development of boys and girls in the literature, it is often found that boys are more interested in politics (Prior, 2019). We find no such gender differences. Young girls and young boys seem to develop in much the same way in many aspects of their civic and political engagement. The differences we find are not large. What stands out in this book is the strong orientation of girls toward caring for people and nature. Perhaps the girls' significantly stronger stance of solidarity expresses their more unquestioning choice to shape their civic lives more faithfully to the ideal of an active and humanistic citizenship.

The Eight Original Challenges

In the introductory chapter, we presented the challenges we identified for new research on political socialization. The first was to conceptualize young people as active agents in their own socialization rather than passive objects of socializing institutions. This has been a central theme throughout the book. We believe we have provided strong evidence for this claim of a politically self-directed process.

The second challenge was to take a longitudinal perspective. For the most part, we have focused on adolescence because of the massive changes over time in political interest, feelings about politics, political attitudes, and attention to political information that occur during this developmental period. Compared to the growth over time that occurs for these and other political dimensions in adolescence, early adulthood is characterized more by a flattening of earlier strong developmental trends. Although early adulthood involves a number of transitional events—moving away from home, marriage, and children—and the emergence of new potential socializing agents—new friends, work and study colleagues, and romantic partners—there is a high degree of stability for most of the political dimensions we examined in early adulthood. The third emphasis was on studying processes and mechanisms rather than correlations. This shift in focus from correlational research and cross-sectional designs to a longitudinal design and tests of specific developmental models, moderators, and mediators has allowed us to ask more specific research questions about developmental processes.

The fourth and fifth challenges were to integrate the different contexts of everyday life, rather than studying one context at a time, and to take seriously the ongoing changes in different contexts. We compared adolescents' susceptibility to political communication from parents, teachers, and friends and found greater susceptibility to parents and teachers than to friends. For several other dimensions of political interactions with parents and friends, the role of parents exceeds that of friends. For example, with medium to large effect sizes, adolescents discuss political issues more with their parents than with their friends, know more about their parents' views than about their friends' views, are seen as more knowledgeable than are friends, and parents try to make adolescents more aware of what is going on in the world and of environmental issues than do friends. Given the strong role that parents play in adolescents' political development, we focused many of our research questions in this book on adolescents' political interactions with their parents. This was a deliberate choice. However, we study and compare the political discussions in the home and school contexts and their interplay.

The sixth challenge was to conceptualize political participation broadly, rather than focusing on formal institutions and narrow electoral aspects. Political opinion formation through posting messages on the Internet, cultural expression, and product boycotts are examples of actions that should be included in contemporary analyses of political participation (Ekman & Amnå, 2022), and we included these ways of expressing political participation in our research design.

The seventh challenge was to disentangle general socialization from specific "civic" experiences in explaining differences in civic engagement. Adolescents and parents talk about many different things at home. We argued that discussions about political issues are different from the conversations adolescents and parents have about everyday issues. Political discussions are driven by adolescents' and parents' political interests, but not much by their affective relationships. In contrast, everyday conversations are driven by parent-child affective relations and have little to do with political discussions.

The eighth and final challenge was to develop new theoretical explanations of political socialization. We developed new theoretical ideas about the early motivational sources of future political involvement for politically interested adolescents, the future political activities of gaining a reputation as politically skilled, why adolescents believe that their parents have similar broad values as they do (and why they are wrong), and how politically interested adolescents perceive their political interactions with other people.

Young People's Political Interest Can Be Thought of in Many Ways

The best summary of contemporary definitions of political interest is reported in Mark Prior's book *Hooked: How Politics Captures People's Interest* (2019). Here he shows that political interest has cognitive, affective, and motivational underpinnings. We would like to add to this summary.

Intrinsic Motivation

Many definitions of political interest converge on the conclusion that political interest attracts people's attention to political information before many other things in their lives (Almond & Verba, 1963; Lane, 1959; Levy & Akiva, 2019; Lupia & Philpot, 2005; van Deth, 2000; Prior, 2019). But why do politically interested youth feel it is more important than other youth to keep up with political issues and what is happening in the world? One explanation is that they have a stronger intrinsic motivation to keep up with political information. Intrinsic motivation is about experiencing political information as thrilling and exciting. We measured adolescents' intrinsic and extrinsic motivation based on self-determination theory (see Pelletier et al., 1995). As described in Chapter 3, confirmatory factor analyses supported the two-dimensional solution.

The three statements measuring intrinsic motivation were "Because it is fun to know a lot about the world we are living in," "Because it is a good way to develop myself," and "For the joy of learning new things." The four statements assumed to measure extrinsic motivation (external-social regulation) were "To get respect of others," "When I know a lot about what is going on, it makes people who are important to me happy," "Because people around me think that it is important to be well informed," and "So that others regard me as a person who knows a lot about what is going on in the world." Confirmatory factor analyses showed that a two-dimensional model (intrinsic and extrinsic motivation) was preferred to the one-dimensional at all ages.

We calculated correlations between political interest on the one hand and extrinsic and intrinsic motivations on the other in the different age groups (Table 13.1). In general, the correlations between intrinsic motivation and political interest were significantly higher than the correlation between extrinsic motivation and political interest among both adolescents and young adults. One answer to the question of why politically interested youth and young adults feel it is more important than other young people to keep up with what is happening in the world is simply that they find these issues exciting and thrilling, rather than following issues that are championed by others - more so in earlier ages than later.

Personality

Each of us is a unique individual. But each of us shares some basic personality dimensions with others. Political interest can potentially be explained by the Big Five framework of personality theory. For the three early adulthood cohorts, we included a measure of the Big Five in the questionnaire. This scale is a translation into Swedish of the Big Five Inventory (John & Srivastava, 1999), which consists of 44 items. We correlated the young adults' five personality traits—extraversion, agreeableness, conscientiousness, neuroticism, and openness—with their political interest. As shown in Table 13.2, Openness to Experience was the personality factor that was particularly associated with the three measures of political interest. Several earlier and a recent meta-analysis of 47 independent studies also found Openness to Experience to be the personality factor most consistently associated with political interest (Bromme et al., 2022). Apparently, a general, broad trait, Openness to Experience appears to be a personality dimension that facilitates young people's interest in political issues.

TABLE 13.1 Associations between political interest and the intrinsic and extrinsic motivation to stay informed at different ages.

Age	*Associations between extrinsic motivation and political interest*		*Associations between intrinsic motivation and political interest*	
	r	*p*	*r*	*p*
14	.22	<.001	.49	<.001
16	.12	.002	.51	<.001
18	.17	<.001	.41	<.001
20	.10	.024	.30	<.001
22	.03	.484	.30	<.001
24	.08	.048	.24	<.001
26	.13	<.001	.30	<.001
28	.07	.232	.30	<.001

TABLE 13.2 Associations between different aspects of political interest and the Big Five trait dimensions among young adults (ages 20, 22, and 26).

	Extraversion	*Agreeableness*	*Conscientiousness*	*Neuroticism*	*Openness to experience*
Political interest	$.06^{*}$	−.01	.03	−.01	$.27^{***}$
Interest in society	$.12^{***}$	$.11^{***}$	$.17^{***}$	−.05	$.26^{***}$
Feelings about politics	$.14^{***}$	.04	$.07^{*}$	$-.05^{*}$	$.26^{***}$

$^{*}p<.05$, $^{***}p<.001$.

The correlations between the three interest measures ranged from .55 to .69.

Genetic Makeup

Another possible answer is that genetic factors underlie the development of political interest, ideologies, and sociopolitical attitudes and values. Party preference is the measure that has historically provided the strongest evidence that parents transmit their political views to their children. Particularly in the United States, parents' party preference is often their children's party preference. Hatemi and McDermott (2012) aggregated all reported twin and kinship studies on a wide range of political attitudes from 1974 to 2012. They were grouped into 26 domains. Hatemi and McDermott confirmed that the shared environment, which includes but is not limited to being raised in the same family, accounted for the lion's share of variation in party preference. The unique environment also explained a large proportion, and genetic factors accounted for only a few percentage points. *But party preference is an exception.* For each of the other 25 domains covered, genetic factors explained between 40% and 60%, unique variance accounted for about 20% of the variation, and shared environment accounted for about 20%. Thus, party preference appears to be largely socially transmitted, but for all other domains, genetic factors are the primary explanation. For political interest, genetic factors and unique environment—which includes people's personal experiences—each explained almost half of the variation, while shared environment explained only a few percentage points. These findings contradict a basic assumption in political socialization research: that parents largely shape young people's political interest through political discussions at home.

Other studies have found roughly the same results, that shared environment has limited explanatory power. A study using the Swedish Twin Registry examined genetic variability in political interest (Dawes et al., 2014). Genetic factors accounted for 50% of the variation in political interest, while unique environment accounted for 44%. Shared environment accounted for only 4%. Very similar genetic and environmental estimates have been reported for American samples (Arceneaux et al., 2012). Similarly, in a study of two independent samples of twins, York (2019b) found that the frequency of discussing political issues with others was explained to roughly the same extent by genetic traits and unique environmental effects, with the shared environment effect close to zero.

The limited role of shared environment in explaining people's political interest and parent-adolescent political discussions is noteworthy and may explain the lack of agreement between adolescents' and parents' views on sociopolitical issues, as well as the lack of agreement between adolescents' and parents' perceptions of their shared political interactions that we document in this book. Because these studies involved middle-aged people, it is unclear whether their findings can be generalized to young people. Nevertheless, the fact that genetic factors account for most of the individual differences in political interest and various aspects of sociopolitical issues and that shared environmental factors account for only a small proportion may explain the lack of agreement between parents' and adolescents' political interest.

Overall, these findings are only the first attempts to understand the role of genetic factors in young people's engagement with political issues, a strong candidate for explaining individual differences in political interest. Gene-environment interaction analyses and molecular genetic studies will provide further insights.

Implications for Research and Policy

What are the research and policy implications of the findings reported in this book? One obvious implication for research is to pay attention to different research approaches that can complement each other.

The Diverse Youth Population

Our sample of young people is as diverse as their parents. As should be clear from Chapters 11 and 12, we believe that standard variable-oriented methods should be complemented by person-oriented designs. Results from cluster analysis, latent class analysis, and other person-oriented methods should be informative about what is true for homogeneous subgroups of individuals. Variable-oriented approaches examine the relative position of an individual within a group and draw conclusions about the sample as a whole. *t*-tests, correlations, and regressions are examples of methods used. Person-oriented approaches examine individual patterns of behavior and draw conclusions about subgroups within the sample.

A key question in person-oriented research is, Are people with one configuration different from other people with other configurations? This question can be used effectively to test specific theoretical questions, such as the heterogeneity among politically interested youth: Do highly politically interested youth with high levels of concern for the welfare of others differ in their attitudes, values, and behaviors from other highly politically engaged youth with lower levels of concern (Chapter 12)? Person-oriented research represents the idea that individuals develop as integrated organisms and should be studied in terms of their characteristic patterns relevant to the problem under consideration. Whereas variable-oriented methods formulate problems and discuss results in terms of relationships among variables, person-oriented research uses individuals rather than variables as the organizing principle: How do they differ from people with other pattern configurations? There are reasons to believe that sometimes it is the pattern as a whole, rather than the individual variables in that pattern, that may drive development and carry the primary explanatory value for the individual's future personal and social behavior.

We also want to highlight other implications.

When Parents Attempt to Politically Socialize Their Children

Given our design, it is presumptuous to suggest if, when, and how parents should introduce information about political issues to their children. Nor whether their attempts are effective (c.f. Hess, 2004; Patterson & Pahlke, 2021). What this longitudinal project can contribute is information about the timing of parents' more general attempts to influence their adolescents politically. Comparing 13- and 16-year-olds, we found that parents tried to politically socialize their 13-year-olds more than their 16-year-olds. Parent reports showed that they were more likely to give their younger adolescents information about activities or organizations to contact or get involved with than their older adolescents. Youth reports showed that 13-year-olds were more likely to report that their parents tried to influence them politically by suggesting newspapers, books, or websites. They were also more likely to report that their parents tried to make them aware of environmental issues and tried to make them aware of what was going on in the world. As well, political discussions with parents had a more positive effect on the political interest of early adolescents than on the political interest of late adolescents and young adults. Furthermore (Chapter 8), for 13-year-olds but not for 16-year-olds, their perceptions of the frequency of political conversations with parents positively predicted their own political interest two years later. We concluded that early adolescence seems to be the time when many Swedish parents think their children are most formative.

We Lack the Mechanisms

Although opinions differ on how active a citizen should be, the vibrancy and survival of democracies depend on civic activity. However, mechanisms for translating young people's political interest into political action are lacking. Fewer than 1 in 20 adolescents and young adults in our study were formally involved in a political, environmental, peace, or human rights organization. Participants did not consider it particularly important to be politically involved. Political interest increased with age, but political and civic activities and membership in associations remained at the same low level from early adolescence to adulthood. Only online political activity showed an increase in later adolescence. National studies show that social media play an increasingly important role in young people's engagement (MUCF, 2021).

As in many other countries, civic and political participation has declined significantly. In Sweden, with a population of 10.5 million, youth political parties experienced a significant loss of membership between 1972 and 1995, from 220,000 to 50,000 members (Rothstein, 2001), and this loss continued between 2005 and 2011 (Karlsson & Lundberg, 2011). In the past decade, this trend has leveled off, with membership fluctuating between 25,000 and 40,000 (Bolin & Backlund, 2021).

The loss of membership in youth political parties can also be seen in the parliamentary parties. Today, political parties have less than 50% of the number of members they had in the early 1990s (https://sv.wikipedia.org/wiki/Riksdagspartiernas_medlemsutveckling). At present 270,000 persons or 3% of the Swedish citizens are members of a political party. By way of comparison, there are 300,00 licensed hunters in Sweden and the sports movement is one of the largest popular movements in Sweden, with three million Swedes being members of a sports club. In our sample, 52% of parents (mother, father, or both) belonged to a sports club, but only 3% were members of a political association. Voter turnout in Sweden has declined slightly over time, from 91% in 1976 to 84% in 2022, and is high by international standards. But just as important are citizens' civic and political activities between elections. Only 15% of citizens feel able to influence political decisions at the national level between elections (Demokratiutredningen, 2016). How this translates to the local level is unknown. However, if few parents feel they do not have this influence, this could be a signal to their children that political participation is not particularly important.

In our study, we asked parents of members of the first and second cohorts two questions: "When the family talks about political or social issues, do you mostly talk about the positive or negative sides?" and "When the family talks about political or social issues, how do you talk about opportunities to influence?" They responded on seven-point scales.

As shown in Figure 13.3, a higher percentage of parents reported that they mostly talked about the negative side when discussing political or social issues than about the positive side (32% vs. 16%). As shown in Figure 13.4, parents were more likely to say that it is possible to have an impact (37%) than to say that there are few ways to have an impact on political or social issues (24%). However, the strong parental message that it is important to participate and influence political decisions is missing. Perhaps the lack of this strong message from parents with their more political experience is reflected in young people's perceptions. It may lead young people to feel that their attempts to influence are out of their hands, leading to powerlessness and alienation, or that it is not important to influence, leading to weakened civic norms. The fact that one in four parents report that they do not see much opportunity to influence political decisions may leave children with the message that it is best to leave politics to politicians. Parents' reports about their political discussions with their children in countries other than Sweden may be very different from what our Swedish parents report. We look forward to an international comparison of how parents in different countries report their political discussions with their children and how children perceive the possibilities to influence political decisions and the issue of trust in the political system. We also look forward to analyses that compare common news sites in terms of their focus on positive and negative political news and how young people respond to this news.

The Role of the Socialization Agents

Parents, friends, and teachers are classically considered the primary socialization agents in political socialization research. Undoubtedly, they are important in young people's political lives. In designing this longitudinal study, initially we did not have clear ideas about the relative roles of parents, friends, and teachers in adolescents' political development. Because parents consistently were found to be the most important socializing agents for adolescents—and, for the most part, for young adults as well—we have primarily examined and reported on participants' political interactions with their parents. A few observations need to be made to qualify the influence of parents. They all tap into young people's political interest.

First, we find bidirectional relationships between the frequency of political discussions in the family and young people's political interest. It seems that the role of political discussions with parents is more important for young people's political interest in adolescence, while political interest influences political discussions more in early adulthood. Note that these relationships are based on adolescents' and young adults' perceptions of how often political discussions take place. If we had swapped adolescents' reports with parents' reports of how often political discussions occur, we would only occasionally find significant relationships between discussions and interest. Thus, it is only when young people report on their political interest and political discussions that these systematic bidirectional relationships emerge.

Second, it is far from certain that adolescents recognize their parents' political messages because parents' political messages have to be filtered through adolescents' perceptions. One example. Adolescents who correctly perceive their parents' high political sophistication are more receptive to their parents' political messages than adolescents who do not perceive their parents' high political sophistication. The former adolescents are more politically interested than the latter.

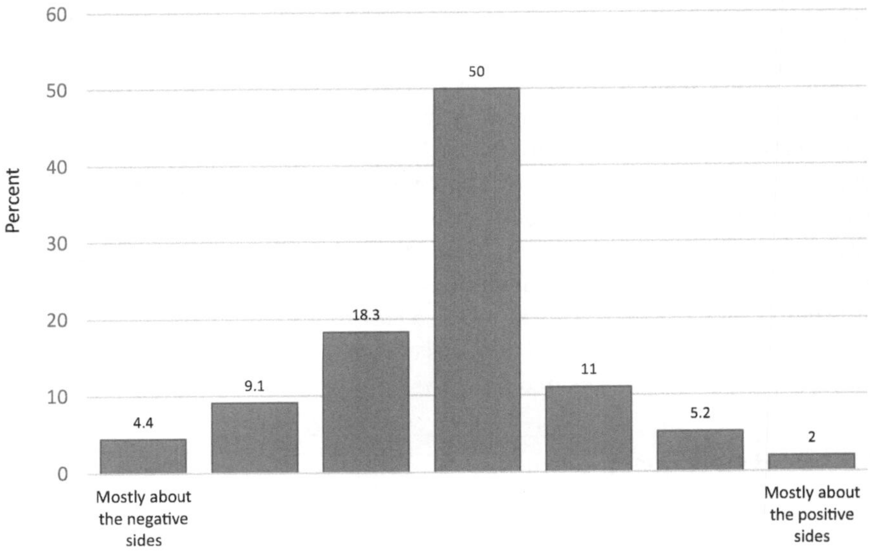

FIGURE 13.3 Responses to the question "When the family talks about politics or societal issues, do you talk mostly about the positive sides or the negative sides?"

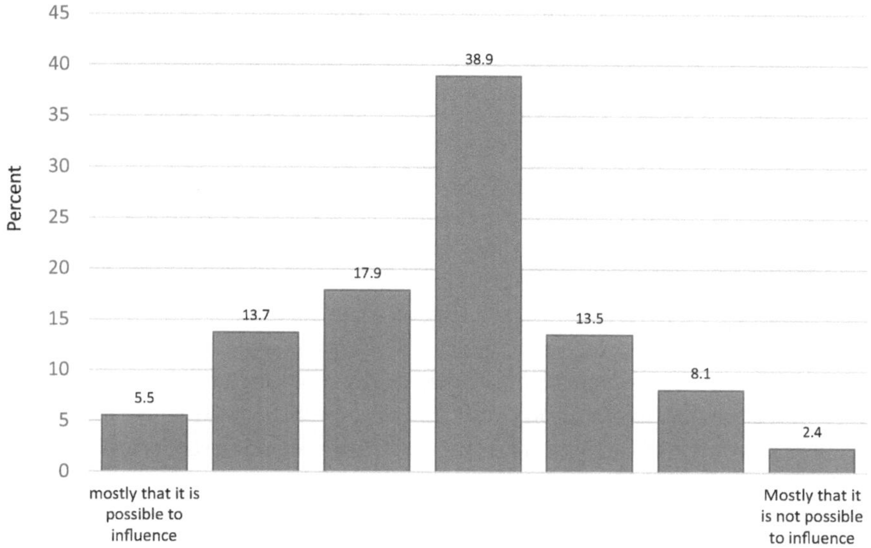

FIGURE 13.4 Responses to the question "When the family talks about politics or societal issues, how do you talk about opportunities to exert influence?"

Third, adolescents' political interest makes them open to the political influence of others. Rather than expecting, from a learning perspective, that perceptions of influence and support from important others would lead to political interest, our results suggest that the causal directions are the opposite. Politically interested adolescents welcome the influence and support of important others and are receptive to their political communication. Above all, our research clearly demonstrates the pervasive importance of a young person's political interest for most aspects of his or her political life. In order to deepen and develop democratic political systems, therefore, nothing seems more crucial for parents, teachers, youth leaders and others than to positively stimulate and support young people's interest in politics during the formative years of adolescence.

Comparing Perceptions of Political Issues Between Parents and Children

Sociopolitical issues and shared political interactions reveal weak correspondences between parents and adolescents. This lack of correspondence, which has been known for 50 years, challenges familiar theoretical ideas in political socialization research. If there is strong intergenerational transmission and if children adopt their attitudes and values from their everyday communication with parents, we should expect adolescents to have similar attitudes and values as their parents. They do not. The correspondence in values, attitudes, and perceptions of shared political interactions between parents and adolescents is low to modest at best.

A perceptual bias, projection, has been one explanation for this lack of correspondence. This bias affects not only the adolescents. It also affects their parents. The idea is that adolescents think that their view of the world is their parents' view of the world. They project their own views onto their parents. Parents do the same. They project their worldview onto their adolescents. But both adolescents and parents are wrong in their beliefs. Their views are not similar. It is their own political interest that leads adolescents to believe that their political interactions with parents are frequent and that their parents are politically supportive, and it is parents' political interest that leads them to believe that their political interactions with their adolescents are frequent and that they are politically supportive.

Projection is one explanation for the lack of correspondence in attitudes and values between adolescents and parents. Other explanations are possible. What makes projection a credible explanation is that this hypothesis both explains the low factual accuracy in values and attitudes that exists between adolescents and provides explanations for why adolescents perceive themselves as accurately recognizing parents' values and attitudes. Potentially the more explicit parents are about politics, the more effective messages and socialization efforts will be. In other words, if parents want to impose their political values and attitudes on their children, they should try to explain their political beliefs as clearly as possible in order to avoid the risk of misinterpretation by their children.

School's Role

Aside from the role that a political reputation plays in political activity, our interest in the role of school was to try to understand what motivates students to be politically active in their classes. We found little empirical evidence that adolescents' views of their teachers' initiative in raising political and social issues in class, their susceptibility to teachers' political communication, or adolescents' emotional bonding to school affected their willingness to be politically active in class. It was very much a matter of whether they were politically interested or not.

We should expect adolescents' knowledge of politics and society to grow as a result of learning more about political issues and formal processes in school. For many adolescents this is likely to go unnoticed because it is just another school assignment to deal with. Our design focused on individual differences, not differences between classes or schools. Ultimately, to determine whether school can make a difference in adolescents' political development, intervention designs are needed that differentiate between classes in which information and discussion about political events occur frequently and classes in which these issues are rarely addressed. Differences in future political interest between the two types of classes is a strong argument for the role of school in adolescent political development. Schools are, in fact, the only institution at our collective disposal that can compensate for inequalities in upbringing and contribute to the survival and development of our democracy.

In the End

Some of you readers of this book have probably wondered why we devoted our energy to finding out what happens from early adolescence to late adolescence—and highlighting the first two cohorts out of five. The answer is simple. This is the time when many changes occur that have powerful consequences later in life. Yes, things happen in early adulthood, too. But from our perspective, the field of political socialization needs to recognize that what happens in early to late adolescence has strong implications for what happens later.

Science is constantly in motion. Perhaps not always forwards. As Daisy Schalling (1923–1997) said, research goes forward and backward by storm. The overarching position of social learning theory became a long-term setback that prevented the development of new ideas about young people's political agency in the field of political socialization for many decades. Young people's self-directed political development is an issue that has only emerged in recent decades.

In this book we have shown how young people's interest in politics drives their understanding of the world and their political interactions with other people. Political interest does not automatically lead to political action, but young people's political interest and genuine concern for others can make these young people willing to act and promote democratic ideals. This is the agency perspective that we hope will move the field of political socialization forward.

REFERENCES

All references marked with * are the published studies that make up this book.

Achen, C. H. (1975). Mass political attitudes and the survey response. *The American Political Science Review*, *69*(4), 1218–1231. https://doi.org/10.2307/1955282

Acock, A. C., & Bengtson, V. L. (1980). Socialization and attribution processes: Actual versus perceived similarity among parents and youth. *Journal of Marriage and the Family*, *42*(3), 501–515. https://doi.org/10.2307/351895

Ajzen, I. (1985). From intentions to actions: A theory of planned behavior. In J. Kuhl & J. Beckman (Eds.), *Action control: From cognition to behavior* (pp. 11–39). Springer-Verlag.

Ajzen, I. (1991). The theory of planned behavior. *Organizational Behavior and Human Decision Processes*, *50*(2), 179–211.

Akers, R. (2009). *Social learning and social structure. A general theory of crime and deviance*. Routledge.

Aleva, A. E., Goossens, F. A., Dekker, P. H., & Laceulle, O. M. (2017). The reliability and validity of a modified revised class play examined in Dutch elementary-school children. *European Journal of Psychological Assessment*, *33*(6), 475–485. https://doi.org/10.1027/1015-5759/a000301

Allen, M., Wicks, R. H., & Schulte, S. (2013). Online environmental engagement among youth: Influence of parents, attitudes and demographics. *Mass Communication and Society*, *16*(5), 661–686. https://doi.org/10.1080/15205436.2013.770032

Almond, G. A., & Verba, S. (1963). *The civic culture: Political attitudes and democracy in five nations*. Sage Publications.

Althaus, S. L. (2003). *Collective preferences in democratic politics: Opinion surveys and the will of the people*. Cambridge University Press.

Amnå, E. (2012). How is civic engagement developed over time?: Emerging answers from a multidisciplinary field. *Journal of Adolescence*, *35*(3), 611–627. https://doi.org/10.1016/j.adolescence.2012.04.011.

Amnå, E., & Ekman, J. (2014). Standby citizens: Diverse faces of political passivity. *European Political Science Review*, *6*(2), 261–281. https://doi.org/10.1017/S175577391300009X

Anderson, C. D., & Goodyear-Grant, E. (2008). Youth turnout: Adolescents' attitudes in Ontario. *Canadian Journal of Political Science/Revue Canadienne De Science Politique*, *41*(3), 697–718. https://doi.org/10.1017/S0008423908080773

Andolina, M. W., Jenkins, K., Zukin, C., & Keeter, S. (2003). Habits from home, lessons from school: Influences on youth civic engagement. *PS: Political Science and Politics*, *36*(2), 275–280. https://doi.org/10.1017/S104909650300221X

ANES. (2014). *User's guide and codebook for the ANES 2012 time series study*. The University of Michigan and Stanford University.
Ansolabehere, S., & Hersh, E. (2012). Validation: What Big Data reveal about survey misreporting and the real electorate. *Political Analysis*, *20*(4), 437–459. www.jstor.org/stable/23359641
Aquilino, W. S. (1997). From adolescent to young adult: A prospective study of parent-child relations during the transition to adulthood. *Journal of Marriage and the Family*, *59*(3), 670–686. https://doi.org/10.2307/353953
Arceneaux, K., Johnson, M. V., & Maes, H. H. (2012). The genetic basis of political sophistication. *Twin Research and Human Genetics*, *15*(1), 34–41. https://doi.org/10.1375/twin.15.1.34
Ardenghi, S., Rampoldi, G., Bani, M., & Strepparava, M. G. (2021). Personal values as early predictors of emotional and cognitive empathy among medical students. *Current Psychology: A Journal for Diverse Perspectives on Diverse Psychological Issues*, *42*, 253–261. https://doi.org/10.1007/s12144-021-01373-8
Arensmeier, C. (2018). Different expectations in civic education. *Journal of Social Science Education*, *17*(2), 5–20. https://doi.org/10.4119/jsse-868
Aseltine, R. H., & Gore, S. (1993). Mental health and social adaptation following the transition from high school. *Journal of Research on Adolescence*, *3*(3), 247–270. https://doi.org/10.1207/s15327795jra0303_3
Bacovsky, P., & Fitzgerald, J. (2023). Raising a politically engaged generation: When parental influence matters most. *Youth & Society*, *55*(1), 44–60. https://doi.org/10.1177/0044118X211029976
Bandura, A. (2006). Guide for constructing self-efficacy scales. In F. Pajares & T. Urdan (Eds.), *Self-efficacy beliefs of adolescents* (pp. 307–337). Information Age.
Bardi, A., & Schwartz, S. H. (2003). Values and behavior: Strength and structure of relations. *Personality and Social Psychology Bulletin*, *29*(10), 1207–1220. https://doi.org/10.1177/0146167203254602
Barni, D., Ranieri, S., Scabini, E., & Rosnati, R. (2011). Value transmission in the family: Do adolescents accept the values their parents want to transmit? *Journal of Moral Education*, *40*(1), 105–121. https://doi.org/10.1080/03057240.2011.553797
Barrett, M. (2016). *Competences for democratic culture. Living together as equals in culturally diverse democratic societies*. Council of Europe Publishing.
Barrett, M., & Brunton-Smith, I. (2014). Political and civic engagement and participation: Towards an integrative perspective. *Journal of Civil Society*, *10*(1), 5–28. https://doi.org/10.1080/17448689.2013.871911
Baumeister, R. F., Zhang, L., & Vohs, K. D. (2004). Gossip as cultural learning. *Review of General Psychology*, *8*(2), 111–121. https://doi.org/10.1037/1089-2680.8.2.111
Beck, P. A., & Jennings, M. K. (1982). Pathways to participation. *The American Political Science Review*, *76*(1), 94–108. https://doi.org/10.2307/1960445
Beck, P. A., & Jennings, M. K. (1991). Family traditions, political periods, and the development of partisan orientations. *The Journal of Politics*, *53*(3), 742–763. https://doi.org/10.2307/2131578
Berger, B. (2009). Political theory, political science, and the end of civic engagement. *Perspectives on Politics*, *7*(2), 335–350. www.jstor.org/stable/40406934
Bergman, L. R., & El-Khouri, B. (1987). EXACON: A Fortran 77 program for the exact analysis of single cells in a contingency table. *Educational and Psychological Measurement*, *47*(1), 155–161. https://doi.org/10.1177/0013164487471024
Bergman, L. R., Magnusson, D., & El-Khouri, B. (2003). *Studying individual development in an interindividual context: A person-oriented approach* (Vol. 4). Lawrence Erlbaum Associates.
Berti, A. E. (2005). Children's understanding of politics. In M. Barrett & E. Buchanan-Barrow (Eds.), *Children's understanding of society* (pp. 69–104). Psychology Press.
Blais, A., & Labbé St-Vincent, S. L. (2011). Personality traits, political attitudes and the propensity to vote. *European Journal of Political Research*, *50*(3), 395–417. https://doi.org/10.1111/j.1475-6765.2010.01935.x.

Bloemraad, I., & Trost, C. (2008). It's a family affair. Intergenerational mobilization in the Spring 2006 protests. *American Behavioral Scientist*, *52*(4), 507–532. https://doi.org/10.1177/0002764208324604

Boehnke, K., & Schwartz, S. H. (1997). Fear of war: Relations to values, gender, and mental health in Germany and Israel. *Peace and Conflict: Journal of Peace Psychology*, *3*(2), 149–165. https://doi.org/10.1207/s15327949pac0302_3

Bolin, N., & Backlund, A. (2021). De politiska ungdomsförbundens medlemmar [Members of the political youth associations]. In MUCF (Ed.), *Vilja att förändra: Drivkrafter, hinder och utmaningar för ungas samhällsengagemang*. [Willingness to change. Drivers, barriers and challenges for young people's civic engagement] (pp. 97–130). Myndigheten för ungdoms- och civilsamhällesfrågor.

Boyd, M. J., Zaff, J. F., Phelps, E., Weiner, M. B., & Lerner, R. M. (2011). The relationship between adolescents' news media use and civic engagement: The indirect effect of interpersonal communication with parents. *Journal of Adolescence*, *34*(6), 1167–1179. https://doi.org/10.1016/j.adolescence.2011.07.004

Bromme, L., Rothmund, T., & Azevedo, F. (2022). Mapping political trust and involvement in the personality space—A meta-analysis and new evidence. *Journal of Personality*, *90*(6), 846–872. https://doi.org/10.1111/jopy.12700

Bukowski, W. M., & Newcomb, A. F. (1984). Stability and determinants of sociometric status and friendship choice: A longitudinal perspective. *Developmental Psychology*, *20*(5), 941–952. https://doi.org/10.1037/0012-1649.20.5.941

Butterfield, R. D., Silk, J. S., Lee, K. H., Siegle, G. S., Dahl, R. E., Forbes, E. E., Ryan, N. D., Hooley, J. M., & Ladouceur, C. D. (2021). Parents still matter! Parental warmth predicts adolescent brain function and anxiety and depressive symptoms 2 years later. *Development and Psychopathology*, *33*(1), 226–239. https://doi.org/10.1017/S0954579419001718

Cameron, K. A. (2009). A practitioner's guide to persuasion: An overview of 15 selected persuasion theories, models and frameworks. *Patient Education and Counseling*, *74*(3), 309–317. https://doi.org/10.1016/j.pec.2008.12.003

Campbell, A., Gurin, G., & Miller, W. E. (1954). *The voter decides*. Row, Peterson.

Chaffee, S. H., McLeod, J. M., & Wackman, D. B. (1973). Family communication patterns and adolescent political participation. In J. Dennis (Ed.), *Socialization to politics: A reader* (pp. 349–364). Wiley.

Chambré, S. M. (2020). Has volunteering changed in the United States? Trends, styles, and motivations in historical perspective. *Social Service Review*, *94*(2), 373–421. https://doi.org/10.1086/708941

Clement, R. W., & Krueger, J. (2000). The primacy of self-referent information in perceptions of social consensus. British Journal of Social Psychology, 39(2), 279–299. https://doi.org/10.1348/014466600164471

Clement, R. W., & Krueger, J. (2002). Social categorization moderates social projection. *Journal of Experimental Social Psychology*, *38*(3), 219–231. https://doi.org/10.1006/jesp.2001.1503

Cohen, J. (1988). *Statistical power analysis for the behavioral sciences* (2nd ed.). Lawrence Erlbaum Associates.

Collins, W. A., Raby, K. L., & Causadias, J. M. (2011). Transformations in close relationship networks. Parent—child relationships and their social extensions. In B. Laursen & W. A. Collins (Eds.), *Relationship pathways: From adolescence to young adulthood* (pp. 3–22). SAGE Publications.

Connell, R. W. (1972). Political socialization in the American family: The evidence reexamined. *The Public Opinion Quarterly*, *36*(3), 323–333. www.jstor.org/stable/2747440

Converse, P. E., & Niemi, R. (1971). Non-voting among young adults in the United States. In W. J. Crotty, D. M. Freeman, & D. S. Gatlin (Eds.), *Political parties and political behavior* (pp. 443–466). Allyn and Bacon.

Cotton, J. L., & Hieser, R. A. (1980). Selective exposure to information and cognitive dissonance. *Journal of Research in Personality*, *14*(4), 518–527. https://doi.org/10.1016/0092-6566(80)90009-4

Craig, S. C., Niemi, R. G., & Silver, G. E. (1990). Political efficacy and trust: A report on the NES pilot study items. *Political Behavior*, *12*(3), 289–314. https://doi.org/10.1007/BF00992337

Crano, W. D. (1983). Assumed consensus of attitudes the effect of vested interest. *Personality and Social Psychology Bulletin*, *9*(4), 597–608. https://doi.org/10.1177/0146167283094009

Cronbach, L. J. (1955). Processes affecting scores on "understanding of others" and "assumed similarity." *Psychological Bulletin*, *52*(3), 177–193. https://doi.org/10.1037/h0044919

Dahlgaard, J., Hansen, J., Hansen, K., & Bhatti, Y. (2019). Bias in self-reported voting and how it distorts turnout models: Disentangling nonresponse bias and overreporting among Danish voters. *Political Analysis*, *27*(4), 590–598. https://doi.org/10.1017/pan.2019.9

D'Alessio, D., & Allen, M. (2002). Selective exposure and dissonance after decisions. *Psychological Reports*, *91*(2), 527–532. https://doi.org/10.2466/PR0.91.6.527-532

Dawes, C., Cesarini, D., Fowler, J. H., Johannesson, M., Magnusson, P. K. E., & Oskarsson, S. (2014). The relationship between genes, psychological traits, and political participation. *American Journal of Political Science*, *58*(4), 888–903. https://doi.org/10.1111/ajps.12100

Deci, E. L., & Ryan, R. M. (1991). A motivational approach to self: Integration in personality. In R. A. Dienstbier (Ed.), *Nebraska symposium on motivation, 1990: Perspectives on motivation* (pp. 237–288). University of Nebraska Press.

Deci, E. L., & Ryan, R. M. (2000). The "what" and "why" of goal pursuits: Human needs and the self-determination of behavior. *Psychological Inquiry*, *11*, 227–268. https://doi.org/10.1207/S15327965PLI1104_01

Deci, E. L., & Ryan, R. M. (Eds.). (2002). *Handbook of self-determination research*. University Rochester Press.

Deci, E. L., & Ryan, R. M. (2008). Facilitating optimal motivation and psychological wellbeing across life's domains. *Canadian Psychology*, *49*(1), 14–23. https://doi.org/10.1037/0708-5591.49.1.14.

Deci, E. L., & Ryan, R. M. (2013). The importance of autonomy for development and well-being. In B. W. Sokol, F. M. E. Grouzet, & U. Müller (Eds.), *Self-regulation and autonomy. Social and developmental dimensions of human conduct* (pp. 19–46). Cambridge University Press. https://doi.org/10.1017/CBO9781139152198.005

Delli Carpini, M. X., & Keeter, S. (1996). *What Americans know about politics and why it matters*. Yale University Press.

De Los Reyes, A. (2013). Strategic objectives for improving understanding of informant discrepancies in developmental psychopathology research. *Development and Psychopathology*, *25*(3), 669–682. http://dx.doi.org/10.1017/S0954579413000096

De Los Reyes, A., Augenstein, T. M., Wang, M., Thomas, S. A., Drabick, D. A. G., Burgers, D. E., & Rabinowitz, J. (2015). The validity of the multi-informant approach to assessing child and adolescent mental health. *Psychological Bulletin*, *141*(4), 858–900. http://dx.doi.org/10.1037/a0038498

Demokratiutredningen [Democracy Inquiry]. (2016). *Statens Offentliga Utredningar, 2016:5*. www.regeringen.se/rattsliga-dokument/statens-offentliga-utredningar/2016/01/sou-20165/

Döring, A. K., Schwartz, S. H., Cieciuch, J., Groenen, P. J. F., Glatzel, V., Harasimczuk, J., Janowicz, N., Nyagolova, M., Scheefer, E. R., Allritz, M., Milfont, T. L., & Bilsky, W. (2015). Cross-cultural evidence of value structures and priorities in childhood. *British Journal of Psychology*, *106*(4), 675–699. https://doi.org/10.1111/bjop.12116

Dostie-Goulet, E. (2009). Social networks and the development of political interest. *Journal of Youth Studies*, *12*(4), 405–421. https://doi.org/10.1080/13676260902866512

Dubas, J. S., & Petersen, A. C. (1996). Geographical distance from parents and adjustment during adolescence and young adulthood. *New Directions for Child and Adolescent Development, 71*(3), 3–19. https://doi.org/10.1002/cd.23219967103.

Dunkel, C. S., & Decker, M. (2012). Using identity style and parental identification to predict political orientation. *Current Psychology, 31*(1), 65–78. https://doi.org/10.1007/s12144-012-9131-8

Eckstein, K., Noack, P., & Gniewosz, B. (2013). Predictors of intentions to participate in politics and actual political behaviors in young adulthood. *International Journal of Behavioral Development, 37*(5), 428–435. https://doi.org/10.1177/0165025413486419

Ekman, J., & Amnå, E. (2022). Civic engagement. In M. Giugni & M. Grasso (Eds.), *The Oxford handbook of political participation* (pp. 381–395). Oxford University Press.

Emler, N. (1990). A social psychology of reputation. *European Review of Social Psychology, 1*, 171–193. https://doi.org/10.1080/14792779108401861

Emler, N. (2013). La réputation comme instrument social. *Communications, 93*(1), 85–100. https://doi.org/10.3406/comm.2013.2718

Emler, N. (2019). Human sociality and psychological foundations. In F. Giardini & R. Wittek (Eds.), *The Oxford handbook of gossip and reputation* (pp. 47–68). Oxford University Press. https://doi.org/10.1093/oxfordhb/9780190494087.013

Emler, N., & Reicher, S. (1995). *Adolescence and delinquency: The collective management of reputation*. Blackwell Publishing.

Epley, N., Keysar, B., van Boven, L., & Gilovich, T. (2004). Perspective taking as egocentric anchoring and adjustment. *Journal of Personality and Social Psychology, 87*(3), 327–339. https://doi.org/10.1037/0022–3514.87.3.327

Erentaité, R., Zukauskiené, R., Beyers, W., & Pilkauskaité-Valickiené, R. (2012). Is news media related to civic engagement? The effects of interest in and discussions about the news media on current and future civic engagement of adolescents. *Journal of Adolescence, 35*(3), 587–597. https://doi.org/10.1016/j.adolescence.2011.12.008

Eveland Jr, W. P., & Scheufele, D. A. (2000). Connecting news media use with gaps in knowledge and participation. *Political Communication, 17*(3), 215–237. https://doi.org/10.1080/105846000414250

Festinger, L. A. (1957). *A theory of cognitive dissonance*. Stanford University Press.

Fieldhouse, E., Tranmer, M., & Russel, A. (2007). Something about young people or something about elections? Electoral participation of young people in Europe: Evidence from a multilevel analysis of the European Social Survey. *European Journal of Political Research, 46*(6), 797–822. https://doi.org/10.1111/j.1475-6765.2007.00713.x

Finkel, S. E. (1985). Reciprocal effects of participation and political efficacy: A panel study. *American Journal of Political Science, 29*(4), 891–913. https://doi.org/10.2307/2111186

Fishbein, M., & Ajzen, I. (1975). *Belief, attitude, intention and behavior: An introduction to theory and research*. Addison-Wesley.

Fishbein, M., & Ajzen, I. (2010). *Predicting and changing behavior. The reasoned action approach*. Psychology Press, Taylor & Francis group. https://doi.org/10.4324/9780203838020

Fitzgerald, J. (2013). What does 'political' mean to you? *Political Behavior, 35*(3), 453–479. https://doi.org/10.1007/s11109-012-9212-2

Fitzgerald, M. A., & Caughlin, J. P. (2002). Interpersonal communication in family relationships. In M. L. Knapp & J. A. Daly (Eds.), *Handbook of interpersonal communication* (pp. 726–777). Sage Publications.

Flanagan, C. A. (2013). *Teenage citizens: The political theories of the young*. Harvard University Press.

Flanagan, C. A., & Sherrod, L. R. (1998). Youth political development: An introduction. *Journal of Social Issues, 54*, 447–456. https://doi.org/10.1111/j.1540-4560.1998.tb01229.x

Foster, E. K. (2004). Research on gossip: Taxonomy, methods, and future directions. *Review of General Psychology, 8*(2), 111–121. https://doi.org/10.1037/1089-2680.8.2.78

Friedlmeier, M., & Trommsdorff, G. (2011). Are mother—child similarities in value orientations related to mothers' parenting? A comparative study of American and Romanian mothers and their adolescent children. *European Journal of Developmental Psychology, 8*(6), 661–680. https://doi.org/10.1080/17405629.2011.590649

Furmark, T., Tillfors, M., Everz, P-O., Marteinsdottir, I., Gefvert, O., & Fredrikson, M. (1999). Social phobia in the general population: Prevalence and sociodemographic profile. *Social Psychiatry and Psychiatric Epidemiology, 34*(8), 416–424. https://doi.org/10.1007/s001270050163

Gage III, R. L., & Thapa, B. (2012). Volunteer motivations and constraints among college students: Analysis of the volunteer function inventory and leisure constraints models. *Nonprofit and Voluntary Sector Quarterly, 41*(3), 405–430. https://doi.org/10.1177/0899764011406738

Gagne', F. M., & Lydon, J. E. (2004). Bias and accuracy in close relationships: An integrative review. *Personality and Social Psychology Review, 8*(4), 322–338. https://doi.org/10.1207/s15327957pspr0804_1

Galambos, N. L., & Kotylak, L. A. (2011). Transformations in parent-child relationships from adolescence to adulthood. In B. Laursen & W. A. Collins (Eds.), *Relationship pathways: From adolescence to young adulthood* (pp. 23–42). SAGE Publications.

Geißler, R. (1996). Politische sozialisation in der familie [Political socialization in the family]. In B. Claußen & R. Geißler (Eds.), *Die politisierung des menschen. Instanzen der politischen sozialisation. Ein handbuch* [The politicization of people. Instances of political socialisation. A handbook] (pp. 51–69). VS Verlag für Sozialwissenschaften/GWV Fachverlage GmbH.

Gerber, A. S., Green, D. P., & Shachar, R. (2003). Voting may be habit-forming: Evidence from a randomized field experiment. *American Journal of Political Science, 47*(3), 540–550. https://doi.org/10.1111/1540-5907.00038

Gifford, R., & Nilsson, A. (2014). Personal and social factors that influence pro-environmental concern and behaviour: A review. *International Journal of Psychology, 49*(3), 141–157. https://doi.org/10.1002/ijop.12034

Gniewosz, B., & Noack, P. (2006). Intergenerationale transmissions und projektionsprozesse intoleranter einstellungen zu ausländern in der familie [Intergenerational transmission and projection processesof intolerant attitudes towards foreigners in the family]. *Zeitschrift für Entwicklungspsychologie und Pädagogische Psychologie, 38*(1), 33–42. https://doi.org/10.1026/0049-8637.38.1.33

Gniewosz, B., Noack, P., & Buhl, M. (2009). Political alienation in adolescence: Associations with parental role models, parenting styles, and classroom climate. *International Journal of*Behavioral *Development, 33*(4), 337–346. https://doi.org/10.1177/0165025409103137

Gniewosz, B., Noack, P., Wentura, D., & Funke, F. (2008). Adolescents' attitudes towards foreigners: Associations with perceptions of significant others' attitudes depending on sex and age. *Diskurs Kindheits-und Jugendforschung Heft, 3*(3), 321–337. https://nbn-resolving.org/urn:nbn:de:0168- ssoar-269419

Goodenow, C. (1993). Classroom belonging among early adolescent students. *The Journal of Early Adolescence, 13*(1), 21–43. https://doi.org/10.1177/0272431693013001002

Grusec, J. E., & Davidov, M. (2021). *Socializing children.* Cambridge University Press.

Grusec, J. E., & Goodnow, J. J. (1994). Impact of parental discipline methods on the child's internalization of values: A reconceptualization of current points of view. *Developmental Psychology, 30*(1), 4–19. https://doi.org/10.1037/0012-1649.30.1.4

Grusec, J. E., & Kuczynski, L. (1997). *Parenting and children's internalization of values: A handbook of contemporary theory.* John Wiley & Sons Inc.

Görtz, C., Zorell, C. V. & Fitzgerald, J. (2023). Casting light on citizens' conceptions of what is 'political'. *Acta Politica, 58*(1-2), 57–78. https://doi.org/10.1057/s41269-022-00233-y

Harmon-Jones, E. (2002). A cognitive dissonance theory perspective on persuasion. In J. P. Dillard & M. Pfau (Eds.), *The persuasion handbook: Developments in theory and practice* (pp. 99–116). Sage.

Hatemi, P. K., & McDermott, R. (2012). The genetics of politics: Discovery, challenges, and progress. *Trends in Genetics*, *28*(10), 525–533. https://doi.org/10.1016/j.tig.2012.07.004

Haynie, D. L., & Osgood, D. W. (2005). Reconsidering peers and delinquency: How do peers matter? *Social Forces*, *84*(2), 1109–1130. www.jstor.org/stable/3598492

Hays, A. D. (2017). *Mediation, moderation, and conditional process analysis. A regression-based approach.* Guilford Press.

Heath, A. F., Lindsay, R., & Jungblut, J. (2022). Political values and political participation. In M. Giugni & M. Grasso (Eds.), *The Oxford handbook of political participation.* Oxford University Press.

Heider, F. (1958). *The psychology of interpersonal relations*. Wiley.

Hess, D. E. (2002). Discussing controversial public issues in secondary social studies classrooms: Learning from skilled teachers. *Theory & Research in Social Education, 30*(1), 10–41. https://doi.org/10.1080/00933104.2002.10473177

Hess, D. E. (2004). Discussion in social studies: Is it worth the trouble? *Social Education, 68*(2). https://doi.org/10.4324/978020384127

Hess, D. E., & McAvoy, P. (2014). *The political classroom: Evidence and ethics in democratic education.* Routledge.

Hidi, S., & Renninger, K. A. (2006). The four-phase model of interest development. Educational Psychologist, 41(2), 111–127. https://doi.org/10.1207/s15326985ep4102_4

Higher Educations in Sweden. (2018). *UKÄ Årsrapport 2018.* Internationella jämförelser [2018 Status report. International comparisons]. Rapport 2018:5.

Highton, B., & Wolfinger, R. E. (2001). The first seven years of the political life cycle. *American Journal of Political Science*, *45*(1), 202–209. https://doi.org/10.2307/2669367

Hogg, M. A., & Mullin, B. A. (1999). Joining groups to reduce uncertainty: Subjective uncertainty reduction and group identification. In D. Abrams & M. A. Hogg (Eds.), *Social identity and social cognition* (pp. 249–279). Blackwell Publishers.

Holmes, D. S. (1968). Dimensions of projection. *Psychological Bulletin, 69*(4), 248–268. https://doi.org/10.1037/h0025725

Hooghe, M., & Dejaeghere, Y. (2007). Does the 'monitorial citizen' exist? An empirical investigation into the occurrence of postmodern forms of citizenship in the Nordic countries, *Scandinavian Political Studies*, *30*(2), 115–129. https://doi.org/10.1111/j.1467-9477.2007.00180.x

Hou, Y., Benner, A. D., Kim, S. Y., Chen, S., Spitz, S., Shi, Y., & Beretvas, T. (2020). Discordance in parents' and adolescents' reports of parenting: A meta-analysis and qualitative review. *American Psychologist*, *75*(3), 329–348. https://doi.org/10.1037/amp0000463

Hunter, F. T. (1985). Adolescents' perception of discussions with parents and friends. *Developmental Psychology*, *21*(3), 433–440. https://doi.org/10.1037/0012-1649.21.3.433

Janmaat, J. G., & Hoskins, B. (2022). The changing impact of family background on political engagement during adolescence and early adulthood. *Social Forces*, *101*(1), 227–251. https://doi.org/10.1093/sf/soab112

Janssen, L. H., Verkuil, B., van Houtum, L. A., Wever, M. C., & Elzinga, B. M. (2021). Perceptions of parenting in daily life: Adolescent-parent differences and associations with adolescent affect. *Journal of Youth and Adolescence*, *50*(12), 2427–2443. https://doi.org/10.1007/s10964-021-01489-x

Jennings, M. K., & Niemi, R. G. (1968). The transmission of political values from parent to child. *American Political Science Review*, *62*(1), 169–184. https://doi.org/10.2307/1953332

Jennings, M. K., & Niemi, R. G. (1974). *The political character of adolescents: The influence of families and schools*. Princeton University Press.

Jennings, M. K., & Niemi, R. G. (1981). *Generations and politics: A panel study of young adults and their parents*. Princeton University Press.

Jennings, M. K., Stoker, L., & Bowers, J. (2009). Politics across generations: Family transmission reexamined. *The Journal of Politics*, *71*(3), 782–799. https://doi.org/10.1017/S0022381609090719

John, O. P., & Srivastava, S. (1999). The Big Five Trait taxonomy: History, measurement, and theoretical perspectives. In L. A. Pervin & O. P. John (Eds.), *Handbook of personality: Theory and research* (pp. 102–138). Guilford Press.

Jugert, P., Greenaway, K., Barth, M., Büchner, R., Eisentraut, S., & Fritsche, I. (2016). Collective efficacy increases pro-environmental intentions through increasing self-efficacy. *Journal of Environmental Psychology, 48*, 12–23. https://doi.org/10.1016/j.jenvp.2016.08.003

Jussim, L., & Osgood, D. W. (1989). Influence and similarity among friends: An integrative model applied to incarcerated adolescents. *Social Psychology Quarterly*, *52*(2), 98–112. https://doi.org/10.2307/2786910

Kahneman, D. (1973). *Attention and effort*. Prentice Hall.

Kandel, D. B. (1978). Homophily, selection, and socialization in adolescent friendships. *American Journal of Sociology*, *84*(2), 427–436. www.jstor.org/stable/2777857

Kapetanovic, S., & Boson, K. (2022). Discrepancies in parents' and adolescents' reports on parent-adolescent communication and associations to adolescents' psychological health. *Current Psychology*, *41*(7), 4259–4270. https://doi.org/10.1007/s12144-020-00911-0

Karlsson, M., & Lundberg, E. (2011). *Mot medlemslösa partier. Partiföreträdare om orsaker, konsekvenser och strategier kring en svikande medlemskår* [Party representatives on the causes, consequences and strategies for a declining membership]. Sektor3.

Katz, D. (1960). The functional approach to the study of attitudes. *Public Opinion Quarterly*, *24*(2), 163–204. www.jstor.org/stable/2746402

Katz, D., & Allport, F. H. (1931). *Student attitudes*. Craftsmen Press.

Kenny, D. A., & Acitelli, L. K. (2001). Accuracy and bias in the perception of the partner in a close relationship. *Journal of Personality and Social Psychology*, *80*(3), 439–448. https://doi.org/10.1037/0022-3514.80.3.439

Kerr, M., & Stattin, H. (2000). What parents know, how they know it, and several forms of adolescent adjustment: Further evidence for a reinterpretation of monitoring. *Developmental Psychology*, *36*(3), 366–380.

*Kim, Y., & Stattin, H. (2019). Parent-youth discussions about politics from age 13 to 28. *Journal of Applied Developmental Psychology*, *62*(201), 249–259 https://doi.org/10.1016/j.appdev.2019.04.001 [chapter 6]

Kinder, B. N., Curtiss, G., & Kalichman, S. (1991). Cluster analyses of headache-patient MMPI scores: A cross-validation. *Psychological Assessment*, *3*(2), 226–231. https://doi.org/10.1037/1040-3590.3.2.226.

Kiousis, S., McDevitt, M., & Wu, X. (2005). The genesis of civic awareness: Agenda setting in political socialization. *Journal of Communication*, *55*(4), 756–774. https://doi.org/10.1111/j.1460-2466.2005.tb03021.x

Knafo, A., & Schwartz, S. H. (2003). Parenting and adolescents' accuracy in perceiving parental values. *Child Development*, *74*(2), 595–611. https://doi.org/ 10.1111/1467-8624.7402018

Knafo, A., & Schwartz, S. H. (2009). Accounting for parent-child value congruence: Theoretical considerations and empirical evidence. In U. Schönpflug (Ed.), *Cultural transmission: Developmental, psychological, and methodological perspectives* (pp. 240–268). Cambridge University Press.

Koerner, A. F., & Fitzpatrick, M. A. (2002). Toward a theory of family communication. *Communication Theory*, *12*(1), 70–91. https://doi.org/10.1111/j.1468-2885.2002.tb00260.x

Koolstra, C. M., & Lucassen, N. (2004). Viewing behavior of children and TV guidance by parents: A comparison of parent and child reports. *Communications, The European Journal of Communication Research*, *29*(2), 179–198. https://doi.org/10.1515/comm.2004.012

Korelitz, K. E., & Garber, J. (2016). Congruence of parents' and children's perceptions of parenting: A meta-analysis. *Journal of Youth and Adolescence*, *45*(10), 1973–1995. https://doi.org/10.1007/s10964-016-0524-0.

Koskimaa, V., & Rapeli, L. (2015). Political socialization and political interest: The role of school reassessed, *Journal of Political Science Education*, *11*(2), 141–156. https://doi.org/10.1080/15512169.2015.1016033

Kraemer, H. C., Measelle, J. R., Ablow, J. C., Essex, M. J., Boyce, W. T., & Kupfer, D. J. (2003). A new approach to integrating data from multiple informants in psychiatric assessment and research: Mixing and matching contexts and perspectives. *American Journal of Psychiatry*, *160*(9), 1566–1577.

Krapp, A. (2007). An educational–psychological conceptualization of interest. International Journal for Educational and Vocational Guidance, 7, 5–21. https://doi.org/10.1007/s10775-007-9113-9.

Krosnick, J. A., & Alwin, D. F. (1989). Aging and susceptibility to attitude change. *Journal of Personality and Social Psychology*, *57*(3), 416–425. https://doi.org/10.1037/0022-3514.57.3.416.

Krueger, J. (1998). On the perception of social consensus. *Advances in Experimental Social Psychology*, *30*, 163–240. https://doi.org/10.1016/S0065-2601(08)60384-6

Kuntz, A., Davidov, E., Schwartz, S. H., & Schmidt, P. (2015). Human values, legal regulation, and approval of homosexuality in Europe: A cross-country comparison. *European Journal of Social Psychology*, *45*(1), 120–134. https://doi.org/10.1002/ejsp.2068

Lake Snell Perry & Associates. (2002). *Short-term impacts, long-term opportunities: The political and civic engagement of young adults in America*. Analysis and Report for The Center for Information and Research in Civic Learning & Engagement (CIRCLE) and The Center for Democracy & Citizenship and The Partnership for Trust in Government at the Council for Excellence in Government. www.higher-ed.org/resources/pp_circle_0302.pdf

Landberg, M., Eckstein, K., Mikolajczyk, C., Mejias, S., Macek, P., Motti-Stefanidi, F., Enchikova, E., Guarino, A., Rämmer, A., & Noack, P. (2018). Being both—A European and a national citizen? Comparing young people's identification with Europe and their home country across eight European countries. *European Journal of Developmental Psychology*, *15*(3), 270–283. https://doi.org/10.1080/17405629.2017.1391087

Lane, R. E. (1959). *Political life: Why people get involved in politics*. The Free Press.

Lee, N. J., Shah, D. V., & McLeod, J. M. (2012). Process of political socialization: A communication mediation approach to youth civic engagement. *Communication Research*, *40*(5), 669–697. https://doi.org/10.1177/0093650212436712

Lefkowitz, E. S. (2005). Things have gotten better developmental changes among emerging adults after the transition to university. *Journal of Adolescent Research*, *20*(1), 40–63. https://doi.org/10.1177/0743558404271236

Lemay, E. P., Jr., Clark, M. S., & Greenberg, A. (2010). What is beautiful is good because what is beautiful is desired: Physical attractiveness stereotyping as projection of interpersonal goals. *Personality & Social Psychology Bulletin*, *36*(3), 339–353. https://doi.org/10.1177/0146167209359700

Levinsen, K., & Yndigegn, C. (2015). Political discussions with family and friends: Exploring the impact of political distance. *The Sociological Review*, *63*(S2), 72–91. https://doi.org/10.1111/1467-954X.12263

Levy, B. L. M. (2013). An empirical exploration of factors related to adolescents' political efficacy. *Educational Psychology*, *33*(3), 357–390. https://doi.org/10.1080/01443410.2013.772774

Levy, B. L. M., & Akiva, T. (2019). Motivating political participation among youth: An analysis of factors related to adolescents' political engagement. *Political Psychology*, *40*(5), 1039–1055. https://doi.org/10.1111/pops.12578

Levy, B. L. M., Solomon, B. G., & Collet-Gildard, L. (2016). Fostering political interest among youth during the 2012 presidential election: Instructional opportunities and challenges in a swing state. *Educational Researcher*, *45*, 483–495. https://doi.org/10.3102/0013189X16683402

Liebes, T., & Ribak, R. (1992). The contribution of family culture to political participation, political outlook, and its reproduction. *Communication Research*, *19*(5), 618–641. https://doi.org/10.1177/009365092019005004

Liu, J., Bullock, A., & Coplan, R. J. (2014). Predictive relations between peer victimization and academic achievement in Chinese children. *School Psychology Quarterly*, *29*(1), 89–98. https://doi.org/10.1037/spq0000044

Luskin, R. C. (1990). Explaining political sophistication. *Political Behavior*, *12*(4), 331–361. https://doi.org/10.1007/BF00992793

Lupia, A., & Philpot, T. S. (2005). Views from inside the net: How websites affect young adults' political interest. *The Journal of Politics*, *67*(4), 1122–1142. https://doi.org/10.1111/j.1468-2508.2005.00353.x

Magnusson, D., & Stattin, H. (2006). The person in the environment: Towards a general model for scientific inquiry. In R. M. Lerner (Ed.), *Theoretical models of human development* (Vol. 6, pp. 400–464) (Volume 1 of Handbook of child psychology). John Wiley & Sons.

Maner, J. K., Kenrick, D. T., Becker, D. V., Robertson, T. E., Hofer, B., Neuberg, S. L., & Schaller, M. (2005). Functional projection: How fundamental social motives can bias interpersonal perception. *Journal of Personality and Social Psychology*, *88*(1), 63–78. https://doi.org/10.1037/0022-3514.88.1.63

Marks, G., & Miller, N. (1987). Ten years of research on the false-consensus effect: An empirical and theoretical review. *Psychological Bulletin*, *102*(1), 72–90. https://doi.org/10.1037/0033-2909.102.1.72

Marsh, B., Todd, P. M., & Gigerenzer, G. (2004). Cognitive heuristics: Reasoning the fast and frugal way. In J. P. Leighton & R. J. Sternberg (Eds.), *The nature of reasoning* (pp. 273–287). Cambridge University Press.

Masche, J. G. (2008). Reciprocal influences between developmental transitions and parent—child relationships in young adulthood. *International Journal of Behavioral Development*, *32*(5), 401–411. https://doi.org/10.1177/0165025408093658

Mayer, J. D., & Schmidt, H. M. (2004). Gendered political socialization in four contexts: Political interest and values among junior high school students in China, Japan, Mexico, and the United States, *The Social Science Journal*, *41*(3), 393–407. https://doi.org/10.1016/j.soscij.2004.04.024

McArdle, J. J., & Nesselroade, J. R. (1994). Structuring data to study development and change. In S. H. Cohen & H. W. Reese (Eds.), *Life-span developmental psychology: Methodological innovations* (pp. 223–268). Erlbaum.

McCall, G. J., & Simmons, J. L. (1978). *Identities and interactions*. Free Press.

McDevitt, M. (2006). The partisan child: Developmental provocation as a model of political socialization. *International Journal of Public Opinion Research*, *18*(1), 67–88. https://doi.org/10.1093/ijpor/edh079

McDevitt, M. (2015). Political socialization. In C. R. Berger & M. E. Roloff (Eds.), *International encyclopedia of interpersonal communication* (pp. 1333–1341). International Communication Association/Wiley-Blackwell. https://doi.org/10.1002/9781118540190.wbeic215

McDevitt, M., & Chaffee, S. H. (2000). Closing gaps in political communication and knowledge effects of a school intervention. *Communication Research*, *27*(3), 259–292. https://doi.org/10.1177/009365000027003001

McDevitt, M., & Chaffee, S. H. (2002). From top-down to trickle-up influence: Revisiting assumptions about the family in political socialization. *Political Communication*, *19*(3), 281–301. https://doi.org/10.1080/01957470290055501

McIntosh, H., Hart, D., & Youniss, J. (2007). The influence of family political discussion on youth civic development: Which parent qualities matter? *PS: Political Science & Politics*, *40*(3), 495–499. https://doi.org/10.1017/S1049096507070758

McLeod, J. M., & Chaffee, S. R. (1972). The social construction of reality. In J. Tedeschi (Ed.), *The social influence processes* (pp. 50–99). Aldine-Atherton.

Meadowcroft, J. M. (1986). Family communication patterns and political development. The child's role. *Communication Research*, *13*(4), 603–624. https://doi.org/10.1177/009365086013004005

Meeusen, C. (2014). The intergenerational transmission of environmental concern: The influence of parents and communication patterns within the family. *The Journal of Environmental Education, 45*(2), 77–90. https://doi.org/10.1080/00958964.2013.846290

Miklikowska, M. (2015). Like parent, like child? Development of prejudice and tolerance towards immigrants. *British Journal of Psychology, 107*(1), 95–116. https://doi.org/10.1111/bjop.12124

Miller, D. (1978). Democracy and social justice. *British Journal of Political Science, 8*(1), 1–19. https://doi.org/10.1017/S0007123400001198

Miller, W. E., Miller, H., & Schneider, E. J. (1980). *American national election studies data sourcebook 1952–1978*. Harvard University Press.

Moeller, J., Shehata, A., & Kruikemeier, S. (2018). Internet use and political interest: Growth curves, reinforcing spirals, and causal effects during adolescence. *Journal of Communication, 68*(6), 1052–1078. https://doi.org/10.1093/joc/jqy062

MUCF. (2021). *Vilja att förändra. Drivkrafter, hinder och utmaningar för ungas samhällsengagemang* [Willingness to change. Drivers, barriers and challenges for young people's civic engagement]. Myndigheten för ungdoms- och civilsamhällesfrågor.

Murray, S. L., Holmes, J. G., & Griffin, D. W. (1996). The benefits of positive illusions: Idealization and the construction of satisfaction in close relationships. *Journal of Personality and Social Psychology, 70*(1), 79–98. https://doi.org/10.1037/0022-3514.70.1.79

Musso, P., Lo Cricchio, M. G., Lo Coco, A., Tani, F., Ingoglia, S., & Rubin, K. H. (2020). A revised short form of the extended Class Play among Italian early adolescents. *Psychological Reports, 123*(5), 1986–2016. https://doi.org/10.1177/00332

Mussweiler, T. (2003). Comparison processes in social judgment: Mechanisms and consequences. *Psychological Review, 110*(3), 472–489. https://doi.org/10.1037/0033-295X.110.3.472

Muthén, L. K., & Muthén, B. O. (1998–2017). *Mplus user's guide* (8th ed.). Muthén & Muthén.

Nabatchi, T. (2014). Deliberative civic engagement in public administration and policy. *Journal of Public Deliberation, 10*(1). https://doi.org/10.16997/jdd.195

Neisser, U. (1967). *Cognitive psychology*. Appleton-Century-Crofts.

Neundorf, A., Smets, K., & García-Albacete, G. M. (2013). Homemade citizens: The development of political interest during adolescence and young adulthood. *Acta Politica, 48*(1), 92–116. https://doi.org/10.1057/ap.2012.23

Niemi, R. G., & Hepburn, M. A. (1995). The rebirth of political socialization. *Perspectives on Political Science, 24*(1), 7–16. https://doi.org/10.1080/10457097.1995.9941860

Noack, P. (2001). Fremdenfeindliche einstellungen vor dem hintergrund familialer und schulischer sozialisation [Xenophobia against the background of familial and school socialization]. Zeitschrift *für Politische Psychologie, 9*, 67–80.

Norris, P. (2003). *Democratic phoenix: Reinventing political activism*. Cambridge University Press. https://doi.org/10.1017/CBO9780511610073

Ojala, M. (2010). *Survey on young people's thoughts and feelings about climate issues*. Unpublished research instrument. Örebro University.

Ojeda, C., & Hatemi, P. K. (2015). Accounting for the child in the transmission of party identification. *American Sociological Review, 80*(6), 1150–1174. https://doi.org/10.1177/0003122415606101

Oser, J. (2021). Protest as one political act in individuals' participation repertoires: Latent class analysis and political participant types. *American Behavioral Scientist, 66*(4), 510–532. https://doi.org/10.1177/00027642211021633

Oswald, H., & Schmid, C. (1998). Political participation of young people in East Germany. *German Politics, 7*(3), 147–164. https://doi.org/10.1080/09644009808404531

Oswald, H., & Schmid, C. (2006). The influence of parents and peers on political participation of adolescents in the new states of Germany. In A. Sliwka, M. Diedrich, & M. Hofer (Eds.), *Citizenship education in youth—theory, research, and practice* (pp. 85–97). Waxmann.

Pacheco, J. S. (2008). Political socialization in context: The effect of political competition on youth voter turnout. *Political Behavior*, *30*(4), 415–436. https://doi.org/10.1007/s11109-008-9057-x

Pancer, S. M. (2015). *The psychology of citizenship and civic engagement*. Oxford University Press.

Patterson, M. M., Bigler, R. S., Phalke, E., Brown, C. S., Hayes, A. R., Ramirez, M. C., & Nelson, A. (2019). Toward a developmental science of politics. *Monographs of the Society for Research in Child Development*, *84*(3), 334. https://doi.org/10.1111/mono.12410

Patterson, M. M., & Pahlke, E. (2021). The elephant (and donkey) in the room: Parents' approaches to political socialization surrounding the 2020 US election. *Analyses of Social Issues and Public Policy*, *21*(1), 121–148. https://doi.org/10.1111/asap.12260

Pelletier, L. G., Tuson. K. M., Fortier, M. S., Vallerand, R. J., Brikre, N. M., & Blais, M. R. (1995). Toward a snew measure of intrinsic motivation, extrinsic motivation, and amotivation in sports: The Sport Motivation Scale (SMS). *Journal of Sport & Exercise Psychology*, *17*(1), 35–53. https://doi.org/10.1123/jsep.17.1.35

Pickard, S. (2019). *Politics, protest and young people: Political participation and dissent in 21st century Britain*. Palgrave Macmillan. https://doi.org/10.1057/978-1-137-57788-7

Prior, M. (2010). You've either got it or you don't? The stability of political interest over the life cycle. *The Journal of Politics*, *72*, 747–766. https://doi.org/10.1017/S0022381610000149.

Prior, M. (2019). *Hooked: How politics captures people's interest*. Cambridge University Press.

Putnam, R. D. (2000). *Bowling alone: The collapse and revival of American community*. Simon & Schuster. https://doi.org/10.1145/358916.361990

Quintelier, E. (2015). Engaging adolescents in politics: The longitudinal effect of political socialization agents. *Youth & Society*, *47*(1) 51–69. https://doi.org/10.1177/0044118X13507295

Quintelier, E., & Hooghe, M. (2012). Political attitudes and political participation: A panel study on socialization and self-selection effects among late adolescents. *International Political Science Review*, *33*(1), 63–81. https://doi.org/10.1177/0192512111412632

Quintelier, E., & van Deth, J. W. (2014). Supporting democracy: Political participation and political attitudes. Exploring causality using panel data. *Political Studies*, *62*(S1), 153–171. https://doi.org/10.1111/1467-9248.12097

Rapeli, L. (2022). What is the best proxy for political knowledge in surveys? *PLOS ONE*, *17*(8), 1–18. https://doi.org/10.1371/journal.pone.0272530

Rauscher, E. A., Schrodt, P., Campbell-Salome, G., & Freytag, J. (2020). The intergenerational transmission of family communication patterns: (In)consistencies in conversation and conformity orientations across two generations of family. *Journal of Family Communication*, *20*(2), 97–113. https://doi.org/10.1080/15267431.2019.1683563

Rice, K. G., & Mulkeen, P. (1995). Relationships with parents and peers: A longitudinal study of adolescent intimacy. *Journal of Adolescent Research*, *10*(3), 338–357. https://doi.org/10.1177/0743554895103003

Rill, L. A., & McKinney, M. S. (2011). Talking politics: Young citizens' interpersonal interaction during the 2008 presidential campaign. In M. S. McKinney & M. C. Banwart (Eds.), *Communication in the U.S. 2008 election. Digital natives elect a president* (pp. 51–70). Peter Lang Publishing.

Ritchie, L. D. (1991). Family communication patterns: An epistemic analysis and conceptual reinterpretation. *Communication Research*, *18*(4), 548–565. https://doi.org/10.1177/009365091018004005

Ritchie, L. D., & Fitzpatrick, M. A. (1990). Family communication patterns: Measuring intrapersonal perceptions of interpersonal relationships. *Communication Research*, *17*(4), 523–544. https://doi.org/10.1177/009365090017004007

Roeser, R. W., Midgley, C., & Urdan, T. C. (1996). Perceptions of the school psychological environment and early adolescents' psychological and behavioral functioning in school: The mediating role of goals and belonging. *Journal of Educational Psychology*, *88*(3), 408–422. https://doi.org/10.1037/0022-0663.88.3.408

Roest, A. M. C., Dubas, J. S., & Gerris, J. R. M. (2009). Value transmissions between fathers, mothers, and adolescent and emerging adult children: The role of the family climate. *Journal of Family Psychology*, *23*(2), 146–155. https://doi.org/10.1037/a0015075

Ross, L., Greene, D., & House, P. (1977). The false consensus effect: An egocentric bias in social perception and attribution processes. *Journal of Experimental Social Psychology*, *13*(3), 279–301. https://doi.org/10.1016/0022-1031(77)90049-X

Rothstein, B. (2001). Social capital in the social democratic welfare state. *Politics & society*, *29*(2), 207–241. https://doi.org/10.1177/0032329201029002003

Rotolo, T., & Wilson, J. (2004). What happened to the "Long Civic Generation"? Explaining cohort differences in volunteerism. *Social Forces*, *82*(3), 1091–1121. https://doi.org/10.1353/sof.2004.0051

*Russo, S., & Stattin, H. (2017). Stability and change in youths' political interest. *Social Indicators Research*, *132*(2), 643–658. https://doi.org/10.1007/s11205-016-1302-9 [chapter 1]

*Russo, S., & Stattin, H. (2017). Self-determination theory and the role of political interest in adolescents' sociopolitical development. *Journal of Applied Developmental Psychology*, *50*, 71–78. https://doi.org/10.1016/j.appdev.2017.03.008 [chapter 3]

Ryan, R. M., & Deci, E. L. (2000). Self-determination theory and the facilitation of intrinsic motivation, social development, and well-being. *American Psychologist*, *55*(1), 68–78. https://doi.org/10.1037/0003066X.55.1.68

Ryan, R. M., & Deci, E. L. (2006). Self-regulation and the problem of human autonomy: Does psychology need choice, self-determination, and will? *Journal of Personality*, *74*(6), 1557–1586. https://doi.org/10.1111/j.1467-6494.2006.00420.x

Sagiv, L., & Schwartz, S. H. (1995). Value priorities and readiness for out-group social contact. *Journal of Personality and Social Psychology*, *69*(3), 437–448. https://doi.org/10.1037/0022-3514.69.3.437

Saphir, M. N., & Chaffee, S. H. (2002). Adolescents' contributions to family communication patterns. *Human Communication Research*, *28*(1), 86–108. https://doi.org/10.1111/j.1468-2958.2002.tb00799.x

Scheufele, D. A. (2000). Talk or conversation? Dimensions of interpersonal discussions and their implications for participatory democracy. *J & MC Quarterly*, *77*(4), 727–743. https://doi.org/10.1177/107769900007700402

Schmid, C. (2012). The value 'social responsibility' as a motivating factor for adolescents' readiness to participate in different types of political actions, and its socialization in parent and peer contexts. *Journal of Adolescence*, *35*(3), 533–547. https://doi.org/10.1016/j.adolescence.2012.03.009

Schönpflug, U. (2001). Intergenerational transmission of values. The role of transmission belts. *Journal of Cross-Cultural Psychology*, *32*(2), 174–185. https://doi.org/10.1177/0022022101032002005

Schudson, M. (1997). Why conversation is not the soul of democracy. *Critical Studies in Mass Communication, 14*, 297–309. https://doi.org/10.1080/15295039709367020

Schudson, M. (1998). *The good citizen: A history of American civic life*. Martin Kessler Books.

Schul, Y., & Vinokur, A. D. (2000). Projection in person perception among spouses as a function of the similarity in their shared experiences. *Personality and Social Psychology Bulletin*, *26*(8), 987–1001. https://doi.org/10.1177/01461672002610008

Schulz, W., Ainley, J., Fraillon, J., Kerr, D., & Losito, B. (2010). *ICCS 2009 International Report: Civic knowledge, attitudes, and engagement among lower secondary school students in 38 countries*. 2010 International Association for the Evaluation of Educational Achievement (IEA). ISBN/EAN: 978-90-79549-07-8

Schulz, W., Ainley, J., Fraillon, J., Losito, B., Agrusti, G., & Friedman, T. (2017). *Becoming citizens in a changing world: IEA International civic and citizenship education study 2016 international report*. IEA Secretariat.

Schwartz, S. H. (1992). Universals in the content and structure of values: Theoretical advances and empirical tests in 20 countries. *Advances in Experimental Social Psychology*, *25*(1), 1–65. https://doi.org/10.1016/S0065-2601(08)60281-6

Schwartz, S. H. (1994). Are there universal aspects in the structure and contents of human values? *Journal of Social Issues*, *50*(4), 19–45. https://doi.org/10.1111/j.1540-4560.1994.tb01196.x

Schwartz, S. H. (2016). Basic individual values: Sources and consequences. In T. Brosch & D. Sander (Eds.), *Handbook of value: Perspectives from economics, neuroscience, philosophy, psychology and sociology* (pp. 63–84). Oxford University Press.

Schwartz, S. H., & Butenko, T. (2014). Values and behavior: Validating the refined value theory in Russia. *European Journal of Social Psychology*, *44*(7), 799–813. https://doi.org/10.1002/ejsp.2053

Schwartz, S. H., Cieciuch, J., Vecchione, M., Davidov, E., Fischer, R., Beierlein, C., Ramos, A., Verkasalo, M., Lönnqvist, J-E., Demirutku, K., Dirilen-Gumus, O., & Konty, M. (2012). Refining the theory of basic individual values. *Journal of Personality and Social Psychology*, *103*(4), 663–688. https://doi.org/10.1037/a0029393

Schwartz, S. H., & Rubel-Lifschitz, T. (2009). Cross-national variation in the size of sex differences in values: Effects of gender equality. *Journal of Personality and Social Psychology*, *97*(1), 171–185. https://doi.org/10.1037/a0015546

Schwartz, S. H., Sagiv, L., & Boehnke, K. (2000). Worries and values. *Journal of Personality*, *68*(2), 309–346. https://doi.org/10.1111/1467-6494.00099

Sears, D. O. (1983). The persistence of early political predispositions: The roles of attitude object and life stage. *Review of Personality and Social Psychology*, *4*(1), 79–116.

Šerek, J., & Jugert, P. (2018). Young European citizens: An individual by context perspective on adolescent European citizenship. *European Journal of Developmental Psychology*, *15*(3), 302–323. https://doi.org/10.1080/17405629.2017.1366308

Shah, D. V., McLeod, J. M., & Lee, N-J. (2009). Communication competence as a foundation for civic competence: Processes of socialization into citizenship. *Political Communication*, *26*(1), 102–117. https://doi.org/10.1080/10584600802710384

Shani, D. (2009). *On the origins of political interest* [PhD dissertation, Princeton University].

Shehata, A., & Amnå, E. (2017). The development of political interest among adolescents: A communication mediation approach using five waves of panel data. *Communication Research*, *46*(8), 1055–1077. https://doi.org/10.1177/0093650217714360

Sherif, M., & Hovland, C. I. (1961). *Social judgment: Assimilation and contrast effects in communication and attitude change*. Yale University Press.

Sherrod, L. R. (2007). Civic engagement as an expression of positive youth development. In R. Silbereisen & R. Lerner (Eds.), *Approaches to positive youth development* (pp. 59–75). SAGE Publications Ltd.

Silvia, P. J. (2006). *Exploring the psychology of interest*. Oxford University Press.

Silvia, P. J. (2008). Interest – the curious emotion. *Current Directions in Psychological Science*, *17*, 57–60. https://doi.org/10.1111/j.1467-8721.2008.00548.x.

Slater, M. D. (2007). Reinforcing spirals: The mutual influence of media selectivity and media effects and their impact on individual behavior and social identity. *Communication Theory*, *17*(3), 281–303. https://doi.org/10.1111/j.1468-2885.2007.00296.x

Slater, M. D. (2015). Reinforcing spirals model: Conceptualizing the relationship between media content exposure and the development and maintenance of attitudes. *Media Psychology*, *18*(3), 370–395. https://doi.org/10.1080/15213269.2014.897236

Smetana, J. G., Metzger, A., & Campione-Barr, N. (2004). African American late adolescents' relationships with parents: Developmental transitions and longitudinal patterns. *Child Development*, *75*(3), 932–947. https://doi.org/10.1111/j.1467-8624.2004.00715.x

Statistics Sweden. (2010). *Statistics database*. www.statistikdatabasen.scb.se/pxweb/sv/ssd/START__BE

Statistics Sweden. (2018). *General elections, Electoral participation survey*. www.scb.se/hitta-statistik/statistik-efter-amne/demokrati/allmanna-val/allmanna-val-valdeltagandeundersokningen/

*Stattin, H., & Amnå, E. (2022). Basic values transform political interest into diverse political values, attitudes and behaviors. *Journal of Youth and Adolescence*. https://doi.org/10.1007/s10964-022-01654-w (see license https://creativecommons.org/licenses/by/4.0/) [chapter 12]

*Stattin, H., Amnå, E., & Russo, S. (2022a). Setting societal engagement goals during adolescence amplifies the impacts of political interest on political activities during young adulthood. *International Journal of Behavioral Development, 47*(2). https://doi.org/10.1177/01650254221113465 [chapter 2]

*Stattin, H., Eckstein, K., & Amnå, E. (2022b). Why some adolescents are open to their parents' political communication. *Journal of Youth and Adolescence*, *51*(11), 2235–2247. https://doi.org10.1007/s10964-022-01653-x [chapter 11]

*Stattin, H., Hussein, O., Özdemir, M., & Russo, S. (2017). Why do some adolescents encounter everyday events that increase their civic interest whereas others do not? *Developmental Psychology*, *53*(2), 306–318. https://doi.org/10.1037/dev0000192 [chapter 3]

*Stattin, H., & Kim, Y. (2018). Both parents and adolescents project their own values when perceiving each other's values. *International Journal of Behavioral Development*, *42*(1), 106–115. https://doi.org/10.1177/0165025417713728 [chapter 9]

Stattin, H., & Korol, L. (2021). Is love politically blind? The role that the romantic partner plays for young adults' sociopolitical interest. *Journal of Youth Studies*, *24*(4), 481–498. https://doi.org/10.1080/13676261.2020.1742301

Stattin, H., & Russo, S. (2023). The political reputation of students in upper secondary school: Consequences for their collective political activities four years later. *Political Psychology, 44*(4), 693-708. https://doi.org/10.1111/pops.12879 [chapter 4]

*Stattin, H., & Russo, S. (2022b). Youth's own political interest can explain their political interactions with important others. *International Journal of Behavioral Development*, *46*(4), 297–307. https://doi.org/10.1177/01650254221095843 [chapter 10]

*Stattin, H., Russo, S., & Arensmeier, C. (2022c). Characteristics and consequences of having a political reputation at class. *Political Psychology*, *43*(2), 635–650. https://doi.org/10.1111/pops.12784 [chapter 4]

*Stattin, H., & Russo, S. (2023). The political reputation of students in upper secondary school: Consequences for their collective political activities four years later. *Political Psychology*, *44*(4), 693–708. https://doi.org/10.1111/pops.12879 [chapter 4]

Stiff, J. (1994). *Persuasive communication*. Guilford Press.

Stoker, L., & Jennings, M. K. (1995). Life-cycle transitions and political participation: The case of marriage. *American Political Science Review*, *89*(2), 421–433. https://doi.org/10.2307/2082435

Stone, V. A., & Chaffee, S. H. (1970). Family communication patterns and source-message orientation. *Journalism Quarterly*, *47*(2), 239–246. https://doi.org/10.1177/107769907004700203

Strohmeier, D., Barrett, M., Bora, C., Caravita, S. C. S., Donghi, E., Dragoti, E., Fife-Schaw, C., Gómez-López, M., Kapéter, E., Mazzone, A., Rama, R., Ros, G., Ortega-Ruiz, R., Steiner, H., Trip, S., Tenenbaum, H., Urhahne, D., & Viejo, C. (2017). The Importance of visions and worries for the future of Europe. *Zeitschrift für Psychologie*, *225*(4), 313–323. https://doi.org/10.1027/2151-2604/a000314

Strömbäck, J., Djerf-Pierre, M., & Shehata, A. (2013). The dynamics of political interest and new media consumption: A longitudinal perspective. *International Journal of Public Opinion Research*, *25*, 414–435. https://doi.org/10.1093/ijpor/eds018

Strömbäck, J., & Shehata, A. (2010). Media malaise or a virtuous circle? Exploring the causal relationships between news media exposure, political news attention and political interest. *European Journal of Political Research*, *49*, 575–597. https://doi.org/10.1111/j.1475-6765.2009.01913.x

Stryker, S., & Burke, P. J. (2000). The past, present, and future of an identity theory. *Social Psychology Quarterly*, *63*(4), 284–297. https://doi.org/10.2307/2695840

Taris, T. W., & Semin, G. R. (1997). Passing on the faith: How mother-child communication influences transmission of moral values. *Journal of Moral Education*, *26*(2), 211–21. https://doi.org/10.1080/0305724970260208

Taylor, S. E., & Brown, J. D. (1988). Illusion and well-being: A social psychological perspective on mental health. *Psychological Bulletin*, *103*(2), 193–210. https://doi.org/10.1037/0033-2909.103.2.193

Tedin, K. L. (1974). The influence of parents on the political attitudes of adolescents. *American Political Science Review*, *68*(4), 1579–1592. https://doi.org/10.2307/1959943

Tedin, K. L. (1980). Assessing peer and parent influence on adolescent political attitudes. *American Journal of Political Science*, *24*(1), 136–154. https://doi.org/10.2307/2110929

ter Bogt, T. F. M., Meeus, W. H. J., Raaijmakers, Q. A. W., & Vollebergh, W. A. M. (2001). Youth centrism and the formation of political orientations in adolescence and young adulthood. *Journal of Cross-Cultural Psychology*, *32*(2), 229–240. https://doi.org/10.1177/0022022101032002009

Thomas, F., Shehata, A., Otto, L. P., Moeller, J., & Prestele, E. (2021). How to capture reciprocal communication dynamics: Comparing longitudinal statistical approaches in order to analyze within- and between-person effects. *Journal of Communication*, *71*(2), 187–219. https://doi.org/10.1093/joc/jqab003

Thornton, A., Orbuch, T. L., & Axinn, W. G. (1995). Parent-child relationships during the transition to adulthood. *Journal of Family Issues*, *16*(5), 538–564. https://doi.org/10.1177/019251395016005003

Thorson, K., Xu, Y., & Edgerly, S. (2018). Political inequalities start at home: Parents, children, and the socialization of civic infrastructure online. *Political Communication*, *35*(2), 178–195. https://doi.org/10.1080/10584609.2017.1333550

Tims, A. R., & Masland, J. L. (1985). Measurement of family communication patterns. *Communication Research*, *12*(1), 35–57. https://doi.org/10.1177/009365085012001002

Tsai, K. M., Telzer, E. H., Gonzales, N. A., & Fuligni, A. J. (2015). Parental cultural socialization of Mexican-American adolescents' family obligation values and behaviors. *Child Development*, *86*(4), 1241–1252. https://doi.org/10.1111/cdev.12358

Tversky, A., & Kahneman, D. (1973). Availability: A heuristic for judging frequency and probability. *Cognitive Psychology*, *5*(2), 207–232. https://doi.org/10.1016/0010-0285(73)90033-9

van den Bulck, J., & van den Bergh, B. (2005). The child effect in media and communication research: A call to arms and an agenda for research. *Annals of the International Communication Association*, *29*(1), 35–48. https://doi.org/10.1080/23808985.2005.11679043

van Deth, J. W. (1990). Interest in politics. In M. K. Jennings & J. W. van Deth (Eds.), *Continuities in political action: A longitudinal study of political orientations in three western democracies* (pp. 275–312). de Gruyter.

van Deth, J. W. (2000). Interesting but irrelevant: Social capital and the saliency of politics in Western Europe. *European Journal of Political Research*, *37*(2), 115–147. https://doi.org/10.1111/1475-6765.00507

van Deth, J., Abendschön, S., & Vollmar, M. (2011). Children and politics: An empirical reassessment of early political socialization. *Political Psychology*, *32*(1), 147–174. https://doi.org/10.1111/j.1467-9221.2010.00798.x

van Deth, J., & Elff, M. (2000). *Political involvement and apathy in Europe 1973–1998*. Working paper, Mannheimer Zentrum für Europäische Sozialforschung, 33.

Vecchione, M., Caprara, G. V., Schoen, H., Castro, J. L. G., & Schwartz, S. H. (2012). The role of personal values and basic traits in perceptions of the consequences of immigration: A three-nation study. *British Journal of Psychology*, *103*(3), 359–377. https://doi.org/10.1111/j.2044-8295.2011.02079.x.

Vecchione, M., Schwartz, S. H., Davidov, E., Cieciuch, J., Alessandri, G., & Marsicano, G. (2020). Stability and change of basic personal values in early adolescence: A 2-year longitudinal study. *Journal of Personality*, *88*(3), 447–463. https://doi.org/10.1111/jopy.12502

Verba, S., Schlozman, K. L., & Brady, H. E. (1995). *Voice and equality: Civic voluntarism in American politics*. Harvard University Press.

Veugelers, W. (2021). A moral perspective on citizenship education and on IEA's international civic and citizenship education studies. In B. Malak-Minkiewicz & J. Torney-Purta (Eds.), *Influences of the IEA civic and citizenship education studies: Practice, policy, and research across countries and regions* (pp. 291–301). Springer International Publishing.

Vollebergh, W. A. M., Iedema, J., & Raaijmakers, Q. A. W. (2001). Intergenerational transmission and the formation of cultural orientations in adolescence and young adulthood. *Journal of Marriage and the Family*, *63*(4), 1185–1198. https://doi.org/10.1111/j.1741-3737.2001.01185.x

Voorpostel, M., & Coffé, H. (2010). Transitions in partnership and parental status, gender, and political and civic participation. *European Sociological Review*, *28*(1), 28–42. https://doi.org/10.1093/esr/jcq046

Warner, B. R., & Warner Colander, C. W. (2016). Talking politics at the dinner table: The effects of family political communication on young citizens' normative political attitudes. In M. S. McKinney, E. Thorson, & D. Shah (Eds.), *Political socialization of young citizens* (pp. 195–211). Peter Lang.

West, T. V., & Kenny, D. A. (2011). The truth and bias model of judgment. *Psychological Review*, *118*(2), 357–378. https://doi.org/10.1037/a0022936

Westholm, A. (1999). The perceptual pathway: Tracing the mechanisms of political value transfer across generations. *Political Psychology*, *20*(3), 525–551. www.jstor.org/stable/3792160

Whitbeck, L. B., & Gecas, V. (1988). Value attributions and value transmission between parents and children. *Journal of Marriage and the Family*, *50*(3), 829–840. https://doi.org/10.2307/352651

Wray-Lake, L. (2019). How do young people become politically engaged? *Child Development Perspectives*, *13*(2), 127–132. https://doi.org/10.1111/cdep.12324

Wray-Lake, L., Arruda, E. H., & Schulenberg, J. E. (2020). Civic development across the transition to adulthood in a national U.S. sample: Variations by race/ethnicity, parent education, and gender. *Developmental Psychology*, *56*(10), 1948–1967. https://doi.org/10.1037/dev0001101

Wray-Lake, L., & Sloper, M. A. (2016). Investigating general and specific links from adolescents' perceptions of ecological assets to their civic actions. *Applied Developmental Science*, *20*(4), 250–266. https://doi.org/10.1080/10888691.2015.1114888

Wu, N., Hou, Y., Wang, Q., & Yu, C. (2018). Intergenerational transmission of educational aspirations in Chinese families: Identifying mediators and moderators. *Journal of Youth and Adolescence*, *47*(6), 1238–1251. https://doi.org/10.1007/s10964–018–0820-ys

York, C. (2019a) Is it top-down, trickle-up, or reciprocal? Testing longitudinal relationships between youth news use and parent and peer political discussion. *Communication Studies*, *70*(4), 377–393. https://doi.org/10.1080/10510974.2019.1614965

York, C. (2019b). Genetic influence on political discussion: Results from two twin studies. *Communication Monographs*, *86*(4), 438–456. https://doi.org/10.1080/03637751.2019.1597274

Young, J. T., Rebellon, C. J., Barnes, J. C., & Weerman, F. M. (2014). Unpacking the Black box of peer similarity in deviance: Understanding the mechanisms linking personal behavior, peer behavior, and perceptions. *Criminology: An Interdisciplinary Journal*, *52*(1), 60–86. https://doi.org/10.1111/1745-9125.12029

Zeglovits, E., & Zandonella, M. (2013). Political interest of adolescents before and after lowering the voting age: The case of Austria. *Journal of Youth Studies*, *16*, 1084–1104. https://doi.org/10.1080/13676261.2013.793785.

Zelezny, L. C., Chua, P-P., & Aldrich, C. (2000). Elaborating on gender differences in environmentalism. *Journal of Social Issues*, *56*(3), 443–457. https://doi.org/10.1111/0022-4537.00177

Zhu, J., Kuang, X., Kennedy, K. J., & Mok, M. M. C. (2018). Previous civic experience and Asian adolescents' expected participation in legal protest: Mediating role of self-efficacy and interest, *Asia Pacific Journal of Education*, *38*(3), 414–431.

AUTHOR INDEX

SUBJECT INDEX